Substance Use and Misuse: Nature, Context and Clinical Interventions

Edited by

G. Hussein Rassool

MSc, BA, RN, FETC, RCNT, RNT, ENB (934), Cert. Ed.,
Cert. Couns., Cert. in Supervision and Consultation

Senior Lecturer in Addictive Behaviour and Nursing,
Department of Psychiatry of Addictive Behaviour,
Centre for Addiction Studies,
St. George's Hospital Medical School (University of London),
London, UK

Blackwell
Science

D0267462

© 1998 by Blackwell Science Ltd, a Blackwell Publishing Company

Editorial Offices:
Blackwell Science Ltd, 9600 Garsington Road, Oxford OX4 2DQ, UK
  Tel: +44 (0)1865 776868
Blackwell Publishing Inc., 350 Main Street, Malden, MA 02148-5020, USA
  Tel: +1 781 388 8250
Blackwell Science Asia Pty, 550 Swanston Street, Carlton, Victoria 3053, Australia
  Tel: +61 (0)3 8359 1011

First published 1998
Reprinted 2003, 2004

Library of Congress Cataloging-in-Publication Data
Rassool, G. Hussein.
  Substance use & misuse: nature, context, and clinical interventions/G. Hussein Rassool.
    p. cm.
  Includes bibliographical references and index.
  ISBN 0-632-04884-0 (pb)
  1. Substance abuse—Prevention. 2. Substance abuse—Treatment.
3. Substance abuse—Nursing. 4. Drug abuse—Prevention. 5. Drug abuse—Treatment.
6. Drug abuse—Nursing.
  I. Title.
  [DNLM: 1. Substance-Related Disorders —nursing. 2. Substance-Related
Disorders—prevention & control. 3. Substance-Related Disorders—therapy.
WY 160 R228s 1998]
RC564.R37 1998
616.86—dc21
DNLM/DLC
for Library of Congress
                                                                          98-2838
                                                                          CIP

ISBN 0-632-04884-0

A catalogue record for this title is available from the British Library

Set in 10/12pt Palatino
by DP Photosetting, Aylesbury, Bucks
Printed and bound in India
by Replika Press Pvt Ltd, Kundli 131028

The publisher's policy is to use permanent paper from mills that operate a sustainable forestry policy, and which has been manufactured from pulp processed using acid-free and elementary chlorine-free practices. Furthermore, the publisher ensures that the text paper and cover board used have met acceptable environmental accreditation standards.

For further information on Blackwell Publishing, visit our website:
www.blackwellpublishing.com

Dedicated to Julie, Yasmin Soraya, Adam Ali Hussein,
Reshad Hassan and Hassim Rassool.

Contents

Contributors   xiii
Foreword   xv
Preface   xix
Acknowledgements   xxi

Part 1   Understanding Substance Use and Misuse

1   Introduction   3
    G. Hussein Rassool
    Historical overview   5
    The drug scenes of yesterday and today   10
    Conclusions   10
    References   11

2   Concepts and Models   13
    G. Hussein Rassool
    Introduction   13
    Drug misuse   13
    Substance use and abuse   14
    Problem drug user   14
    Addictive behaviour   15
    Drug dependence   15
    The dependence syndrome   17
    Routes of drug administration   17
    The drug experience   18
    Patterns of substance misuse   19
    Why do people take drugs?   20
    An overview of models of substance misuse   20
    Conclusions   23
    References   23

3   Tobacco Smoking   27
    G. Hussein Rassool & Julie Winnington
    Introduction   27
    The Health of the Nation and smoking   27
    Nicotine addiction   29
    Harmful constituents of tobacco smoke   29
    Medical and psychological effects of smoking   30

Health gains and benefits of smoking cessation   33
Smoking cessation   33
Conclusions   35
References   35

4 An Overview of Psychoactive Drugs   **38**
G. Hussein Rassool
Introduction   38
Opiates   38
Cannabis   40
Stimulants   41
Hypnosedatives   43
LSD and other hallucinogens   44
Ecstasy   45
Anabolic steroids   47
Amyl and butyl nitrite   48
Volatile substances   49
Over-the-counter drugs   50
Other drugs on the UK drug scene   51
References   52

5 Alcohol and Alcohol Related Problems   **54**
Julie Winnington & G. Hussein Rassool
Introduction   54
Concepts of alcohol dependence and problem drinking   55
Pattern and extent of use   57
Use of health services   58
Chemical nature and production of alcohol   58
Metabolism of alcohol   58
General effects of alcohol   59
Alcohol dependence and withdrawal   61
Sensible and controlled drinking   63
How much is moderate?   64
Conclusions   64
References   65

**6 It's Everybody's Business: The Responses of Health
Care Professionals**   **68**
G. Hussein Rassool
Introduction   68
Rationale for working with substance misusers   68
Attitudes towards substance mususers   69
Health care professionals' roles   71
Generic interventions with substance misusers   72
Conclusions   77
References   78

Part 2 Prevention, Recognition and Intervention

7 Prevention and Health Education **83**
G. Hussein Rassool
Introduction 83
Nursing and health education 83
Health education and prevention 84
General interventions 87
Community approach 88
Rational use of psychoactive substances 88
Health promoting institutions 89
Health promotion: substance misuse and the work place 91
Personal health education of nurses 91
Conclusion 92
References 93

8 Screening and Generic Assessment **96**
G. Hussein Rassool
Introduction 96
Context and setting for screening substance use history 96
Screening for high risk behaviour 97
Screening methods for alcohol and drugs 98
Nursing assessment 100
Assessment and history taking 100
Assessment of current prescribed medication of
psychoactive drugs 102
Conclusions 102
References 104

9 An Overview of Intervention Strategies **106**
G. Hussein Rassool & Bridget Kilpatrick
Introduction 106
Principles of clinical intervention 107
Intervention strategies 107
Conclusions 113
References 114

10 Service Provision for Substance Misusers **116**
G. Hussein Rassool
Introduction 116
Non specialist services 117
Specialist services 118
Conclusions 121
References 121

Part 3   Generic Responses: Different Contexts and Settings

11   Drug Use, Pregnancy and Care of the New-Born   **125**
Faye Macrory
        Introduction   125
        Women, drug use and pregnancy   126
        Antenatal care   127
        Intrapartum care   130
        Postpartum care   131
        Discharge   132
        Social services and child protection issues   132
        Case vignette   133
        Conclusions   134
        References   134

12   Health Visiting and Substance Misuse   **136**
Julie Gafoor
        Introduction   136
        Nature of problems in parents who are substance misusers   137
        Summary of problems   138
        Role of the health visitor in substance use and misuse   138
        Health visiting interventions   138
        Case vignette   141
        Conclusions   142
        References   143

13   Practice Nurse: Recognition and Early Interventions   **145**
Claire Cowan
        Introduction   145
        General practice versus specialist services   146
        Why the practice nurse?   147
        Patient presentation   147
        Assessment   148
        Planning care and interventions   150
        Raising health awareness   151
        Health education and provision of information   151
        Effecting changes of behaviour   152
        Support   152
        Clinical management   152
        Shared care   153
        Evaluation   153
        Case vignette 1   154
        Case vignette 2   155
        Conclusions   156
        References   157

14 School Nursing and Substance Misuse   **159**
    Pat Jackson & Judy McRae
        Introduction   159
        Nature and extent of substance use and misuse   159
        School health service   160
        The National Curriculum   160
        Role of the school nurse   161
        School nurse interventions   162
        Health education   163
        School policies   164
        Smoking policies   164
        Drug policies: alcohol and illicit substances   165
        Case vignettes   165
        Conclusions   166
        References   166

15 Substance Misuse in the Accident & Emergency Department   **168**
    Fiona Jeffcock
        Introduction   168
        Perception of health care professionals   168
        Dealing with an emergency   169
        Presenting at the A&E department   169
        Types of patients   170
        Nursing care   172
        Case vignette 1   173
        Case vignette 2   174
        Conclusions   174
        References   175

16 HIV, Hepatitis and Substance Misuse   **176**
    Helen Pritchitt & Andy Mason
        Introduction   176
        Nature and extent of HIV infection   176
        HIV disease   177
        Hepatitis   181
        Care of drug users in an acute general ward   184
        Health education   184
        Palliative/terminal care   185
        Case vignette   185
        Conclusions   186
        References   187

Part 4   Addiction Nursing: Specialist Responses

17 Alcohol: Community Detoxification and Clinical Care   **191**
    Mike Gafoor & G. Hussein Rassool
        Introduction   191

What is detoxification?   191
Rationale for community alcohol detoxification   192
The alcohol withdrawal syndrome   193
Assessment of community detoxification   193
Lay and professional roles   194
Clinical care and management   195
The importance of follow-up care   196
Nursing model for community detoxification   196
Case vignette   196
Conclusions   197
References   198

18   Benzodiazepines: Clinical Care and Nursing Interventions   200
Mike Gafoor
Introduction   200
Nature and extent   201
Nature of problems   202
Summary of problems   203
Clinical care and nursing interventions   203
Case vignette   205
Conclusions   206
References   206

19   Stimulants: Clinical Care and Nursing Interventions   208
Mike Flanagan
Introduction   208
Background and nature of stimulant misuse   208
Problems and issues   209
Stimulant withdrawal   210
Clinical care and therapeutic interventions   211
Case vignette   214
Conclusions   215
References   215

**20   Opiate and Polydrug Use: Clinical Care and
Nursing Interventions   217**
Mike Gafoor
Introduction   217
Nature and extent   217
Nature of problems   218
Problems of dependence and withdrawal   220
Assessment   220
Medical management   221
Psycho-social support   222
Case vignette   223
Conclusions   223
References   224

21 Nicotine Addiction: Health Care Interventions   **225**
Carole Mills
    Introduction   225
    A smoking cessation service   225
    One to one intervention   226
    Case vignette 1: One to one counselling   228
    Group interventions   229
    Case vignette 2: Group counselling   231
    Smokers' clinics   233
    Conclusions   233
    Acknowledgements   234
    References   234

22 Working with Diverse Special Populations   **236**
G. Hussein Rassool & Bridget Kilpatrick
    Introduction   236
    Ethnic minorities   236
    The elderly   239
    Young people   241
    The homeless   244
    References   246

23 Working with Dual Diagnosis Clients   **249**
Mike Gafoor & G. Hussein Rassool
    Introduction   249
    What is dual diagnosis?   249
    Nature and extent   250
    Problems and issues for mental health nurses   251
    Working with dual diagnosis patients   252
    Assessment and screening   253
    Shared care   254
    Case vignette   254
    Implications for nursing   255
    Conclusions   257
    References   257

24 Contemporary Issues in Addiction Nursing   **260**
G. Hussein Rassool
    Introduction   260
    Concept of addiction nusing   261
    Nursing roles   262
    Nursing diagnosis   262
    Education and training   264
    Clinical supervision   265
    Nursing research   266
    Conclusions   267
    References   267

Appendices   **271**

1   UK Self-Help Groups and Helplines   273
2   International Organisations: Professional Information and
    Resources   275
3   UK Education and Training Resources (Addiction Studies)   277

Index   *279*

Contributors

C. Cowan, Practice Nurse Lecturer, Reading University Health Centre, University of Reading.

M. Flanagan, Community Psychiatric Nurse (Substance Misuse), Department of Psychiatry, Epsom General Hospital, Epsom, Surrey.

J. Gafoor, Health Visitor, Doddington Health Centre, Cornwallis House, Oxford.

M. Gafoor, Chief Executive, Addiction Counselling Trust, Aylesbury, Buckinghamshire.

P. Jackson, School Nurse Co-ordinator and Lecturer-Practitioner Optimum Health Services, Elizabeth Blackwell House, London.

F. Jeffcock, Ward Sister, Accident and Emergency Department, Kingston Hospital, Surrey.

B. Kilpatrick, Research Nurse, Centre for Addiction Studies, Department of Addictive Behaviour, St George's Hospital Medical School (University of London), London.

F. Macrory MBE, Drug Liaison Midwife, Manchester Drug Service, The Bridge, Manchester.

A. Mason, Community Psychiatric Nurse (Community Drug Team) Merton, Sutton and Wandsworth, London.

J. McRae, School Nurse Team Leader, New Salomons Clinic, Guy's Hospital, London.

C. Mills, Clinical Nurse Specialist (Smoking), St George's Hospital, London.

H. Pritchitt, Ward Sister, Clinical Infection Unit, St George's Hospital, Knightbridge Wing, London.

G. Hussein Rassool, Senior Lecturer in Addictive Behaviour and Nursing, Department of Psychiatry of Addictive Behaviour, Centre for Addiction Studies, St George's Hospital Medical School (University of London), London.

J. Winnington, Staff Nurse (Addiction) Bethlem and Maudsley NHS Trusts, Wickham Park House, Kent.

Foreword

Alcohol, drugs and tobacco use and misuse have now become major public health concerns that cannot be ignored by policy makers, service planners and providers, professionals of all disciplines or the community at large. The publication of the second white paper, *Drugs Misuse – To Building a Better Britain – A Ten-Year Strategy for Substance Misuse* (1998), emphasises the present government's policies following on from the previous *Tackling Drugs Together* (1995–98) white paper. Three forthcoming white papers on alcohol strategy, tobacco control and public health, not to mention the Testing and Treatment Order, will no doubt help to synchronise policy and planning issues relating to substance misuse in general.

It is now widely accepted that substance use and misuse simply cannot be tackled by specialist drug and alcohol agencies alone. With *Tackling Drugs Together* (1995–98), Drug Action Teams (DATs) were set up to co-ordinate the process of planning and provision of drug services at local level. Many of these Drug Action Teams responded to local needs and views by incorporating alcohol misuse as part of their overall Substance Misuse Strategy and Action Plan. The establishment of DATs has been welcomed as a positive way forward. The domain of service developments and provisions, however, continues to remain to a large extent with specialist drug and alcohol agencies; this is still very obvious within the National Health Service.

Within both generic services, that is general hospital and primary care settings, and within mainstream psychiatric services, the move to integrate drug and alcohol services into their overall service provisions has been met with less enthusiasm. That is not to say that examples of good practice concerning the integration of drug and alcohol services into these service provisions do not exist; of course they do. Often, however, these initiatives are led by the motivation of dedicated individuals rather than through policy dictum.

One of the arguments put forward quite often by generic and non-specialist services is that they are not trained and therefore lack the competency to look after this client group, or that there are few readily available materials, in terms of treatment guidelines, for this client group. Well, times are changing rapidly. ANSA (Association of Nurses in Substance Abuse), for example, recently produced guidelines for good clinical practice in dealing with substance misuse clients, which were supported by the Department of Health. The review of good clinical practice guidelines for doctor clinicians is awaited this year. Over the last few years, there has been an increase in the amount of drug and alcohol information available to professionals, service planners, generic and specialist substance misuse agencies, and the public. Information ranges from basic health promotion resources to specific prevention initiatives, training packages, treatment approaches, after care provision, developing outcome measures and effective purchasing. We are now much better informed on drug and alcohol misuse than we were a decade ago.

Nurses have been one of the leading groups of professionals whose contribution to this field has been increasing steadily. Many nurses are specialists in their own domain, working as clinical nurse specialists, academics, researchers, managers, commissioners and freelance consultants. Many of them have been at the cutting edge of development and involved in introducing new ideas and concepts in substance misuse service provisions.

In this textbook: *Substance Use and Misuse*, the editor details the nature, context and clinical interventions of addiction from a range of angles, describing its historical perspectives and relevance, cultural context and norms, and types of treatment approaches. In brief, it gives the reader a broad picture of substance misuse, from a historical view of addiction to today's knowledge and skills for its treatment and care.

Addiction nursing as a concept of nursing applied to the field of substance misuse is discussed. This is now becoming increasingly relevant in this country, whereas in the United States and elsewhere it has already been acknowledged as a nursing speciality in its own right.

The clinical aspects of healthcare issues faced by clients and practitioners in treatment settings are well detailed and hopefully will encourage the reader to become interested in the treatment and care of the substance user/misuser. To me this is one of the key objectives of this book.

The book is written in simple terms, is easy to read and is well referenced. Both the generic nurse and nurse specialist dealing with drug and alcohol misuse clients daily during their clinical work will find this book very relevant.

Although written primarily for nurses, *Substance Use and Misuse* should be equally useful for other professionals with an interest in substance misuse. The contributors are practitioners in the field; amongst them are clinical nurse specialists, community psychiatric nurses, health visitors, A&E nurses, midwives and others, all of whom are actively involved in providing direct care to the substance users and misusers. What better way for nurses working or interested in this field to learn about the subject matter than from their own colleagues? Especially given the fact that the vast majority of drug treatment and generic health care agencies, both within the health service and outside, are staffed by nurses.

The editor is to be congratulated for bringing these skilled staff together and making their knowledge and experience available to the nursing profession. The book illustrates the rich resources within the nursing profession and is a celebration of nursing skills!

Leckraj Boyjoonauth
Clinical Development Manager
& Deputy Director
Substance Misuse Directorate
Riverside Mental Health Trust, London
and
Member of ACMD.
Executive. Member of ANSA

Preface

For the past decade there has been a growing call for generic health care professionals to play a key role in the early recognition and management of substance misusers. Dealing with substance misuse and addictive behaviour is everyone's responsibility rather than the sole domain of specialist addiction nurses.

The theme of this book is about substance use and misuse in both acute and primary health care settings. The book is written by experienced nurse clinicians, academics and managers practising in generic settings and specialist substance misuse agencies. The contributors include addiction nurses, a midwife, health visitor, practice nurse, school nurse and general nurses.

The book provides an introduction to the theoretical, clinical and practical issues in working with substance misusers. It will assist student and practising nurses, and other health care practitioners, to understand the extent and nature of substance use and misuse and the clinical practice of generic health care professionals and addiction nurses. In addition, it will provide a framework for practitioners and so enable them to provide effective management and care when dealing with those who misuse tobacco, alcohol and drugs.

The complexities of substance misuse and addictive behaviour are illustrated by case vignettes. A section of the book also covers clinical perspectives of addiction nurses. It is acknowledged that addiction nursing is still in the relatively early stage of knowledge development, and many issues and aspects of theoretical and clinical practice require further and extensive development and investigation. While the book addresses issues related to nursing and substance misuse, it is envisaged that it will also provide an excellent resource for other health and social care professionals and for those who are unfamiliar with the substance misuse field.

Structure of the book

The book is presented in four sections. Part 1 provides an understanding of substance use and misuse and examines the extent and effects of tobacco, psychoactive drugs and alcohol misuse, and the responses of health care professionals working with substance misusers in both residential and community settings.

Part 2 examines the role of prevention and health education in substance use and misuse. It also covers screening and generic assessment, intervention strategies in generic and specialist settings, and service provision for substance misusers.

Part 3 deals with the generic responses to substance misuse in a variety of different settings and contexts, including pregnancy and care of the newborn, health visiting, school nursing, practice nursing, accident and emergency nursing and general nursing.

Part 4 deals with specialist responses to substance misusers by addiction nurses. These include community or home detoxification of alcohol and the clinical and nursing management of benzodiazepine, stimulant (amphetamines and cocaine), opiate and nicotine addiction. The issues, problems and nursing interventions relating to special populations – ethnic minorities, elderly, young people and the homeless – are examined. In addition, the co-existence of psychiatric disorders and substance misuse is examined and the final chapter focuses on contemporary issues in addiction nursing such as nursing roles, nursing diagnosis, clinical supervision, professional development and research.

Acknowledgements

I would like to thank all the staff at the academic department, clinical staff, past and present students and patients who stimulated and taught me about substance misuse and addictive behaviour. I am also particularly grateful to all contributors who facilitated completion of this book in a relatively short time. My special thanks are extended to Professor James P. Smith and to Professor A. Hamid Ghodse whose wisdom and guidance have inspired me in my personal and professional development. My particular thanks must be reserved for Griselda Campbell, Lisa Field and the rest of the team at Blackwell Science Ltd, for their unswerving support and encouragement. Finally, I am indebted to my family, Julie, Yasmin, Adam and Reshad; without their love and support this book would never have been completed.

'Knowledge by itself does not give any excellence. It is the use to which it is put that determines its quality. For extolling moral values, it is like a faithful friend; for serving baser objectives of life, it is like a serpent'

Maulana Jalalu'din Rumi (1207–1273)

Part 1
Understanding Substance Use and Misuse

Chapter 1
Introduction

G. Hussein Rassool

Substance misuse and addictive behaviour are universal phenomena and are regarded, in the twentieth century, as a major public health problem. Historical evidence suggests that, since ancient times, living with psychoactive substances seems to be part of the fabric of our lives. In some ways, there has always been a love/hate relationship with or a sense of ambivalence towards the use of a psychoactive substance. According to Gossop (1993),

> 'the desire to experience some altered state of consciousness seem to be an intrinsic part of the human condition ... and we are surrounded by drugs ... the cup of tea and coffee, the glasses of beer, wine and whisky, the cigarettes, the snorts of cocaine, the joints, the tablets of acid, the fixes of heroin, and the ubiquitous tranquillisers and sleeping pills.'

That is, the use addictive substances has become part of our psychological and cultural consciousness.

However, the ways in which a particular society determines which drugs should be made legal is not contingent upon the pharmacological properties or therapeutic values of the drugs, but rather based on the influence of the political climate, socio-cultural contexts, historical development and religious considerations. For example, tea, coffee and tobacco have all been illegal in this country at various points in history (Whitaker 1987). With time, increasing availability and more widespread use, opinions may change and a formerly illegal drug may be 'normalised'. Edwards (1971) stated that

> 'a drug which is permissible yesterday might tomorrow be prohibited; a drug which for one society was of importance in religious sacrament might in another place be preached against. You could conclude that one of the main businesses in the world was to cultivate, manufacture, advertise, legislate on, tax, consume, adulate and decry mind-altering substances. The complexity of the matter is overwhelming, its ramifications endless.'

In the European Union (EU), it has been suggested that Britain is second only to Italy in the misuse of psychoactive substances in proportion to the population (Clutterbuck 1995). In the UK it is estimated that 6% of the population, around 3 million people, take at least one illegal drug in any one year (Tackling Drugs Together, 1995). In addition, it was estimated that between 2.5 million and 5 million people take illegal drugs at some time in their lives (Institute for the Study of Drug Dependence (ISDD) 1993). Consumption of drugs is increasing year by year, particularly cocaine (crack), amphetamines, Ecstasy (methylenedioxymethamphetamine or (MDMA) and LSD. It is estimated that about half a million people spent 200 million on Ecstasy at raves in the UK in 1993 at about 18 per dose (*The Economist* 1993). There has been a dramatic rise in the number of young people who have tried drugs or volatile substances. By the age of 20, one third of young men and one fifth of young women have abused drugs (ISDD 1993). The World Health Organization (1991) targeted addiction as one of the major health problems to be solved by the year 2000. In Europe, Target 17 in the policy document 'Health for All' (HFA) of the World Health Organization (1991) states that 'by the year 2000, the health-damaging consumption of dependence-producing substances such as alcohol, tobacco and psychoactive drugs should have been significantly reduced in all member states.'

Although we are noticing a positive approach to tackling drug misuse, in reality the impact of alcohol, tobacco and prescription and over-the-counter drugs is being virtually disregarded. The health and social costs of the misuse of these psychoactive substances, unfortunately, reflect most disturbing morbidity and mortality figures (Rassool & Gafoor 1997a). The sequelae of the harm – physical, social, psychological and economic – derived from the misuse of psychoactive substances not only affect the individual user but also the family or significant others and the whole community. Some of the health related problems include:

- higher risks of premature death
- risk of acquiring blood borne viruses such as hepatitis B and C, and HIV
- overdose
- respiratory failure
- obstetric complications
- suicide and mental health problems

Substance use and misuse is unique as it impinges on all aspects of the five key areas of *The Health of the Nation document* (Department of Health 1992):

- coronary heart disease and stroke
- cancers
- mental illness
- accidents
- HIV and sexual health

In all key areas, alcohol, drugs and tobacco smoking are important contributory and risk factors.

The magnitude of the health and other related problems emphasised the need for greater involvement of those in the helping professions. Community psychiatric nurses, health visitors, practice nurses, district nurses, family planning nurses, school nurses, occupational health nurses and midwives, etc., are increasingly coming into contact with clients with health-related problems in various settings. Members of the primary health care team and community workers are in an ideal position to identify, intervene and manage individuals with substance misuse problems, as substance misusers are more likely to use primary health care services (Pollak 1989). It is everyone's business rather than the responsibility and domain of a single health professional group. The changing and ever increasing health needs of the general population require statutory, non statutory and voluntary organisations to play a key role in effective preventive strategies, early recognition and management of substance misuse.

Historical overview

Substance use dates back thousands of years and records of ancient civilisations provide evidence of the use of alcohol and plants with psychoactive properties. From the earliest time, alcohol, tobacco and other psychoactive substances have been used for medicinal, religious, cultural and recreational purposes and as a social lubricant.

Alcoholic beverages are believed to have been used as early as 6000 BC. However, the use of alcohol was profoundly affected by the discovery of the process of distillation by Razi (or Rhazzes, AD 850–922), a Persian physician. This discovery made it easier to transport alcohol and to become drunk (Ghodse 1995). The earliest reference to the misuse of alcohol appears in the Old Testament, referring to Noah's plantation of a vineyard and his drunkenness. Drinking bouts and excessive drinking were common in ancient Egypt and Assyria for religious rituals and festive occasions. In Ancient Greece, habitual drunkenness was uncommon because of the social etiquette attached to drinking and drinking behaviour. At the height of the Roman Empire, the shift from ceremonial drinking – confined to banquets and special occasions – to casual, everyday drinking was accompanied by an increase in chronic drunkenness, which today would be labelled alcoholism (Babor 1986).

With the collapse of the Roman Empire, religious institutions, particularly the monasteries, became the repositories of the brewing and wine making techniques developed in the ancient world (Babor 1986). It is argued that the early ritualisation of alcohol in Christian Europe and the church's revultion of mind altering psychoactive substances helped alcohol to achieve dominance in European nations (Gossop 1993). The harm of purified drugs seems even more apparent when the psychoactive substance is consumed outside its historical and cultural context. Whitaker (1987) suggested that distilled alcohol inflicted more havoc on North

American Indians and Australian Aborigines than any other drug throughout history.

Plants such as the opium poppy were used by Middle Eastern and Asian cultures, and were brought to Europe through the opening of trade routes, wars and expeditions. References to the juice of the poppy occur in the Assyrian medical tablets of the seventh century BC, and in Sumerian ideograms of about 4000 BC the poppy is called 'plant of joy' (Berridge & Edwards 1987). The Arab physicians such as Ibn-Sina (or Avicenna, AD 980–1037) used opium extensively. They wrote special treatises on its preparations and recommended the plant especially for diarrhoea and diseases of the eye. In England, opium was chiefly used as a narcotic and a hypnotic. The drug's soporific and narcotic qualities were described in Chaucer's *Canterbury Tales* and Shakespeare's *Othello*.

In the nineteenth century, laudanum, a mixture of alcohol solution and tincture of opium, could be bought over the counter at any grocer's shop and for decades it was every family's favourite remedy for minor aches and pains (Royal College of Psychiatrists 1989). In effect, opium was used in preference to alcohol and in various forms for endemic conditions such as malaria. Subsequently, the identification of the active alkaloids of opium and the development of the process of acetylation by which morphine is converted to heroin changed the whole pattern of opiate use, not only in the West where the discovery was made, but also in the East, where the parent drug originated (Ghodse 1995).

Cannabis sativa (or Indian hemp), more commonly known as cannabis or marijuana, was one of the first plants to be cultivated for its non food properties, and was primarily harvested for its fibre. The plant grows freely throughout the world, but is indigenous to Central Asia and the Himalayan region and is cultivated widely in Africa, India, North America and the Caribbean region. It is thought to have originated in China, around 2700 BC. It was recommended for its pharmacological properties by the Emperor Shen Nung to his citizens for the treatment of pain, illness, gout, absent-mindedness and other ailments (Maisto *et al.* 1995). In addition, it has been speculated that cannabis was also used for countering evil spirits and for its psychoactive properties (Abel 1980). With the spread of cannabis to neighbouring countries, this psychoactive substance was regarded as a sacred plant and used for religious functions and rituals. While marijuana comes from the leafy top portion of the plant, hashish, made from the resin, was used by Arabs around the tenth century (Abel 1980).

The use of the drug for its recreational and intoxicating effects appears to stem from the Middle East and North Africa. The drug most probably first reached European countries in the nineteenth century, following the Arab invasion of Spain. The exposure of cannabis to Europe was also influenced by the printed literature describing personal experiences in the use of hashish. The medical profession began to show an interest in the use of cannabis by the middle of the nineteenth century. An Irish physician, William O'Shaughnessy, who described the medical application of cannabis while in India, introduced cannabis into Great Britain (Bloomquist 1971). In France, the use and effects of hashish were described by a small group of writers, intellectuals and artists. In the 1840s, Le Club Des Hachishins (The Hashish Club) was founded in an exclusive hotel in Paris. The splendours of their hallucinatory experiences and the elements of mystery, joy, ecstasy, fear, and paranoia were described by French authors such as Bauderlaire and Gautier (Gautier 1966). Despite its attraction as a recreational or intoxicating drug, it did not immediately spread throughout Europe. The widespread use of cannabis or hashish for its psychoactive properties seems to have occurred in Europe in the 1960s as a result of the 'peace culture' – a young generation movement – in the USA. Cannabis still remains the most frequently used illicit drug in the UK.

The coca plant is indigenous to the Andean highlands of Bolivia, Columbia and Peru. The use of the coca leaf dates back to the Inca civilisations and their descendants. The Inca people apparently learned the practice of chewing the coca leaf from the Aymara Indians of Bolivia, whose own use dates back to around 300 BC. (Grinspoon & Bakalar 1976). For centuries, the coca leaf has been chewed by the Andean Indians of Peru and other South American countries. The coca plant was used for medicinal purposes, religious ceremonies, rituals, burials and other special occasions. The Peruvian Indians used coca to increase their physical strength, to lessen fatigue and to prevent hunger. After the Spanish conquistadors conquered the Incas, they encouraged the use of the coca leaf in the belief that it helped the Incas to work longer and harder. In fact, because of its social importance, the Spanish eventually took over coca production and distribution and used coca as a tool to control the conquered population (Petersen 1977).

It was not until the early 1800s that Europeans started to experiment with the use of coca. In the 1850s European chemists were able to isolate the far more potent ingredient in the leaf which they called cocaine. The extraction of cocaine from the leaf led to a whole new era in the history of stimulant drug use and misuse. Freud, in his first major publication, *On Coca*, advocated the therapeutic and recreational use of cocaine. He also thought that cocaine was an aphrodisiac (Byck 1974). He recommended the use of cocaine as a local anaesthetic and as a treatment for drug addiction, alcoholism, depression, various neuroses, indigestion, asthma and syphilis.

By the 1880s cocaine was widely available in patent medicines without prescription. These included Mariani's Coca Wine, a best seller in Europe, and Coca-Cola. Cocaine became very popular and was also sold in cigarettes, in nose sprays and in chewing gum (Gossop 1993). It was not until the 1980s that the USA, and to a lesser extent the UK, experienced a 'cocaine epidemic.' However, the acceptance of cocaine has been fostered by an association with glamorous image and compounded by the idea of the 'non addictive' nature of the drug. Coca leaves and other psychoactive substances such as coffee, tea and tobacco were introduced to Europe from South America.

Hallucinogenic drugs come into the category of psychoactive substances which have caused intense controversy in their use in the past, and still continue to do so. Originally called 'phantastica' (Lewin 1964), during the 1960s the drugs were referred to as 'psychedelics' (Stevens 1987). The Indian peoples of Central and South America used the naturally occuring psychoactive plant as part of religious rituals and practices and in predicting the future. The medicine man or 'shaman' also used the substances in healing the sick. It has been suggested that the psilocybin mushroom, regarded as a sacred mushroom, was used by the Mayan civilisation even before 1000 BC. (Schultes 1976). Mexico has been the source of hallucinogenic mushrooms and the cactus plant (peyote) and both have played an important role in cultural and religious traditions. The use of sacred mushrooms and morning glory seeds (whose psychoactive components are ergine and isoergine) still persists in parts of Mexico today in rituals for healing and divination (Schultes 1976).

These hallucinogenic psychoactive plants had very little impact on the European culture, despite its long history of drug use, until the 1960s. It was then the synthetic hallucinogens such as LSD (lysergic acid diethylamide) that came under scientific and medical scrutiny. LSD was discovered in 1943 by Albert Hofmann, a chemist working at Sandoz laboratories in Switzerland. Initially, LSD was primarily used as an adjunct to psychotherapy and later in the treatment of alcoholism, drug dependence, sexual problems and psychotic and neurotic disorders. By the early 1960s the drug was used by the emerging 'hippie' subculture for spiritual enlightenment and for mystical peak experiences. Throughout the 1980s in the UK there was a decline in the use of LSD, but it resurfaced in the late 1980s together with other hallucinogens in the 'Rave' subculture. Ecstasy, although not a new drug, appeared on the scene in 1985 and since then there has been an increase in the consumption of both Ecstasy and LSD by young people. The drug was first synthesised in Germany to be used as an appetite suppressant.

Another psychoactive substance that was synthesised in 1887 was amphetamine. It was marketed in the form of a benzedrine inhaler for use in the treatment of nasal congestion, mild depression, schizophrenia, alcoholism and obesity. During the Second World War, amphetamines were widely used by the armed forces to keep the troops functioning under stressful and physically demanding conditions. More recently, amphetamines have also been used in the treatment of narcolepsy and hyperactivity in children. The use of the stimulant was also widespread among athletes and sports men and women to enhance their performance.

During the 1950s there was overprescription of amphetamines by doctors for use in the treatment of common conditions. It was not until the 1960s that amphetamine misuse erupted in the UK among young people and subsequently resulted in an epidemic of injection of methampthetamine. It is argued that, in the UK, the largest positive influence limiting amphetamine misuse has been the slow growth in medical awareness of the danger of these drugs, leading to changes in medical prescribing, as well as a growing realisation among the general population that 'pep pills' are none-too-wise a prop (Royal College of Psychiatrists 1987).

Since ancient times, plants that contain caffeine and other methylxanthines have been used to make beverages. Caffeine is the world's most popular psychoactive substance. Coffee was known to the Arab travellers in the sixth century and was used medicinally and for religious purposes, particularly by the Dervishes to keep themselves awake during long religious practices and rituals (Ghodse 1995). During the seventeenth century, coffee drinking spread from the Arab world and Persia to Britain and other European countries and in eighteenth-century England, coffee was seen as an alternative to sex and as a cure for alcohol intoxication. In the 1840s the 'Bohemians' of Paris took drugs as part of their life-style, which shocked public opinion at that time. The drug was coffee. Coffee is the major source of caffeine and other familiar psychoactive substances such as tea, cocoa and chocolate also contain caffeine. During the last three decades, soft drinks have risen dramatically as a significant source of caffeine. Brazil is the world's leading producer of coffee and the major producers of tea are China and the Indian subcontinent. Cocoa is primarily produced in Africa and Switzerland has the highest per capita consumption of cocoa (James 1991).

This brief overview has covered only a few drugs that have been used over the years and in different cultures for their psychoactive properties. There seems to be a parallel development in the therapeutic use of psychoactive substances and the non medical or recreational use of these drugs. Most of the 'old' drugs such as cannabis, tobacco and alcohol have been used for religious or medicinal purposes. In modern times, these drugs have been primarily used as part of recreational and social activities. It is argued that England's emergence as a colonial power in the seventeenth century was based chiefly upon tobacco and the development of the European market for tobacco was seen as being essential to England's economic future (Harrison 1993). However, in the 1920s Britain had its first notable drug panics. The detection of a drug underground of cocaine and heroin provided an opportunity to initiate debates about women, race, sex and the nation's place in the world. In addition, the outlawing of drugs was the consequence not of their pharmacology, but of their association with ethnic and social groups that were perceived as potentially dangerous (Kohn 1992). In reality, it was the British who promoted the use of psychoactive substances such as opium to the Chinese and the Opium Wars safeguarded the opium trade. In addition, the remnants of this belief still remain in the public consciousness. Contrary to popular mythology, most of the biggest drug importers and criminal gangs in Britain are led, not by Blacks, but by White businessmen or criminals who have the necessary capital (Clutterbuck 1995).

The drug scenes of yesterday and today

In the twentieth century there has been no dovetailing of interest in the use of psychoactive substances and plants. In the 1880s few restrictions were placed on psychoactive drugs such as opium, morphine, marijuana, cocaine and heroin, and these drugs were fairly accessible. However, in the 1990s the above mentioned drugs are all under legal or medical restrictions. Patterns of drug use and misuse frequently change as a result of political and socio-economic conditions and the same 'old' drugs may reappear in different forms or as so called 'designer drugs'. One of the recent concerns regarding the use of psychoactive plants is the use of khat. It is a stimulant containing cathine and cathinone, and is taken by chewing the leaves. Khat use is common in Somalia, Ethiopia, Kenya and the Yemeni Republics. Although illegal in most European countries and the USA, it remains legal in the UK. While khat use in its natural form may not present a significant social and health problem, a potent synthetic form of the active ingredients may cause severe social, psychological, physical and economic harm to the individual and to their families and communities.

Synthetic psychoactive drugs that have resurfaced in the 1990s are LSD and Ecstasy. Another drug which has been mentioned with increased frequency as part of the dance culture is ketamine. It is a short acting anaesthetic with hallucinogenic properties and is not related to LSD or Ecstasy. The issue of young people and alcohol is once again a popular topic. The sudden influx of 'alcopops' and designer alcohol drinks on the market targeted at young consumers has evoked widespread concern and extensive media coverage. The principal concerns are related to the high alcohol content of some of the alcopops, the sweet taste of the drink which has an instant appeal to young people and the marketing of the designer drinks for the club scene. However, at present there is no evidence of an increased incidence of alcohol in the young.

Conclusions

New designer drugs will come and go but they have a tendency to be accompanied by inherent dangers with unpredictable effects and consequences. Society has learned to co-exist with psychoactive substances in the past, and currently more efforts are now being generated to combat substance use and misuse at national and international levels. However, it is worth mentioning the health warning advocated by the Royal College of Psychiatrists (1987) who stressed that 'drug problems will not be beaten out of society by yet harsher laws, lectured out of society by yet more hours of "health education", or treated out of society by yet more drug experts'. The need to understand substance use and misuse in its socio-cultural context and respond to the holistic needs of the substance misusers is beyond dispute.

Currently, it is recognised that substance misuse is preventable and that the associated harm can be reduced if proper intervention and treatment are offered (Rassool & Gafoor 1997b). Different intervention strategies are required at different times and for diverse populations in tackling substance misuse. The need for health care professionals, generic and specialist, to respond effectively to substance use and misuse cannot be overemphasised. Innovative strategies are being considered in the access and delivery of services to those with addictive behaviour, and more emphasis is being placed on developing partnerships in care between the patient, carer and health care professionals. It is through a multi-professional approach to care and management of substance misusers that practitioners will best serve the needs of the population.

References

Abel, E.L. (1980) *Marijuana. The First Twelve Thousands Years.* Plenum Press, New York.

Babor, T. (1986) *Alcohol – Customs and Rituals.* Burke Publishing Company, London.

Berridge, V. & Edwards, G. (1987) *Opium and the People. Opiate Use in Nineteenth-Century England.* Yale University Press, New Haven and London.

Bloomquist, E.R. (1971) *Marijuana: The Second Trip,* revised edn. Glencoe Press, Beverly Hills, CA.

Byck, R. (ed.) (1974) *Cocaine Papers by Sigmund Freud.* Stonehill Publishing Company, New York.

Clutterbuck, R. (1995) *Drugs, Crime and Corruption.* Macmillan Press, London.

Department of Health (1992) *The Health of the Nation: A Strategy for Health in England.* HMSO, London.

Edwards, G. (1971) Unreason in an age of reason. Edwin Stevens Lecture for the Laity. Royal Society of Medicine, London.

Gautier, T. (1966) Le club de hasishins. In: *The Marijuana Papers* (Originally published 1844.) (ed. D. Solomon), pp. 121–35. Bobbs-Merrill, New York.

Ghodse, A.H. (1995) *Drugs and Addictive Behaviour. A Guide to Treatment.* Blackwell Science, Oxford.

Gossop, M. (1993) *Living with Drugs,* 3rd ed. Avebury, Aldershot.

Grinspoon, L. & Bakalar, J.B. (1976) *Cocaine: A Drug and its Social Evolutions.* Basic Books, New York.

Harrison, L. (ed.) (1993) *Race, Culture and Substance Problems.* Department of Social Policy and Professional Studies, University of Hull.

Institute for the Study of Drug Dependence (1993) *National Audit of Drug Misuse in Britain,* pp. 20–1. ISDD, London.

James, J.E. (1991) *Caffeine and Health.* Academic Press, New York.

Kohn, M. (1992) *Dope Girls. The Birth of the British Drug Underground.* Lawrence & Wishart, London.

Lewin, L. (1964) *Phantastica–Narcotic and Stimulating Drugs: Their Use and Abuse.* Routledge and Kegan Paul, London.

Maisto, S.A., Galizio, M. & Connors, G.J. (1995) *Drug Use and Abuse,* 2nd edn. The Harcourt Press, Fortworth, Texas.

Petersen, R.C. (1977) History of cocaine. In: *Cocaine* (eds. R.C. Petersen and R.C. Stillman), pp. 17–34. Research Monograph 13. National Institute of Drug Abuse, Washington DC.

Pollak, B. (1989) Primary health care and the addictions: where to start and where to go. *British Journal of Addiction*, **84**, 1425–32.

Rassool, G.H. & Gafoor, M. (1997a) Themes in addiction nursing. In: *Addiction Nursing: Perspectives on Professional and Clinical Practice* (eds G.H. Rassool & M. Gafoor), pp. 3–5. Stanley Thornes, Cheltenham.

Rassool, G.H. & Gafoor, M. (1997b) Health education, prevention and harm-minimization. In: *Addiction Nursing: Perspectives on Professional and Clinical Practice* (eds G.H. Rassool & M. Gafoor), pp. 171–9. Stanley Thornes, Cheltenham.

Royal College of Psychiatrists (1987) *Drug Scenes. A Report on Drugs and Drug Dependence.* Gaskell, London.

Schultes, R.E. (1976) *Hallucinogenic Plants.* Golden Press, New York.

Stevens, J. (1987) *Storming Heaven: LSD and the American Dream.* Atlantic Monthly Press, New York.

Tackling Drugs Together (1995) *A Strategy for England 1995–1998.* HMSO, London.

The Economist, 13 November 1993, pp. 38.

Whitaker B. (1987) *The Global Connection: The Crisis of Drug Addiction.* Jonathan Cape, London.

World Health Organization (1991) *Expert Committee on Drug Dependence. 28th Report.* WHO, Geneva.

Chapter 2
Concepts and Models

G. Hussein Rassool

Introduction

What is a drug? There are various elements to this question, as the concept is heavily influenced by both the socio-cultural context and the purpose of its use. The definition of the term drug is a product of social custom and law, both of which change over time (Smith 1970). According to the World Health Organization (1981), a drug is defined as

> 'any chemical entity or mixture of entities, other than those required for the maintenance of normal health (like food), the administration of which alters biological function and possibly structure'

A drug, in the broadest sense, is a chemical substance which has an effect on bodily systems and behaviour. Drugs can be therapeutic, non therapeutic or both. A psychoactive drug is a drug that affects the central nervous system and alters mood, thinking, perception and behaviour. In this context, alcohol, tobacco and drug (prescribed and illicit) are psychoactive substances. This text is mainly concerned with the non medical use of psychoactive drugs. The fundamental explanation of the above concept brings us to the question of drug use, misuse and abuse.

Drug misuse

The term drug misuse, according to the Institute for the Study of Drug Dependence (ISDD) (1996), may be seen understood as the use of drug in a socially unacceptable way. It can also be taken to mean the use of a drug which carries implications of illegality or harmfulness and which is used without medical approval. The Royal College of Psychiatrists (1987) defines drug misuse as

> 'any taking of a drug which harms or threatens to harm the physical or mental health or social well-being of an individual, or other individuals, or of society at large, or which is legal.'

This broad definition encompasses the misuse of alcohol, prescribed drugs such as temazepan or diazepam and illicit drugs such as heroin or cocaine. The World Health Organization recommends the use of the following terms:

- Unsanctioned use: a drug that is not approved by society
- Hazardous use: a drug leading to harm or dysfunction
- Dysfunctional use: a drug leading to impaired psychological or social functioning
- Harmful use: a drug that is known to cause tissue damage or psychiatric disorders.

Substance use and abuse

The terms substance use and abuse are difficult concepts to define precisely. The operational use of these concepts is heavily dependent on particular ideology and clinical practice. Substance use, in this book, will be defined as the ingestion of a substance which is used for therapeutic purposes or as prescribed by medical practitioners. Substance misuse is the result of a psychoactive substance being consumed in a way that it was not intended and which may cause physical, social and psychological harm. It is also used to represent the pattern of use: experimental, recreational and dependent.

The term substance abuse, often associated with addiction and dependence, is considered to be value laden and has limited use in the addiction literature in the UK. In the USA, practitioners prefer the term substance abuse for problems resulting from the use of alcohol or other mood altering drugs and use addictive disorders when the problems have escalated to dependency (Sullivan 1995). Whether a substance is used or abused depends very much on the social and cultural context, the individual perspective, the pattern and mode of consumption and the perception of the observer.

Terms such as problem drug user and problem drinker are recommended by the Advisory Council for the Misuse of Drugs (ACMD) Advisory Committee on Alcoholism.

Problem drug user

The ACMD report *Treatment and Rehabilitation* (ACMD 1982) defines a problem drug user as

> 'any person who experiences social, psychological, physical or legal problems related to intoxication and/or regular excessive consumption and/or dependence as a consequence of his own use of drugs or other chemical substances.'

This definition was widened to include any form of drug misuse which involves, or may lead to, sharing of injecting equipment (ACMD 1988).

The above definition focuses on the needs and problems of the individual and places less emphasis on the substance oriented approach. It is a holistic definition in acknowledging that the problem drug user has social, psychological, physical and legal needs and the definition could be expanded to incorporate the spiritual needs of the problem drug user or problem drinker.

Addictive behaviour

Addictive behaviour is a complex dynamic behaviour pattern having psychological, physical, social and behavioural components. Addictive behaviour, according to Marlatt *et al.* (1988) is defined as

> 'a repetitive habit pattern that increases the risk of diseases and/or associated personal or social problems. The individual usually has a loss of control, immediate gratification with delayed, deleterious effects, and experiences relapses when trying to quit.'

Addictive behaviour includes the misuse of psychoactive substances and activities leading to excessive behavioural patterns. Individuals who have problems with excessive behaviours such as eating, drinking, drug use, gambling and sexuality present similar descriptions of the phenomenology of their disorders (Wallace 1977; Cummings *et al.* 1980; Orford 1985; Stall & Biernacki 1986).

Drug dependence

The concept of drug dependence is associated with the World Health Organization (WHO) (1969) and has the advantage of a universal definition. The WHO defined drug dependence as

> 'a state, psychic and sometimes also physical, resulting from the interaction between a living organism and a drug, characterised by behavioural and other responses that always include a compulsion to take the drug on a continuous or periodic basis in order to experience its physical effects, and sometimes to avoid the discomfort of its absence. Tolerance may or may not be present. A person may be dependent on more than one drug.'

This comprehensive definition has been widely accepted and highlights the core features of dependence such as tolerance and psychological and physical dependence. These concepts need further explanation.

Tolerance

Tolerance is a behavioural state and refers to the way the body usually adapts to the repeated presence of a drug. Higher doses of the psychoactive substance are required to reproduce the original or similar effects. Tolerance may develop rapidly in the case of LSD or slowly in the case of alcohol or opiate. The drug must be taken on a regular basis and in adequate quantities for tolerance to occur. Tolerance can be subdivided into:

- ❏ Pharmacodynamic tolerance, when higher doses of the drug are needed to produce the desired response or effect
- ❏ Metabolic tolerance, when there is an increased capacity to metabolise a drug
- ❏ cross tolerance – when one is tolerant to one drug, there is also tolerance to other drugs of the same type or classification

Psychological dependence

Psychological dependence can be described as a compulsion or a craving to continue to take a drug because of the need for stimulation, or because it relieves anxiety or depression. Psychological dependence is recognised as the most widespread and the most important (ISDD 1996). This kind of dependence is not only attributed to the use of psychoactive drugs but also to food, sex, gambling, relationships and physical activities.

Physical dependence

Physical dependence is a state of bodily adaptation to the presence of a particular psychoactive drug. This manifests itself in physical disturbances or withdrawal symptoms following cessation of use. The withdrawal symptoms depend on the type or category of drug. For example, for nicotine, the physiological withdrawal symptoms may be relatively slight. In other dependence inducing psychoactive substances, such as opiates and depressants, the withdrawal experience can range from mild to severe. The withdrawal from alcohol, for instance, can cause hallucinations or epileptic fits and may be life threatening. In the case of heroin withdrawal, physical symptoms such as diarrhoea, running nose and cramps, etc., are present. Physical withdrawal syndromes are not, however, the essence of dependence. It is possible to have dependence without withdrawal and withdrawal without dependence (Royal College of Psychiatrists 1987). However, it is argued that many of the supposed signs of physical dependence are sometimes psychosomatic reactions triggered off, not by the chemical properties of the psychoactive drug, but by the user's fears, beliefs and fantasies about what withdrawal entails (Plant 1987).

The dependence syndrome

The original framework of the dependence syndrome was referred specifically to alcohol dependence, but has since been expanded to include other psychoactive substances. According to Edwards and Gross (1976), there are seven components of the syndrome:

- ❑ Increased tolerance to the drug
- ❑ Repeated withdrawal symptoms
- ❑ Compulsion to use the drug (a psychological state known as craving)
- ❑ Salience of drug seeking behaviour (obtaining and using the drug becomes more important in the person's life)
- ❑ Relief or avoidance of withdrawal symptoms (regular use of the drug to relieve withdrawal symptoms)
- ❑ Narrowing of the repertoire of drug taking (the pattern of drinking may become any everyday activity
- ❑ Rapid reinstatement after abstinence

The dependence syndrome has provided a common language for academics and clinicians to talk about the same phenomena. According to Drummond (1991), the dependence concept has helped to sharpen up diagnostic precision, predict treatment needs and has also provided a means of making experiences intelligible to the problem drinker or problem drug user.

Routes of drug administration

The common routes of drug taking are orally and by smoking, inhalation and injection. The route of administration is very important in the speed of influencing the physical and psychological effects of the drug.

Oral

The oral route (swallowing) is the most popular method of drug administration, although effectively the slowest route because of the slow absorption of the drug into the blood stream. It is stated that, unlike the injection or inhalation routes, there is little stigma associated with taking drugs orally either in pills or in the form of beverages containing alcohol or caffeine (Schilit & Lisansky Gomberg 1991)

Injection

The methods of drug injection include intramuscularly, subcutaneously or intravenously. Injection of drugs is less widespread than other routes of drug administration but is also the most hazardous. The major dangers of injecting are risk of overdose because of the concentrated effect of this method. There is also the risk of infection from non sterile injection methods, which includes hepatitis B and HIV infections, abscesses, gangrene and thromboses. The onset of the effects of the drug is rapid when it is administered intravenously and is a major reason why drugs are often self-administered by injecting. Drugs that are mainly injected include heroin, cocaine, amphetamines and some hypno-sedatives.

Inhalation

The inhalation route (sniff) is also used to self-administer drugs. Absorption of the drug is through the mucous membranes of the nose and mouth. The types of drugs that are inhaled include cocaine, tobacco snuff and volatile substances and solvents. Inhalation may also produce rapid absorption and response, as in the case of crack.

Smoking

Smoking is also a very effective route as the drug is inhaled, as in the case of tobacco or heroin smoking (chasing the dragon). Cannabis or marijuana is also smoked in the form of a 'joint', which is usually mixed with tobacco.

The drug experience

It is acknowledged that the effect a psychoactive substance or 'drug experience' will have on a given individual will depend on several other factors beside the pharmacological properties of the drug. The gamut of drug experience involve interrelated sets of non pharmacological and pharmacological factors. The non pharmacological factors include the personality of the individual and the context or setting. The pharmacological factors include the chemical properties or type of drug used. Different drugs have different modes of action on the body due to their pharmacological properties, dosage and route of administration. The effects or actions of a psychoactive drug are influenced by the personal characteristics of the drug user, which include biological makeup, personality, gender, age and drug tolerance. For instance, some individuals may develop a toxic reaction to a single cup of coffee or the normally insignificant elevation of heart rate caused by cannabis can be painful for those suffering from angina pectoris, whereas glaucoma patients may find cannabis beneficial but a few cups of coffee may aggravate their conditions (ISDD 1996). In addition, the knowledge, attitude and expectations (psychological set) about a drug will have an influence on the drug experience.

For example, if an individual believes or expects that a particular substance will produce a certain effect, the desired effect may be experienced. The last set of factors is the setting or context in which a drug is used. This includes the physical environment where the drug is used, the cultural influences of the community where the drug is consumed, the laws related to drug use and the context in which a drug is used.

All three interrelated factors – pharmacological properties, individual differences and context of use – influence the individual's experience of drug taking. According to the Royal College of Psychiatrists (1987)

'It is necessary to see the drug–brain interaction not as a simple chemical event but as a matter of considerable complexity involving the drug, the particular person, and the messages and teachings which come from the environment and which powerfully influence the nature and meaning of the drug experience.'

Patterns of substance misuse

The patterns of drug or alcohol use and misuse for some individuals may vary over a period of time. According to the patterns, substance misusers are often described as experimental, recreational and problematic.

Experimental users

Experimental users are described as those who use drugs, legal or illicit, on a few occasions. By definition, anyone's initial use of a drug is experimental. The main motivation for experimental drug or alcohol use includes curiosity, anticipation of effects and availability. This usually forms part of the desire among adolescents to experiment and try new, risky experiences. There is no pattern in the use of psychoactive substances but the choice of the drug misused is indiscriminate. The choice of drug use depends on factors such as availability, reputation of the drug, subculture, fashion and peer group influence. Experimental use of illicit psychoactive substances is usually a short lived experience and the majority of people may confine the consumption to drugs that are socially acceptable. Experimental users, however, are in the highest category of risk for infections (if injecting), medical complications or overdose due to the indiscriminate use of adulterated psychoactive substances.

Recreational users

Experimental users may or may not become recreational users of illicit psychoactive substances. The term recreational refers to a form of substance use in which pleasure and relaxation are the prime motivations. There is a strict adherence to the pattern of use so that the drug is only used on certain occasions, such as weekends, and less likely on consecutive days. There is usually a preference for a particular drug (drug of choice) – the user has learnt how to use it and appreciate its effects. Drug or alcohol use is one aspect of the user's life and tends to complement social and recreational activities. There are usually no adverse medical or social consequences as a result of the recreational use.

Dependent users

By definition, a dependent user has progressed to regular and problematic use of a psychoactive drug or has become a polydrug user. There is the presence of psychological and/or physical dependence and it may be distinguished from experimental and recreational use. The pattern of use is more frequent and regular but less controlled. The process of obtaining the drug is more important to the user than the quality of the experience. This tends to displace rather than complement social activities. Injecting drugs is common and the frequent use creates problems of intoxication, infections if sharing needle and syringe, and other medical complications. Personal, social, psychological and legal problems may be present in this group.

Why do people take drugs?

Many models and theories have been put forth to explain why people use or misuse psychoactive substances. The theories provide explanations for the initiation into substance misuse, why individuals begin to use drugs and the process of addiction. Some theories explain both initial and continuing use of drugs (Addiction Research Foundation 1986). However, the reason why people start using drugs may not be the same reason why they continue to use drugs.

An overview of models of substance misuse

A number of models of substance misuse have been proposed in an attempt to understand and clarify substance use and misuse:

- ❑ The moral model
- ❑ The medical/disease model
- ❑ The psychological model
- ❑ The sociocultural model

These models have implications in the delivery of care and treatment programmes to substance misusers. For a more detailed discussion of the models see Miller and Hester (1989). An overview of the models, with a brief explanation of the relevant theories appropriate to each, will be presented in this section.

Moral model

According to this model individuals are viewed as responsible for the initiation and development of problems as a result of substance misuse. Addictive behaviours such as drug taking, heavy drinking or gambling are seen as sinful or weak willed. Substance misusers need to exert willpower to refrain from drinking or taking drugs and treatment consists of mainly spiritual intervention.

Medical/disease model

The disease concept of alcoholism was initially proposed by Jellinek (1960). This model views addictive behaviour as a progressive, incurable disorder and the cause of the disease is firmly attributed to the genetic/biological make up of the individual. A number of studies have suggested that substance misuse is the result of genetic or induced biological abnormality of a physiological, structural or chemical nature. There is strong evidence that early onset alcoholism is genetically determined (Cloninger 1987; Blum *et al.* 1990). It also appears that a genetic predisposition may also protect some individuals who have a genetically based metabolic sensitivity to indulging in psychoactive substances such as alcohol (Wolf 1972). In the case of narcotic addiction, vulnerability is explained by an unspecified metabolic deficiency (Dole & Nyswander 1967).

This medical/disease approach also implies the adoption of the sick role by the substance misusers and the individuals are expected to be treated as having a 'disease'. The treatment approach also implies that recovery from drug or alcohol misuse can only be sustained through the goal of total abstinence within the self help group movements such as AA, NA and GA (Alcoholics Anonymous, Narcotics Anonymous, Gamblers Anonymous respectively). The disease concept of addictive behaviour is incorporated in the philosophy underpinning the approaches of NA or AA in the adoption of the Minnesota model (Cook 1988).

Psychological model

The psychological model includes the social learning, family interaction and personality approaches. The social learning theory model proposes that social behaviour is learnt through observation and modelling. It is stated that modelling by parents is an important factor in the initial pattern of consumption of social and illicit psychoactive substances, especially in those with poor social skills (Baer *et al.* 1987). Nathan (1983) described alcohol use as a socially acquired, learned behaviour pattern maintained by cognitive factors, modelling influences, expectancies and cues, reinforcement and the interaction of behavioural and genetic mechanisms.

The family interaction model emphasises the role of parental behaviour in the substance misuse family in the case of alcoholism. Family environment, it seems, plays an important part in determining alcohol consumption; and it is suggested that alcoholism is consistently associated with deficits in parenting, family tension, rejection, emotional distancing and parental alienation (Baer *et al.* 1987; Schilit & Lisansky Gomberg 1991). The most common psychological theory is that many young people try psychoactive substances out of sheer curiosity about the effects and a desire to experiment (Rassool 1993).

The personality characteristics of the substance misuser have also been linked to substance misuse. Several factors, including lack of maturity, interpersonal and intrapersonal conflicts, low self-esteem, underlying depression and anxiety, inability to cope with anger, etc., have been suggested to be the cause of drug and alcohol problems. The term 'addictive personality' has been ascribed to those individuals who have become dependent on drugs or alcohol. Research in the area of personality and substance misuse has partly supported the view that the concept is applicable to all the various addictive behaviours. However, Johns (1990) argued that there is no evidence for an 'addictive personality type' common to substance misusers, although there are indications that they show more neuroticism and hostility than non uses.

Another model of personality traits and addictive behaviour has been proposed by Cloninger (1987), who identified two types of alcohol abuse:

❑ Type 1 is associated with traits of a passive-dependent or anxious personality (alcohol seeking behaviour and psychological dependence).
❑ Type 2 is associated with characteristics of an antisocial personality (novelty seeking behaviour is prominent).

Sociocultural model

Sociocultural explanations of the use and misuse of psychoactive substances emphasise the role of culture, beliefs, values and attitudes held by a community or minority groups in the way individuals will abstain from or take drugs. Cultural attitudes towards the use of psychoactive drugs may also play an important part in shaping individual behaviour. In some culture or ethno-cultural groups abstinence may be the norm, and in others it may be part of religious ritual and ceremonies, or acceptable as a social and recreational drug. For example, a subculture or a minority group may have norms and rules of behaviour that govern the use of cannabis, khat or alcohol. It is asserted that roles such as those of 'skaghead', 'addict', or 'dealer' may be rewarding for some individuals in that they contribute to a sense of personal identity or identification with a cultural subgroup. More recently, the drug Ecstasy has been identified with the subculture of 'ravers'.

Sociological factors such as unemployment, social deprivation, poor environment, etc., may have important effects on whether individuals start to misuse drugs and whether they continue (Peck & Plant 1986). Other social factors such as age, sex, religion, ethnicity, socio-economic class and family background directly influence whether an individual will use psychoactive substances in that way. A number of socio-cultural models have been distinguished by Heath (1988). The socio-cultural framework includes the normative model, the single distribution model, the anxiety model, the social organisation model, the conflict-over-dependency model, the power model, the symbolic interactionist model and the social learning model.

Government interventions tend to sanction and impose legislation on the use of psychoactive substances and medicines. Drugs are classified according to a schedule (see Chapter 4 for the legal aspects of psychoactive substances). Interventions are focused on health and social policy levels including prevention, health education, treatment, taxation and demand reduction.

A summary of a multi-faced model of addiction, according to Checinski (1996) (see Table 2.1).

Conclusions

It is apparent from the literature that no single model or factor is responsible as the cause of substance misuse, rather several factors are involved. A number of models have been presented in order to provide different perspectives of substance misuse from different disciplines. Research in the area of the aetiology of substance misuse and addictive behaviour is flawed due to the lack of objective criteria for measurement and the selected groups of patients or clients in institutions. Substance misuse and human behaviour are complex issues that require a holistic approach in both the understanding of the underlying causes of substance misuse and in the application of clinical practice.

References

Advisory Council on the Misuse of Drugs (1982) *Treatment and Rehabilitation.* HMSO, London.

Advisory Council on the Misuse of Drugs (1988) *Aids and Drug Misuse: Part 1.* HMSO, London.

Table 2.1 Multifaceted model of addiction.

	Moral	Disease	Symptomatic	Learning	Social
Aetiology	Weak or bad character	Biological factors, possibly genetic	Another primary mental disorder	Learned behaviour disorder	Environmental and social factors
Focus of treatment	Control of behaviour through deterrent punishment	Abstinence to stop progression of disease	Improved mental functioning	Learning behaviour alternative to or incompatible with substance misuse	Improved social functioning
Advantages	Responsibility for change lies with the user	Not blaming or punitive	Not blaming or punitive. Emphasis on importance of diagnosing and treating co-existing mental disorders	Not blaming or punitive. Holds user responsible for new learning	Easily integrated into other models
Disadvantages	Punitive	Absolves user of responsibility to change. Ignores psychological, cultural and environmental factors	Implies treatment of mental disorder is sufficient	Tends to ignore personality disability consequences of excessive substance misuse and irrationality of human beings	Implies change of social situation is sufficient

Source: Dr Roger Farmer

Addiction Research Foundation (1986) *Essential Concepts and Strategies.* Canadian Government Publishing Centre, Supply and Services, Toronto.

Baer, P.E., Garmezy, L.B., McLaughlin, R.J., *et al.* (1987) Stress, coping, family conflict and adolescent alcohol use. *Journal of Behavioural Medicine*, **10**, 449–66.

Blum, K., Noble, E.P., Sheridan, P.J., *et al.* (1990) Allelic association of human dopamine D2 receptor gene in alcoholism. *Journal of American Medical Association*, **263**, 2055–60.

Checinski, K. (1996) Models of substance misuse. Department of Addictive Behaviours, St George's Medical School, London (unpublished work).

Cloninger, C.R. (1987) Neurogenetic adaptive mechanisms in alcoholism. *Science*, **236**, 410–15.

Cook, C. (1988) The Minnesota model in the management of drug and alcohol dependency: miracle, method or myth? Part 1. The philosophy and the programme. *British Journal of Addiction*, **83**, 625–34.

Cummings, C., Gordon, J.R. & Marlatt, G.A. (1980) relapse: prevention and prediction. In: *The Addictive Behaviours: Treatment of Alcoholism, Drug Abuse, Smoking and Obesity* (ed. W.R. Miller). Pergamon Press, New York.

Dole, V.P. & Nyswander, M.E. (1967) Rehabilitation of street addict. *Archives of Environmental Health*, **14**, 477–80

Drummond, C. (1991) Dependence on psychoactive drugs: finding a common language. In: *The International Handbook of Addiction Behaviour* (ed. I.B. Glass), Chapter 1. Routledge, London.

Edwards, G. & Gross, M.M. (1976) Alcohol dependence: provisional description of a clinical syndrome. *British Medical Journal*, **1**, 1058–61.

Heath, D.B. (1988) Emerging anthropological theory and models of alcohol use and alcoholism. In: *Theories on Alcoholism* (eds C.D. Chaudron & D.A. Wilkinson). Addiction Research Foundation, Toronto.

Institute for the Study of Drug Dependence (1996) *Drug Abuse Briefings*, 6th edn. ISDD, London.

Jellinek, E.M. (1960) *The Disease Concept of Alcoholism.* Hillhouse Press, New Haven.

Johns, A. (1990)) What is drug dependence? In: *Substance Abuse and Dependence* (eds A.H. Ghodse & D. Maxwell). Macmillan Press, London.

Marlatt, G.A., Baer, J.S., Donovan, D.M. & Kivlahan, D.R. (1988) Addictive behaviours: etiology and treatment. *Annual Review of Psychology*, **39**, 223–52.

Miller, W.R. & Hester, R.K. (1989) Treating alcohol problems: toward an informed eclecticism. In: *Handbook of Alcoholism Treatment Approaches* (eds R.K. Hester & W.R. Miller), pp. 3–14. Pergamon, New York.

Nathan, P.E. (1983) Behavioural theory and behavioural theories of alcoholics. In: *Recent Developments in Alcoholism* (ed. M. Galanter), Vol. 1. Plenum, New York.

Orford, J. (1985) *Excessive Appetites: A Psychological View of Addictions.* Wiley, New York.

Peck, D.F. & Plant, M.A. (1986) Unemployment and illegal drug use. Concordant evidence from a prospective study and national trends. *British Medical Journal*, **293**, 929–32.

Plant, M. (1987) *Drugs in Perspective*, pp. 13–14. Hodder and Stoughton, London.

Rassool, G.H. (1993) Adolescents and street drugs: issues for community nurses. *Professional Care of Mother and Child*, November/December.

Royal College of Psychiatrists (1987) *Drug Scenes. A Report on Drugs and Drug Dependence.* Gaskell, London.

Schilit, R. & Lisansky Gomberg, E.S. (1991) *Drugs and Behaviour.* Sage Publications, Newbury Park.

Smith, J.P. (1970) Society and drugs: a short sketch. In: *Drug Abuse Data and Debate* (ed. P.H. Blachly). Charles C. Thomas, Springfield.

Stall, R. & Biernacki, P. (1986) Spontaneous remission from the problematic use of substances: an inductive model derived from a comparative analysis of the alcohol, opiate, tobacco and food/obesity literatures. *International Journal of the Addications,* **21**, 1–32.

Sullivan, E.J. (1995) *Nursing Care of Clients with Substance Abuse.* Mosby Year Book, Missouri.

Wallace, J. (1977) Alcoholism from the inside out: a phenomenological analysis. In: *Alcoholism: Development, Consequences and Interventions* (eds N.J. Estes & M. Heinemann). Mosby, St Louis.

Wolf, P.H. (1972) Ethnic differences in alcohol sensitivity. *Science,* **175**, 449–50.

World Health Organization (1969) *Sixteenth report of WHO Expert Committee on Drug Dependence.* Technical Report Series No 407. WHO, Geneva.

World Health Organization (1981) Nomenclature and classification of drug-and alcohol-related problems: a WHO memorandum. *Bulletin of the World Health Organization,* **59**, 225–42.

Chapter 3
Tobacco Smoking

G. Hussein Rassool and Julie Winnington

Introduction

Tobacco smoking is probably the single largest preventable cause of serious ill health and premature mortality. It is, without doubt, both a personal and public health issue (Ghodse 1994). Although the prevalence has declined steadily in the UK over the past decade, 28% of adults in England are regular smokers and most started smoking before the age of 18. Among specific groups such as women, teenagers and those in the lower socio-economic groups, the rates of decline are slow (Office of Population Censures and Surveys 1992). Smoking related diseases account for some 150 000 deaths a year in the UK, including about a third of deaths in middle age (Royal College of Physicians 1983; Ghodse 1994). It is estimated that smoking kills about five times more people than all other avoidable deaths put together, including road accidents, fires and other accidents, suicide, murder, AIDS and illicit substance misuse (Department of Health 1990).

The health and risk factors associated with active cigarette smoking include cancer, cardiovascular disease, respiratory diseases, sexual health and maternal health. It is clear that the harmful effects of smoking are not confined to smokers; data on the health effects of cigarette smoking documents the adverse effects of 'second hand' or passive smoking (Kauffmann *et al.* 1983). It is against this background that *The Health of the Nation* document (Department of Health 1992) sets a target for reduction in the prevalence of cigarette smoking to 20% by the year 2000. A framework for action in reducing smoking is set out in the document *Smoke-Free for Health* (Department of Health 1994).

The aims of this chapter are to examine the health of the nation in relation to tobacco smoking and the harmful constituents of tobacco smoke. In addition, aspects of passive smoking and health concerns, health gains and smoking cessation are also addressed.

The Health of the Nation and smoking

The Health of the Nation (Department of Health 1992) is a strategic plan aimed at promoting good health and preventing ill health for everyone in England. The plan, in the context of tobacco smoking, sets out specific targets to reduce the prevalence of smoking in adults and also among the 11–15 year olds. In order to reduce the health related damage caused by tobacco addiction, the government set four main targets:

❑ To reduce the prevalence of cigarette smoking in men and women aged 16 and over to no more than 20% by the year 2000 (a reduction of at least 35% in men and 29% in women, from a prevalence in 1990 of 31% and 28% respectively).
❑ To reduce by at least a third the number of women smoking at the start of their pregnancy, by the year 2000.
❑ To reduce the consumption of cigarettes by at least 40% by the year 2000.
❑ To reduce smoking prevalence among 11–15 year olds by at least 33% by 1994 (from about 8% in 1988 to less than 6%).

Although *The Health of the Nation* was an encouraging initiative, it failed to recognise smoking as a form of addiction and made no recommendations on the need to provide treatment for smokers (Ghodse 1994). However, the government is taking action in five main areas to achieve the targets set in *The Health of the Nation*. This strategy (Department of Health 1995) focuses on:

❑ Raising tobacco taxation in order to reduce accessibility of tobacco products.
❑ Effective health education and prevention campaigns to increase the awareness of health risks and to provide support for smokers who want to give up.
❑ Ensuring effective controls on advertising and promotion of tobacco products.
❑ Protecting non smokers from passive smoking by regulations covering smoking in work places and in public places, including transport.

Among further improvements the government seeks are:

❑ Patients to be asked routinely about their smoking habits when they visit their GP.
❑ An increase in the number of smokers visiting their GP who receive smoking cessation advice.
❑ An increase in smoking cessation advice given to smokers attending hospital out-patient clinics.
❑ A high priority given to the provision of advice on smoking and support for those wishing to stop.
❑ An increase in the smoking cessation advice given to pregnant women attending hospital and GP antenatal clinics, with support for those wishing to stop.

Nicotine addiction

There is evidence to suggest that tobacco smoking is addictive. The US Department of Health and Human Services (1988) reported that 'the pharmacologic and behavioural processes that determine tobacco addiction are similar to those that determine addiction to drugs such as heroin and cocaine'. Henningfield (1986) compared tobacco dependence to other forms of substance misuse and concluded that there are more commonalities than differences. He concluded that tobacco dependence is a complex process involving interactions between drug and non drug factors and includes the development of tolerance and withdrawal symptoms.

Tobacco, like many psychoactive substances, is subjectively pleasurable and often produces rewarding effects in the relief of stress and in enhancing mood and performance. According to the *Diagnostic and Statistical Manual of Mental Disorders* (DSM-lll-R) (American Psychiatric Association 1987), nicotine dependence is considered to be a psychoactive substance use disorder.

Harmful constituents of tobacco smoke

The burning of tobacco produces different gases and chemicals and the main components include tar, nicotine and carbon dioxide. According to Russell (1989), people smoke mainly for nicotine but die mainly from the effects of carbon monoxide, tar and other constituents.

Tar

Tar comprises 4000 different organic chemicals, including carcinogens, and, on smoke exhalation, the brown sticky substance remains in the lungs causing irritation and damage. According to Mangan and Golding (1984) the various components of tar are cancer initiating and cancer accelerating. The lung cancer risks of smoking are causal and direct and are associated with the tar. There is evidence to suggest that reduction in tar yield has contributed to the decline in lung cancer rates (Department of Health 1994).

Nicotine

Nicotine, a principal toxic component of cigarette smoking, is highly addictive. It is a powerful psychoactive substance which acts on the nervous system and increases the heart rate and blood pressure (Royal College of Physicians 1983). Nicotine can increase the stickiness of the blood platelets and, in patients with established coronary heart disease, it can precipitate an episode of arrhythmia (irregular heart beat). The amount of nicotine in tobacco depends upon the brand and type of cigarette. The average cigarette yields at least 6 to 8 mg of nicotine while a cigar may contain approximately 15 to 40 mg of nicotine. Although nicotine is poisonous it is not delivered rapidly enough to prove fatal to the individual as it is absorbed very slowly when it is inhaled.

Carbon monoxide

Carbon monoxide, a colourless, odourless gas, is one of the harmful gases in tobacco smoke. It rapidly enters the blood stream and its toxicity stems from its ability to bind to haemoglobin to form carboxyhaemoglobin. Thus, habitual smokers have a reduced amount of haemoglobin available and an increased number of red blood cells. It has been reported that carbon monoxide binds not only to haemoglobin but also to many other iron proteins (Goldsmith & Landau 1968). In smokers, where the oxygen carrying capacity of the blood is reduced, disease of the peripheral circulation can have adverse health effects.

Medical and psychological effects of smoking

Cardiovascular disease

- ❑ Coronary heart disease is one the major cause of deaths from tobacco smoking.
- ❑ It is estimated that 18% of coronary heart disease deaths, approximately 26 000 a year, are associated with smoking (Health Education Authority 1992).
- ❑ Coronary heart disease, including acute myocardial infarction and chronic ischemic heart disease, occur frequently in women who smoke.
- ❑ The use of oral contraceptives by women who smoke cigarettes increases the risk of myocardial infarction by a factor of approximately 10.
- ❑ Both nicotine and carbonmonoxide in cigarette smoke can precipitate angina attacks.
- ❑ Smoking is an important risk factor for stroke when it occurs in association with other risk factors such as high blood pressure. About 11% of deaths (approximately 7000 deaths a year) are associated with stroke (Health Education Authority 1992).
- ❑ Smoking also contributes to cerebral, aortic and peripheral vascular disease. (US Department of Health and Human Services 1989).

Respiratory diseases

- ❑ The majority of patients suffering from chronic bronchitis, pulmonary emphysema and bronchial asthma are cigarette smokers (Crowdy & Snowden 1975).

❑ It is estimated that at least 80% of chronic bronchitis and emphysema is associated with smoking, causing around 19 000 deaths a year (Health Education Authority 1992).

❑ There is a close relationship between cigarette smoking and chronic cough and mucus hypersecretion.

Cancer

❑ There is a direct relationship between cigarette consumption and cancer (Doll & Peto 1976).

❑ It is estimated that at least 80% of lung cancer is associated with smoking, with some 27 000 deaths a year (Health Education Authority 1992).

❑ Smokers taking 20 or more cigarettes a day have 20 times the risk of lung cancer than non smokers (Royal College of Physicians 1991).

❑ Smoking has also been associated with cancer of the lung, mouth, pharynx, larynx, bladder, pancreas, kidney, stomach and cervix (US Department of Health and Human Services 1989).

❑ The risk of developing cancer of the larynx is 10 times greater among tobacco smokers who are also problem drinkers.

Sexual health

❑ Tobacco smoking might impair fertility in both women and men. Smokers take longer to conceive than non smokers.

❑ Smokers are more likely to have an early menopause than non smokers (Wald & Baron 1990).

❑ Women smokers who take oral contraceptives have approximately 10 times the risk of a heart attack, stroke or other cardiovascular disease compared to non smokers (Health Education Authority 1991).

Effects of maternal smoking during pregnancy

❑ Maternal smoking during pregnancy is associated with increased fetal and perinatal mortality and low birth weight (Poswillo & Alberman 1992).

❑ Maternal smoking during pregnancy exerts a direct growth retarding effect on the fetus and delays physical and mental development of infants (Poswillo & Alberman 1992).

❑ Women who continue to smoke tobacco in pregnancy have an increased risk of miscarriage (Royal College of Physicians 1992).

❑ Premature labour is twice as common and perinatal mortality is increased by almost a third in women who smoke during pregnancy (Royal College of Physicians 1992).

❑ Smoking in pregnancy may adversely affect the child's long term growth, behavioural characteristics and educational achievement (Poswillo & Alberman 1992).

❑ During pregnancy, female smokers have an increased rate of antenatal problems, reflecting retarded intra-uterine growth (Royal College of Physicians 1983).

Passive smoking and health concerns

One of the more recently published health effects of environmental tobacco smoke (ETS) concerns the uptake of smoke impregnated environment by non smokers (Independent Scientific Committee on Smoking and Health (ISCSH); 1988 EPA 1992). The non smoker breathes sidestream smoke, that is, the smoke which arises from smouldering tobacco and passes directly into the surrounding air. Many potential toxic and carcinogenic compounds at higher concentrations than in mainstream smoke are present in this (International Agency for Cancer Research 1986). When smoking has occurred, an average room has nearly 85% of side stream smoke and about three times the normal carbon monoxide level.

Research on the effects of passive smoking has established the following:

❑ Carcinogenic tars enter the lungs of non smokers and nicotine can be measured in their urine.
❑ Acute effects of passive smoking include irritation of the eyes, nose and throat. This can result in reddening, itching, increased running of the eyes, coughs and sore throats (US Environmental Protection Agency 1992).
❑ Non smokers who are exposed to tobacco smoke for most of their lives have a 10–30% greater risk of lung cancer than non-smokers who are not exposed to passive smoking (HMSO 1988).
❑ Non smoking wives of husbands who smoke have a doubled risk of lung cancer (Hirayama 1981)
❑ Passive smoking may contribute to the development of coronary heart disease (US Department of Health and Human Services 1990).

Parental smoking and child illnesses

❑ The health of the child is impaired: bronchitis and pneumonia are increased in infants and older children suffer more respiratory complaints (US Environmental Protection Agency 1992).
❑ It has been estimated in one study that parental smoking was responsible for at least 17 000 admissions to hospital per year of children under the age of 5 (Royal College of Physicians 1992).
❑ It has been reported that as many as one third of cases of 'glue ear' are attributable to parental smoking and there is strong evidence of a causal

association (Royal College of Physicians 1992; US Environmental Protection Agency 1992).

❑ It has been reported that passive smoking is a risk factor for asthma in children without previous symptoms and that the symptoms of asthma are twice as common in children of smokers (Royal College of Physicians 1992; EPA Report 1993).

❑ Current evidence strongly suggests that infants whose mothers smoke are at an increased risk of cot death (Department of Health 1993).

Psychological effects of tobacco smoking

The main psychological effects of tobacco smoking are summarises below:

❑ Smokers' self-reports indicate that tobacco smoking acts as a mood regulator and increases pleasure.

❑ Smoking acts as a relief in highly stressful situations and periods of strong emotion and reduces aggression and irritability.

❑ Smoking increases performance and concentration on minor tasks.

Health gains and benefits of smoking cessation

❑ An improvement in overall health and other health gains will result from giving up smoking.

❑ The risk of death of former smokers compared to that for continuing smokers begins to decline shortly after giving up until after some 15 years of abstinence (US Department of Health and Human Services 1990).

❑ Smoking cessation substantially reduces the risk of coronary heart disease among men and women (US Department of Health and Human Services 1990).

❑ Smoking cessation reduces the risk of stroke (US Department of Health and Human Services 1990).

❑ A reduction of risk of between 30% and 50% for lung cancer has been reported after 10 years abstinence. Bladder cancer and cervical cancer risks are also substantially lower after a few years of abstinence (US Department of Health and Human Services 1990).

❑ Women who stop smoking before becoming pregnant have infants of the same birth weight as those born to women who have never smoked (ISCSH 1983).

Smoking cessation

In the adult population in the UK there has been a sustained decrease in the number of smokers. Some 29% of men are now smokers, compared to 31%

in 1990; 27% of women now smoke, compared to 28% in 1990 (Office of Population Censuses and Surveys 1992). Many smokes are well motivated to stop smoking and would like to give up but feel unable to do so. When regular smokers cut down or stop their tobacco intake they experience a withdrawal syndrome characterised by craving for nicotine, irritability, frustration or anger, anxiety, difficulty concentrating, restlessness, increased appetite or weight gain and decreased heart rate. Withdrawal symptoms begin within 24 hours of reduction or cessation of nicotine use and usually decrease in intensity over a period of a few days to several weeks. It is estimated that at least 5% of smokers would give up with brief intervention from their GP (Health Education Authority 1992).

A number of approaches have been suggested to help people stop smoking, with different degrees of success. Within these approaches, two broad strategies can be identified: the motivational approaches and the treatment methods. It is suggested that motivational approaches increase the desire and intention to stop, while treatment methods offer specific strategies to overcome dependence (Jarvis & Russell 1989).

Motivational interventions can 'nudge' individuals to change, but this depends on the individual's readiness to change his drug using behaviour. Prochaska and Di Clemente (1983, 1986) have developed a model to assess the individual according to his 'stage and readiness to change'. According to this, there are five stages of change: the precontemplation stage, contemplation stage, decision making and preparation stage, action stage and maintenance stage. Tobacco smokers will be at different stages in this dynamic process at any one time. In the precontemplation stage, the individual smoker is not thinking about stopping and may not be aware of his addiction. In the contemplation stage, individuals are aware of their dependence on nicotine and may consider stopping. In the decision making and preparation stage the individual may decide to stop. The action stage involves the individual in the process of smoking cessation. In the maintenance stage the individual is involved in maintaining the desired change of being drug free and avoiding relapse. According to Prochaska and Di Clemente (1983), many smokers who have succeeded in stopping smoking have tried and failed on previous occasions. The motivational approaches include mass media campaigns and health education activities to persuade smokers to quit. These campaigns have been successful in making many smokers want to stop, but their effectiveness has been limited by the extent to which nicotine dependence constitutes a block for many smokers (Jarvis 1991).

Treatment approaches including nicotine substitutes in the form of nicotine patches, chewing gum or sprays have been used as part of the treatment package for short periods of time. There is evidence to suggest that brief interventions by GPs given as part of routine health checks induce a small percentage of mainly light smokers to give up. GP surgeries can help smokers to give up, particularly when nicotine replacement therapy is used (Russell *et al.* 1979; West 1993). Most researchers agree that both behavioural techniques and one to one counselling, when used in a complementary fashion, can effect long term changes in smoking behaviour (Jarvis & Russell 1989).

The essential features common to most methods of helping smokers to stop, according to Foulds and Jarvis (1995), are that they provide the smoker with a strategy and a rationale, i.e. a plan of what to do and a convincing reason for following that plan of action. Health care professionals can make an impact in this area by providing health education about the risks of smoking, supplemented by brief counselling and support. (See Chapter 21 on the health care interventions in nicotine addiction.)

Conclusions

Tobacco smoking can 'seriously damage your health', causing cancer, cardiovascular disease, respiratory disease and sexual and maternal ill health. Health care professionals need to be aware of the paradox of this legal psychoactive substance. In all specialities, they have a key part to play in preventing serious ill health and premature mortality through self-care programmes and health education activities. However, it is argued that education and other restrictive control measures which are advocated by health education authorities and *The Health of the Nation* will not be effective alone, even though they are crucial to any comprehensive programme. They should be complemented by adequate provision of help and treatment for those who need it and who are ready to accept it (Ghodse 1994). A handbook to help practice and community nurses, health visitors and midwives to offer more comprehensive and practical advice to patients who want to stop smoking and educational programmes aimed at helping health care professionals to organise a stop smoking programme are available from the Health Education Authority.

References

American Psychiatric Association (APA) (1987) *Diagnostic and Statistical Manual of Mental Disorders*, 3rd edn. APA, Washington DC.

Crowdy, J.P. & Snowden, R.R. (1975) Cigarette smoking and respiratory ill-health in the British army. *Lancet*, **1**, 1232.

Department of Health (1990) *OPCS Scottish and Northern Ireland Registrars General; For the Study of Drug Dependence*. HMSO, London.

Department of Health (1992) *The Health of the Nation*. HMSO, London.

Department of Health (1993) *The Sleeping Position of Infants and Cot Death. Report of the Chief Medical Officer's Expert Group*. HMSO, London.

Department of Health (1994) *Smoke-Free for Health*. HMSO, London.

Department of Health (1995) *Fit for the Future: Second Progress Report on the Health of the Nation*. HMSO, London.

Doll, R. & Peto, R. (1976) Mortality in relation to smoking: 20 years observations on male British doctors. *British Medical Journal,* **2,** 1525–36.

Foulds, J. & Jarvis, M.J. (1995) Smoking cessation and prevention. In: *Chronic Pulmonary Disease* (eds P. Calverley & N. Pride). Chapman & Hall, London.

Ghodse, A.H. (1994) Modifying tobacco consumption. In: *Modifying Tobacco Consumption – Psychological and Behavioural Approaches. Conference Proceedings. St George's Hospital Medical School, London, March 1994.*

Goldsmith, J.R. & Landau, S.A. (1968) Carbon monoxide and human health. *Science,* **162,** 1352.

Health Education Authority (1991) *Health Update: 2: Smoking.* Health Education Authority, London.

Health Education Authority (1992) *The Smoking Epidemic – A Manifesto for Action in England.* Health Education Authority, London.

Henningfield, J.E. (1986) How tobacco produces drug dependence. In: *The Pharmacologic Treatment of Tobacco Dependence: Proceedings of the World Congress (ed. J.K. Ockene), pp. 19–31. Institute for the Study of Smoking Behaviour and Policy, Cambridge, MA.*

Hirayama, T. (1981) Non smoking wives of heavy smokers have a higher risk of lung cancer: a study from Japan. *British Medical Journal,* **ii,** 1109–12.

Independent Scientific Committee on Smoking and Health (1983) *Third Report.* HMSO, London.

Independent Scientific Committee on Smoking and Health (1988) *Fourth report.* HMSO, London.

International Agency for Cancer Research (1986) *Tobacco Smoking.* IARC Monograph 38. IARC, Lyon.

Jarvis, M.J. (1991) Tobacco smoking: an everyday drug addiction. In: *The International Handbook of Addiction Behaviour* (ed. I.B. Glass), pp. 97–9. Tavistock/Routledge, London.

Jarvis, M.J. & Russell, M.A.H. (1989) Treatment for the cigarette smoker. *International Review of Psychiatry,* **1,** 139–47.

Kauffmann, F., Tessier, J.F. & Oriol, P. (1983) Adult passive smoking in the home environment: a risk factor for chronic airflow limitation. *American Journal of Epidemiology,* **117, 269.**

Mangan, G.L. & Golding, J.F. (1984) *The Psychopharmacology of Smoking.* Cambridge University Press, Cambridge.

Office of Population Censuses and Surveys (1992) *General Household Survey 1990.* HMSO, London.

Poswillo, D. & Alberman, E. (eds) (1992) *Effects of Smoking on the Fetus, Neonate and Child.* Oxford University Press, Oxford.

Prochaska, J.O. & DiClemente, C.C. (1983) Stages and processes of self-change of smoking: toward an integrative model of change. *Journal of Consulting and Clinical Psychology,* **51,** 390–95.

Prochaska, J.O. & DiClemente, C.C. (1986) Towards a comprehensive model of change. In: *Treating Addictive Behaviours: Process of Change* (eds W.R. Miller & N. Heather) pp. 3–27. Plenum Press, New York.

Royal College of Physicians (1992) *Smoking and the Young. A Report of a Working Party of the Royal College of Physicians.* RCP, London.

Royal College of Physicians (1991) *Preventive Medicine. A Report of a Working Party of the Royal College of Physicians.* RCP, London.

Royal College of Physicians (1983) *Health or Smoking? Follow-up Report of the Royal College of Physicians.* Churchill Livingstone, London.

Russell, M.A.H. (1989) 'The addiction research unit at the Institute of Psychiatry – II. The work of the unit's smoking section. *British Journal of Addiction*, **84**, 853–64.

Russell, M.A.H., Wilson, C., Taylor, C. & Baker, C.D. (1979) Effects of general practitioners' advice against smoking. *British Medical Journal*, **2**, 231–5.

US Department of Health and Human Services (1988) *Nicotine Addiction: A Report of the Surgeon General*. USDHHS, Washington DC.

US Department of Health and Human Services (1989) *Reducing the Health Consequences of Smoking. 25 years of progress. A report of the Surgeon General*. USDHHS, Washington DC.

US Department of Health and Human Services (1990) *The Health Benefits of Smoking Cessation. A Report of the Surgeon General*. USDHHS, Washington DC.

US Environmental Protection Agency (1992) *Respiratory Health Effects of Passive Smoking: Lung Cancer and other Respiratory Disorders*. Office of Health and Environmental Assessment, Office of Atmospheric and Indoor Air Programs, Washington DC.

Wald, N. & Baron, J. (eds) (1990) *Smoking and Hormone-Related Disorders*. Oxford University Press, Oxford.

West, R. (1993) Tobacco smoking: the health service and the health of the nation. *Substance Misuse Bulletin*, **4**, 3–4.

Chapter 4

An Overview of Psychoactive Drugs

G. Hussein Rassool

Introduction

This chapter focuses on the nature and effects of psychoactive substances. An overview only is provided on the different drugs that are part of the UK drug scene. Psychoactive substances such as alcohol and tobacco are dealt with in subsequent chapters. More extensive coverage of drugs such as opiates, benzodiazepines and stimulants is included in Section 4 of the book. In this chapter, the classification of psychoactive substances will be examined; these include opiates, hypnosedatives, stimulants, hallucinogens, cannabis, tranquillisers, steroids, the rave drug Ecstasy and other less common psychoactive substances. The use, legal status and effects of the drugs will be described briefly.

Opiates

The term opiate refers to any psychoactive substance, either natural or synthetic, that has an effect similar to morphine. Opiates are derived from the opium poppy although there are a number of psychoactive synthetic substitutes. The drug opium is obtained from scarifying the seed of the poppy; morphine and codeine are extracted from opium and heroin is manufactured chemically from morphine. Some of the more common opiate drugs are codeine, heroin, pethidine, methadone (physeptone), morphine and dipipanone (diconal). The street names for heroin include smack, junk, gear, scag H, scat, tiger, chi, elephant, harry and dragon. There is an increase in the illicit use of opiates, especially heroin, due to widespread availability. In 1995, illicit heroin, averaging 50% purity, was retailed at around £100 per gramme, often with wide regional variations (Institute for the study of Drug Dependence (ISDD) 1996).

Therapeutic and illicit uses

The medical applications of opiates include effective relief of pain, treatment for diarrhoea and vomiting and as a cough suppressant. Morphine, for instance, is widely used for short term acute pain resulting from fractures, burns and the later stages of terminal illnesses. Methadone is often prescribed to heroin addicts for maintenance or withdrawal purposes. Some of the opiates such as pethidine, morphine, dihydrocodeine and methadone are highly addictive.

The most popular of the opiates as an illicit drug is heroin. The drug is swallowed, smoked ('chasing the dragon' — it is heated on silver paper and smoked or inhaled), sniffed or injected either subcutaneously or intravenously. If injected it is generally mixed with water or lemon juice. Habitual users of heroin may well consume from $\frac{1}{2}$ gramme to over 1 gramme per day.

Legal status

Heroin, pethidine, morphine, dihydrocodeine and methadone are class A controlled drugs. Codeine and dihydrocodeine are class B, but class A if prepared for injection. Distalgesics, dextropoxyphene and buprenorphine (temgesic) are class C.

Effects

In moderate doses, opiates produce a range of generally mild physical effects apart from the analgesic effect. The depressant effects reduce the activity of the nervous system including reflex functions such as coughing, respiration and heart rate. They also dilate the blood vessels, thus giving a feeling of warmth. Although stupor, coma and death can occur from overdoses, there is generally little effect on the motor skills and sensation. Heroin users report the ability of the drug to induce a relaxed detachment from pain and anxiety. The user of opiates may appear detached or withdrawn, with contraction of the pupils. However, most complications arise from unsterile injections and adulterated street drugs. Street drugs have sometimes been diluted or mixed with substances such as chalk dust, caffeine, flour, quinine and talcum powder. Heroin, taken by injection, is also a risk factor in contracting hepatitis, HIV and septicaemia.

If the supply of the drug is cut off, withdrawal symptoms may become apparent 8 to 24 hours after the last dose. The drug must have been used daily for at least 2 to 3 weeks for physical withdrawal to occur. Some of the signs and symptom of this are:

❑ Anxiety
❑ Insomnia
❑ Diarrhoea
❑ Aches
❑ Tremor
❑ Sweating

❑ Muscular spasms
❑ Sneezing and yawning

The long term effects of heroin include respiratory complaints and menstrual irregularities, and opiate use during pregnancy may result in smaller babies and withdrawal symptoms after birth (see Chapter 11)

Cannabis

Cannabis is derived from a bushy plant, *Cannabis sativa*, which can be easily cultivated in the UK. The most common form used in the UK is resin, compressed into blocks known as hash or hashish. Herbal cannabis, also known as marihuana, is a weaker preparation of dried plant material. The strongest preparation, cannabis oil, prepared from the resin, is less common in the UK. Usually these substances are mixed with tobacco and smoked in a cigarette or a pipe, brewed in a drink or mixed with food. Smoking allows the user to regulate the dose because the effect is very rapid when used in this way.

Therapeutic and illicit uses

In the past, cannabis has been used as an anaesthetic, anti-convulsant, muscle relaxant, hypnotic, analgesic and rheumatic medicine. Currently, there are a number of research studies examining the beneficial effects of cannabis in the treatment of certain conditions and disorders. The focus of attention is directed towards the use of cannabis in glaucoma, to counter the nauseous effects of chemotherapy in terminal cases, as an appetite stimulant in HIV-positive patients and to control muscle spasm and other conditions in multiple sclerosis. Compared with all other drugs controlled under the Misuse of Drugs Act, cannabis has the greatest non medical usage. It is commonly used as a drug to enhance leisure activity, as a relaxant or a mild intoxicant by large sections of the population. There is evidence that approximately 1 in 20 of the population (as a conservative estimate) has tried cannabis and there are probably about one million cannabis users in the UK. Cannabis is usually retailed in ounces (28 g) or fractions of ounces: $\frac{1}{4}$ ounce (7 grammes), $\frac{1}{2}$ ounce (14 grammes). An eighth of an ounce of resin at a current price of £15 is sufficient for a small number of 'joints' and about $\frac{1}{2}$ gramme of resin is used to make a couple of joints. Cannabis imported into the UK comes from various sources in North Africa, the Middle East and Asia. More recently, a greater percentage being sold in this country is 'home grown'.

Legal status

Cannabis is controlled under the Misuse of Drugs Act (class B), making it illegal to cultivate, produce, supply or possess the drug unless a Home Office licence has been issued for research use or other special purposes. It is an offence to allow any premises to be used for cultivating, producing, supplying, storage or smoking of cannabis.

Effects

The effects of cannabis usually start just a few minutes after smoking and last from about one hour to several hours depending on consumption, expectations, motivation and mood of the user. The following are common effects: talkativeness, bouts of hilarity, relaxation and a greater sensitivity to sound and colour. While under the influence of cannabis, concentration and mental and manual dexterity are impaired, making tasks such as driving or other psycho-motor activities both difficult and dangerous. If the drug is used while an individual is anxious or depressed, these feelings may be accentuated leading to a feeling of panic, but there is no hangover of the type associated with alcohol use.

Opinion varies about the effects of long term cannabis use. Like tobacco, frequently and chronically inhaled cannabis smoke probably causes bronchitis and other respiratory problems and may also contribute to the development of lung cancer. While there is little evidence that cannabis can produce a physical dependence, regular use can produce a psychological need for the drug and some individuals may come to rely on it as a 'social lubricant'. Heavy cannabis users with a personality disturbance or psychiatric problems may precipitate a temporary exacerbation of psychotic symptoms.

Stimulants

Stimulants are synthetic powders available as a variety of tablets and capsules, sometimes in combination with other drugs. Both amphetamine and cocaine are classed as stimulants. Drugs such as methylphenidate (Ritalin) and diethylproprion (Tenuate Dospan, Apisate) have a similar effect to amphetamine, but are less potent. These drugs may be taken orally or sniffed in powder form, smoked or dissolved in water and injected. Cocaine hydrochloride, a powerful stimulant, is a white powder which is usually sniffed or 'snorted' up the nose through a tube and absorbed through the nasal membranes, although the substance is sometimes injected. 'Freebasing' consists of smoking cocaine base (or crack), that is, cocaine that has been treated to remove impurities and adulterants so that it can be smoked. It has the appearance of small crystalline 'rocks'. This is a more potent route of administration than snorting and it produces a 'rush' similar to the experience of injecting cocaine. Cocaine is also known as coke, snow, nose, candy and Charlie; crack is known as freebase, scud and rock. Amphetamine's 'street' names are speed, whizz and sulph.

Therapeutic and illicit uses

In the 1950s and 1960s, amphetamines were widely prescribed for the symtoms of depression and as appetite suppressants. The main recommended use now is in the treatment of pathological sleepiness and, paradoxically, in some cases for treatment of hyperactivity in children. Cocaine was mainly used as a local anaesthetic and in various 'medicinal' tonics. Most street stimulants are illicitly manufactured amphetamine sulphate powder and are heavily diluted with adulterants (often to 10–15% purity), they are readily available and retailing at between £5 and £10 per gramme. The street price for cocaine is £40 to £60 per gramme and 'rocks', about the size of raisins, cost from £15 to £25 each.

Legal status

All amphetamines and similar stimulants are prescription only drugs under the Medicines Act. Most are also controlled under the Misuse of Drugs Act, with the exception of some mild stimulants. Amphetamine, dex-and methyl-amphetamine, phenmetrazine and methylphenidate are in class B, but if prepared for injection the increased penalties of class A apply. Diethylpropion and other amphetamine like stimulants are in class C. Cocaine, its derivative salts and the leaves of the coca plant come under class A of the Misuse of Drugs Act.

Effects

Amphetamines create arousal, making the user feel more energetic, confident and cheerful. There is an increased sense of well-being, power and confidence and an enhanced ability to concentrate and stay awake. The psychological effects include mood swings, agitation, irritability, confusion and anxiety, which may subsequently lead to paranoid delusions and hallucinations.

The effects of a single dose last about 3 to 4 hours, leaving the user feeling tired and depleted, and it may take a couple of days for the body to recover fully. Amphetamines can cause profound psychological dependence, with no major physical withdrawal syndrome.

The short term effects of cocaine are similar to those of amphetamines. Psychological effects include euphoria, sexual arousal, increased energy and a sense of well-being. The physiological effects include hypertension, tachycardia, raised temperature, dilated pupils, suppressed appetite and disturbed sleep. When sniffed, the psychological effects peak after 1 to 4 minutes, leading to the dose being repeated approximately every 20 minutes in order to maintain the effect. When crack is smoked, the effects are more immediate and diminish after 12 minutes. On cessation, the individual is likely to feel deeply depressed, lethargic and very hungry. Amphetamines and other stimulants merely postpone fatigue and hunger without satisfying the need for rest and nourishment.

Hypnosedatives

The hypnosedatives include both hypnotics and minor tranquillisers. The barbiturates are Tuinal, Membutal, Sodium Amytal, Phenobarbitone, etc., and the benzodiazepines: Valium (diazepam), Librium (chlordiazepoxide), Ativan, Mogadon (nitrazepam), tamazepam, etc. Other hypnosedatives include Heminevrin (chlormethiazole), chloral hydrate, etc. The street names are downers, barbs and tranx. Barbiturates come in the form of tablets, ampoules and solution, or in coloured capsules. Those who misuse barbiturates generally take them by mouth, occasionally with alcohol, but may also inject (ISDD 1996). Benzodiazepines are available on the illicit market and retail at about £1 for a 5 mg tablet or capsule.

Therapeutic and illicit uses

Hynosedatives are drugs of misuse not only among the illicit drug population but in the population in general. However, barbiturates are less common as part of the illicit drug culture in the UK. Barbiturates have been used medically in anaesthesia, in the treatment of epilepsy and, rarely nowadays, for insomnia. Benzodiazepines are the most commonly prescribed drugs in Britain and about 80% of benzodiazepines are prescribed for sleeping problems, anxiety or mental distress (ISDD 1996). Benzodiazepines are usually taken by mouth but are sometimes ground up and injected. Temazepam has become a popular drug with substance misusers, especially in Scotland, as a substitute for opiates like heroin.

Legal status

Benzodiazepines and barbiturates are prescription only medicines and are class C and B controlled drugs, respectively, under the Medicines Act. It is illegal to supply these psychoactive substances. It is still not illegal to possess benzodiazepine in non medicinal form without a prescription, with the exception of temazepam (ISDD 1996).

Effects

Barbiturates are depressant drug and their effects are similar to alcohol intoxication: slurred speech, stumbling, confusion, reduction of inhibition, lowering of anxiety and tension and impairment of concentration, judgement and performance. In case of overdose, respiratory failure and death may result if these drugs are mixed with alcohol or with each other. Injecting these drugs is particularly hazardous, with an increased risk of overdose, gangrene and abscesses. Barbiturates are highly addictive and withdrawal symptoms include anxiety, headaches, cramps in the abdomen, pains in the limbs and even epileptic fits. Withdrawal of barbiturates can be dangerous and should always be medically supervised.

Benzodiazepines, in small doses, generally make people drowsy, lethargic and impair driving and other psychomotor skills. High doses or drugs such as mogadon (nitrazepam) and dalmane can act as a hynotic to induce sleep over a long period. Tolerance develops to both the therapeutic and non therapeutic effects and it is estimated that at least half of those continuing to take benzodiazepines for more than a year do so due to dependence (ISDD 1996). Severe withdrawal symptoms occur in 20–40% of long term users and may occur within 2–3 days of stopping (lorazepam, temazepam, etc.) and within 7–10 days of stopping long acting drugs (diazepam, clobazam, etc.). Withdrawal symptoms include insomnia, tremor, nausea, vomiting, anxiety, feeling of panic, feeling of unreality, confusional states and epileptic fits.

LSD and other hallucinogens

This section deals with a group of substances known as hallucinogens or hallucinogenic drugs. Lysergic acid diethylamide, known as LSD, is derived from an alkaloid (ergot) which is a synthetic. LSD, also known as acid, costs between £3 and £5 per tablet; the hallucinogen-containing mushrooms are also known as 'magic mushrooms'. It is suggested that up to 10% of those aged 15–24 might have tried LSD and this psychoactive substance appears to be an historical precursor to Ecstasy (ISDD 1966). Other hallucinogens include psilocybin (from liberty cap mushrooms), *Amanita muscaria* (fly agaric mushrooms) and mescaline, which is derived from the peyote cactus.

Therapeutic and illicit uses

In ancient cultures the plants and their extracts were used during religious rituals and witchcraft and were employed as intoxicants in medicine. In recent times, LSD has been used occasionally in psychotherapy. The widespread experimentation with LSD and other hallucinogens in the subculture of the 1960s resurfaced in the late 1980s. Experimentation with the drug in recent times has been associated with the advent of the rave scene. In its pure form LSD is a white powder, but it is often supplied as an impregnated square of paper or as a drop on a piece of blotting paper and it is nearly always taken orally. LSD is also used in combination with amphetamines and Ecstasy to enhance the perceptual experiences. The effect starts after about half an hour and intensifies over a period of 2 to 6 hours. The effect may last up to 12 hours, depending on the dose. The mushrooms, mentioned above, may be eaten raw, cooked or brewed into a tea.

Legal status

LSD is a class A controlled drug. Psilocybin or psilocybin containing mushrooms are legal in their freshly picked state, but preparing them or growing or possessing them with intent to supply is illegal and restricted by the Misuse of Drugs Act 1971, 1973.

Effects

There is no physical dependence or withdrawal symptoms associated with recreational use of LSD. The effects of the drug depend on the user's prior experience, mood, expectations and setting. It is much stronger in effect than psychedelic mushrooms or mescaline. A moderate dose will produce profound alterations in mood, sensation and consciousness, intensified sensory experiences and perceptual distortions. Confusion of time, space, body image and boundaries can occur with what have been called the blending of sight and sound. The user may 'see' sounds and 'hear' colours. The side-effects and toxicity of the drug may cause panic, confusion, impulsive behaviour, unpleasant illusions ('bad trip' and) flashbacks and may precipitate psychotic reactions. Cases of accidental death due to impaired judgement have occurred but this is extremely rare. The negative and unpleasant effects are much more likely to arise if the user is in a negative mood or situation, or mixes hallucinogens with other drugs or alcohol. Fly agaric mushrooms often cause nausea and stomach pain. However, the greatest danger with hallucinogenic mushrooms is that the user may take a similar looking poisonous species by mistake. There is no physical dependence but tolerance builds up with LSD and mushrooms in so far as the user needs to space out 'trips' to get the desired effects.

Ecstasy

Ecstasy, chemically known as 3, 4-methylenedioxymethamphetamine, or MDMA for short, is often categorised as a hallucinogenic amphetamine. In some respect Ecstasy resembles LSD, leading to changes in states of consciousness, but it does not actually produce a hallucinogenic effect. It is manufactured from the components of methylamphetamine and safrole (a nutmeg derivative). It is usually known as 'E', and comes in tablet form or in capsules. It is sometimes referred to as XTC, 'Dennis the Menace', 'Rhubarb and Custard', 'New Yorkers', 'Love doves', 'Disco Burgers', or 'Phase 4'. The appearance varies considerably depending on the actual content of the drug, ranging from brown to white tablets to pink, red, yellow or clear capsules. A tablet or capsule of Ecstasy retails at £10 to £15.

Therapeutic and illicit uses

Ecstasy was first used as an appetite suppressant, although it was never actually marketed for this purpose, and in a limited way as an adjunct to various types of psychotherapy. In addition, the drug has also been used to some extent with terminally ill patients in order to help them come to terms with their situation and to communicate their feelings more easily. The main illicit use of Ecstasy has been as 'house music' and all night raves.

Legal status

Ecstasy is a class A drug.

Effects

The effects start after about 30–60 minutes, peak in 2–4 hours and can last several hours in total. It is described as having a calming effect with an enhanced perception of colours and sound. With higher doses the user can feel anxious and confused and co-ordination can be impaired, making driving or similar activities very dangerous. If taken regularly over the period of a few days the user can experience temporary paranoia or insomnia. The physical effects include sweating, dry mouth, tight jaw, raised blood pressure, temperature and heart rate and loss of appetite. The Ecstasy users report feeling relaxed, happy and warm and describe a sense of empathy between themselves. Bad experiences are usually associated with high dose use over a period of time and include anxiety, depression, panic, confusion, insomnia and psychosis.

Although Ecstasy is not physically addictive, tolerance to the effects of the drug does build up. There is a high risk of complications for patients with heart conditions, hypertension, a history of seizures or any type of psychiatric disorder. There have been several deaths reported to be associated with the use of Ecstasy. Often these deaths are linked with exhaustion or high body temperature (hyperpyrexia) which have led to collapse, convulsions or renal failure. There is also the danger of the drug being contaminated by other substances such as LSD or ketamine. The side-effects of these contaminants can be potentially alarming and unpredictable.

Anabolic steroids

Steroids are hormones that occur naturally in the body and control the development and functioning of the reproductive system. Anabolic agents are those substances which increase muscle mass and strength and include anabolic steroids, human growth hormone, beta-2-agonists such as clenbuterol and others. Synthetic anabolic steroids, in particular the modified male sex hormone testosterone, form the main market supplies. There are no official statistics on the misuse of steroids but there is some evidence to suggest that steroids are widespread in health clubs and body-building clubs. The cost of 100 tablets is approximately £20, 10 ampoules cost approximately £30; the steroid user spends anything from £20 to £70 per week.

Therapeutic and illicit uses

Only two anabolic steroids are available on prescription in the UK, these are nandrolone (Durabolin) and Stanozol (Stromba). Anabolic steroids have an effect on muscle building and are medically used in the treatment of thrombosis, anaemia and muscle wasting. Illicit anabolic steroids are used mainly by athletes and bodybuilders. The idea behind the use of these steroids is that because they build muscle bulk they will also increase strength. The drug can be taken in tablet form or by injection.

Legal status

Anabolic steroids are not controlled under the Misuse of Drugs Act 1971. They are, however, prescription only drug and intent to supply can be an offence under the Medicines Act. It is not illegal to possess steroids for personal use.

Effects

Anabolic steroids increase the retention of nitrogen by the body, allowing this to be used to build muscle. Steroids also aid in the production of red blood cells and this has led to the belief that they might be helpful in increasing indurance. There is, however, no empirical evidence to support this. As anabolic steroids are modelled chemically on male hormones they can have a masculinizing effect. Women may have an increase in body hair, a deepened voice, enlargement of the clitoris and decrease in breast size. Men may suffer from a decrease in sperm production and testes size and development of breast tissue. Some of these effects may be permanent and therefore irreversible. The increase in aggression is welcomed by athletes, but sometimes the associated 'steroid mania' has been blamed for violent crimes. Physical dependence does not seem to be a problem but users have reported depression and lethargy after stopping their use.

Amyl and butyl nitrite

Amyl and butyl nitrites, known collectively as alkyl nitrites, are chemically related to nitrous oxide or laughing gas. They are clear, yellow, volatile and inflammable liquids with a sweet smell when fresh. When stale, the drug degenerates to a smell often described as 'smelly socks'. Butyl nitrites known as 'poppers' are largely on sale in the UK and sold in bottles, at £5 each, under brand names such as KIX ROCK HARD, TNT, RUSH, etc.

Therapeutic and illicit uses

Medically, amyl nitrite has been used in the treatment of angina and as an antidote to cyanide poisoning. Butyl nitrite has no therapeutic medical use. In the UK, drug such as butyl nitrite are on sale in sex shops, pubs, bars and clubs. As a street drug, butyl nitrite comes in small bottles with screw or plug tops. It is sold mainly, but not exclusively, to the gay community. The drug is widely used for the 'rush' of blood to the brain, to enhance sexual activity.

Legal status

Butyl nitrite is not classified as a drug and has no restrictions on its availability under current medicine or drug legislation. However, other laws such as the Offences Against the Persons Act 1861 or the Intoxication Substances Supply Act 1985, may be used to restrict distributions of these substances.

Effects

Once inhaled, the effects are virtually instantaneous and last for 2–5 minutes. The blood vessels dilate, there is an increase in heart rate and blood rushes to the brain. Those using the drug to enhance sexual pleasure report a slow sense of time, prolonged sensation of orgasm and the prevention of premature ejaculation. Alkyl nitrites are also used for the relaxation of the anal sphincter, easing anal intercourse. Sniffing of nitrites could cause a reduction in blood pressure and contribute to unconsciousness. Anyone with cardiovascular problems, glaucoma or anaemia should avoid using nitrites. The users often experience weakness, headache, facial flushing, nausea and vomiting. Tolerance to the drug develops within 2 to 3 weeks of regular use, but after a few days of abstinence this tolerance is lost. There are no reports of withdrawal symptoms or psychological dependence. There appear to be no serious long term effects of the drug as it is excreted rapidly from the body in healthy individuals.

Volatile substances

Some organic (carbon) based substances produce effects similar to alcohol or anaesthetics when their vapours are inhaled. Some of these are used as solvents in glue, paint, nail varnish removers, dry cleaning fluids, degreasing compounds, thinning fluids, etc. Others are used as propellant gases in aerosols and fire extinguishers or as fuels, such as petrol, cigarette lighter gas, etc. Sniffers of volatile substances heighten the desired effect by increasing the concentration of the vapour and excluding air, for example by sniffing from a bag or by placing a plastic bag over the head while inhalation takes place.

Illicit use

Solvent abuse seems to occur in very localised areas, for example in a particular housing estate, school or group. The age group 12–16 years is mainly concerned and some of these children continue to sniff glue for several years. The government has produced guidelines for retailers to ensure that these products are stocked out of the reach of children and that the sales are restricted to adults. Many youngsters who sniff these substances have accidents while they are intoxicated and suffer serious health consequences. It is reported that deaths from volatile substance abuse increased from 58 in 1994 to 68 in 1995, and that there have been significant falls in the numbers of deaths associated with aerosols and glues, but not in those associated with gas fuels (Taylor *et al.* 1997)

Legal status

The Intoxicating Substances Supply Act, passed in 1985, makes it an offence to supply a young person under 18 years with a substance which the supplier knows or has reason to believe will be used 'to achieve intoxication'. The law is mainly directed to shopkeepers but could also be applied to anyone who sells or gives a young person a sniffable product.

Effects

The effect is similar to alcohol but inhaled solvent vapours are absorbed quickly through the lungs and rapidly reach the brain. Respiratory rate and heart rate are depressed and repeated or deep inhalation can result in an 'overdose', causing disorientation, loss of control and unconsciousness. The experience is similar to being drunk, and experienced sniffers try to achieve a dream-like state. The effects appear quickly and disappear within a few minutes to half an hour of sniffing being stopped. There may be a hangover effect with headache and poor concentration for about a day.

There is a considerable risk of accidental injury or death if the individual becomes intoxicated in a hazardous environment. Most deaths are caused by choking when the user has been intoxicated to the point of unconsciousness. Some volatile substances such as aerosol gases and cleaning fluids can sensitise the heart, causing heart failure, especially if exertion takes place at the same time. Some gases squirted directly into the mouth can cause death from suffocation. Sniffing from small bags held to the mouth or nose have caused fewer deaths than the practice of inhaling butane and similar gases with plastic bags placed over the head.

Long term heavy solvent abuse can result in moderate and lasting impairment of brain function, particularly affecting the control of movement. Chronic misuse of aerosols and cleaning fluids can lead to renal and hepatic damage, weight loss, depression and tremor. The practice of sniffing leaded petrol can cause lead poisoning. Tolerance can develop but physical dependence does not constitute a significant problem. Psychological dependence occurs in susceptible youngsters with concomitant family or personality problems. These individuals are also more prone to become 'lone sniffers' instead of the usual pattern of sniffing in groups.

Over-the-counter-drugs

Several medicinal preparations are available without prescription and are sold in chemist shops and are purchased for their non medical therapeutic effects. These include depressants such as codeine linctus, Collis Browne's mixture, Gee's linctus and kaolin and morphine. The stimulants include Fenox, Mercocaine lozenges, Sinutads, Sudafed and Do-Do Tablets. Travel sickness remedies such as Kwells, which contain hallucinogenic compounds, are also available over the counter.

Therapeutic use

Many of the medical preparations are used for the relief of pain, coughs and the common cold and in the treatment of diarrhoea and respiratory conditions.

Legal status

No prescriptions are required to purchase these substances.

Effects

Some of these substances are taken in large doses and are often combined with other drugs to obtain the desired effects. Antihistamines may be used for their sedative properties and/or mixed with methadone or heroin. The amphetamine derivatives in decongestants may be used as stimulants; cough linctuses and diarrhoea drugs may be used for their opiate content.

Other drugs on the UK drug scene

Several drugs that are less common on the UK drug scene are used mainly by specific groups of people. Drugs such as GHB, ketamine and khat fall outside the control of the Misuse of Drugs Act.

GHB

GHB (or GBH) is an anaesthetic with sedative properties and may be used as a premedication drug before surgical intervention. It is a colourless liquid which is sold in small bottles and is mainly used by bodybuilders and those on the club scene. It is sold in liquid form or capsules and retails at around £10 to £15 for a bottle and at around £15 for 20 capsules. The effects of GBH are similar to alcohol in small doses, as they enhance social interactions and increase libido. At higher doses, the reported effects include nausea, vomiting, stiffening of muscles, disorientation, convulsions and respiratory collapse (Institute for the Study of Drug Dependence (ISDD) 1996). The possible long term consequences are unknown but there may be a potential risk for psychological and physical dependence. GBH is not controlled under the Misuse of Drugs Act and possession is not an offence.

Ketamine

Ketamine is an anaesthetic with analgesic and psychedelic properties related to phencyclidine (PCP or 'angel dust'). The substance can be sniffed and used intravenously and intramuscularly and forms part of the dance youth culture. Prices range from £6 to £25 for a wrap of powder. The speed of effect of ketamine depends on the mode of use, ranging from 20 minutes when taken orally to about 30 seconds if injected (intraveneously). Reported physical effects include an initial cocaine like 'rush', vomiting and nausea, slurring of speech and vision, numbness and ataxia and temporary paralysis. Psychological reactions include euphoria, hallucinations, depersonalisation, confusion and dissociative state. The long term consequences of ketamine may include flashbacks, memory impairment, poor attention, etc. (ISDD 1996). Although there is tolerance to the drug, physical dependence and withdrawal are not part of the use of ketamine. It is reported that frequent use of ketamine may lead to psychological dependence and psychosis (ISDD 1996). Ketamine is not controlled under the Misuse of Drugs Act.

Khat

Khat (qat, chat), *Catha edulis,* is a green leafy plant grown in the Yemen and East Africa, particularly in Kenya (Miri) and Ethopia (Hereri). The active ingredients are cathine and cathinone which are relatively mild stimulants. A typical khat chewing session is said to be the equivalent of ingesting a moderate 5 mg dose of amphetamine sulphate (ISDD 1996). The psychological effects include increased energy, heightened self-confidence and mild euphoria. The physical effects include cardiovascular, digestive, endocrine and genitourinary problems and hypothermia. With prolonged and excessive use there is a risk of spermatorrhoea in men and low birthweight in women. Stomatitis, oral cancer, depression and paranoid behaviour have also been attributed to heavy khat use. Khat is not controlled under the Misuse of Drugs Act, but the active ingredients are class C drugs.

References and further reading

Institute for the Study of Drug Dependence (1996) *Drug Abuse Briefings,* 6th edn. ISDD, London.
Institute for the Study of Drug Dependence (1996) *The Misuse of Drugs Act Explained,* revised ed. ISDD, London.
Royal College of Psychiatrists (1987) *Drug Scenes. A report on drugs and drug dependence.* The Royal College of Psychiatrists, Gaskell, London.
St George's Hospital Medical School. *Addiction Prevention Counsellors – How to help resource pack.* Department of Psychiatry of Addictive Behaviour, Centre for Addiction Studies, London.

Taylor, J.C., Norman, C.L., Bland, J.M., *et al.* (1997) *Trends in Deaths Associated With Abuse of Volatile Substances 1971–1995*. Report No 10. Department of Public Health Sciences and the Toxicology Unit and the Department of Cardiological Sciences, St George's Hospital Medical School, London.
Tyler A. (1995) *Street drugs*. Hodder and Stoughton, London.

Chapter 5

Alcohol and Alcohol Related Problems

Julie Winnington and G. Hussein Rassool

Introduction

Alcohol, the nation's favourite drug (Royal College of Psychiatrists 1986), is regarded as a major public health issue which produces more health-related problems than tobacco and illicit drugs. Alcoholic beverages form part of the social and cultural fabric of most European and North American nations and, unfortunately, alcohol is not generally perceived as a drug, especially as a psychoactive substance, with addictive potential. Alcohol is used variously as a stimulant, tranquilliser, anaesthetic, celebrant, medicine, social lubricant, religious symbol, food and fuel (Health Education Authority 1994).

In the UK, alcohol misuse is associated with approximately 28 000 deaths annually (Anderson 1988), making it the single largest preventable cause of death in the UK. Excessive alcohol consumption or heavy drinking now ranks third as a major public health problem and it is estimated that about 6% of adult males and about 1% of adult females consume alcohol at high risk levels (Goddard & Ikin 1991). The average consumption of alcohol among women is increasing and the trend towards heavy drinking in women is steadily rising (Office of Population Censuses and Surveys (OPCS) 1992).

The epidemiological evidence suggests that there is a wide range of problems associated with alcohol consumption – with the number and kind of disabilities increasing progressively with the amount of alcohol (Edwards *et al.* 1994). Alcohol consumption, especially heavy drinking, can, over a period of time, contribute to physical, psychological and social problems. The physical problems include cardiovascular disease, stroke, cancer, malnutrition, gastro-intestinal disorders, liver disease, dementia, HIV/AIDS, sexual health and accidents. The effects on the psychological and social state of an individual include depression, apathy, isolation, loneliness, relationship problems, absenteeism at work which can lead to unemployment and the narrowing of social circles.

The Health of the Nation documents (Department of Health 1992, 1995a) set out a strategy for health, emphasising disease prevention and health promotion. The specific targets for the reduction in alcohol consumption by the year 2005 are:

❏ To reduce the proportion of men drinking more than 21 units of alcohol per week from 28% to 18%.
❏ To reduce the proportion of women drinking more than 14 units per week from 11% to 7%.

The focus of the strategy, in England, is to reduce the number of adults aged 18 or over drinking in excess of the recommended weekly limits. The Department of Health reports (1995a, 1995b) have also highlighted the need for preventive intervention and the adequate training of nurses, midwives and health visitors in the incidence and problems related to alcohol misuse. It is during routine admission to the general health care system that there is ample opportunity for health care professionals to carry out simple screenings and take a drug and alcohol history. There is evidence to suggest that routine assessment, screening and brief or minimal intervention are effective means to achieve the health targets set by the government (Cole 1990; Department of Health 1995a).

The aims of this chapter are to examine the concepts of alcohol dependence, the alcohol dependence syndrome, the problem drinker and the nature and extent of alcohol use and misuse in the community. In addition, a brief overview of the pharmacology and general effects of alcohol is presented. Guidelines for sensible and controlled drinking are also discussed.

Concepts of alcohol dependence and problem drinking

A variety of health and social constructs, both past and present, have been associated with alcohol. These include: alcohol problem, alcoholism, alcohol dependence, alcoholic, alcohol dependence syndrome, problem drinker, etc. Jellinek (1960) defined alcoholism as 'any use of alcoholic beverages that causes any damage to the individual or society or both'. However, some individuals may display a number of alcohol related problems without necessarily appearing to have an unusual or excessive drinking pattern. For example, certain individuals may have a biological tendency to become easily intoxicated even with a very low alcohol intake, thus increasing the risk of accidents and generally impairing their judgement.

There is no satisfactory universal definition of alcoholism. Dr E. Jellinek described alcoholism as a progressive chronic disease, defining each stage – for example, gamma alcoholism to emphasise the criterion of loss of control, delta alcoholism referred to an inability to abstain from alcohol. Within the disease concept of alcoholism, there is little or no recognition of the psychological, social or environmental contribution and this is consequently a severely limited perspective. The definition of alcohol dependence, according to the International Classification of Disease 10 (ICD 10), (World Health Organization 1992) is:

'A state, psychic and usually also physical resulting from taking alcohol, characterized by behavioural and other responses that always include a compulsion to take alcohol on a continuous or periodic basis in order to experience its psychic effects and sometimes to avoid the discomfort of its absence.'

The above definition stressed the existence of a compulsive behaviour and withdrawal syndrome in alcohol dependence. The 'alcohol dependence syndrome' was described by Edwards and Gross (1976) and the key characteristics are as follows:

❏ Narrowing of drinking repertoire (i.e. reduced ability to decide when, what and how much to drink)
❏ Compulsion to drink
❏ Prominence or salience of drink seeking behaviour
❏ Increased tolerance
❏ Withdrawal symptoms
❏ Relief drinking to reduce withdrawal symptoms
❏ Reinstatement after a period of abstinence

In clinical practice, some individuals with some of the elements of the alcohol dependence syndrome were functioning without apparent harm or alcohol related disabilities, while others with little or no evidence of the syndrome were suffering from the harm and the sequelae of alcohol related problems. In view of this anomaly, two categories of drinkers were suggested by the Royal College of Physicians (1987) heavy drinkers and problem drinkers.

Heavy drinking may be defined as consumption of alcohol resulting in a measurable biochemical abnormality (e.g. raised liver enzymes) without apparent harm to the drinker. Problem drinking is the consumption of alcohol resulting in harm to the drinker or to significant others. The problems may be related to intoxication or to regular heavy drinking. A 'dependent drinker', according to the Royal College of Physicians (1987), is

'someone who has a compulsion to drink; takes roughly the same amount each day; has increased tolerance to alcohol in the early stages and reduced tolerance later; suffers withdrawal symptoms if alcohol is stopped which are relieved by consuming more; in whom drinking takes precedence over other activities and who tends to resume drinking after a period of abstinence.'

Currently, the term problem drinker is used in both the literature and in clinical practice. It refers to individuals with a range of problems, e.g. physical, psychological, social or legal, experienced as a consequence of his or her alcohol use/misuse. This does not necessarily entail tolerance or physiological or psychological dependence on alcohol (Cooper 1994). A problem drinker, then, may be regarded as anyone who experiences difficulties in any sphere of living as a result of his or her alcohol use or misuse.

Pattern and extent of use

In Great Britain, data from the General Household Survey (OPCS 1992) indicated that 38% of men and 40% of women were in the low consumption category, i.e. drinking 1–10 unites per week (men) and 1–7 units per week (women). Men were more likely than women to be in both the moderate consumption (11–21, men; 8–14, women) and higher consumption group categories. Twenty-eight per cent of men but only 11% of women were classified into the high consumption categories (21–50 units per week), indicating they drank more than the recommended sensible limits. It is estimated that this amounts to about 7 million adults in England (Health Education Authority 1994). The proportion of men drinking 51 units per week was 7% and the proportion of women drinking 36+ units per week was 2%.

Alcohol affects individuals to varying degrees and studies have shown trends of higher alcohol use in some cultures, socio-economic groups, professions and geographical areas (Goddard & Ikin 1991; Godfrey 1992; OPCS 1995). However, it is estimated that alcohol misuse is associated with 60% of parasuicides (Platt 1983), 30% of divorces, 40% of cases of domestic violence (Gayford 1975) and 20% of child abuse cases (Creighton 1984). Homelessness can be the result of problematic drinking (Borg 1978) but being homeless seems to increase the risk of heavy drinking (Priest 1976). It is estimated that heavy drinkers are more susceptible to acts of violence, abuse and crime with women being responsible for 7% of all drunkenness offences (Fillmore 1985).

The General Household Survey (OPCS 1995) showed that alcohol consumption in women was higher in non manual than in manual groups; 14% of women in the professional group usually drank more than 14 units a week compared with 6% of women in the unskilled manual group. There are wide regional variations in the UK in the level of alcohol consumption. Among men, consumption levels were highest in the north (32%) and north-west regions (32%) of England compared with the south-east (26%) and south-west (25%). The lowest level was found in East Anglia. There were fewer regional variations in women (OPCS 1992); the proportion drinking more than the sensible weekly limits ranged from 6% in Scotland to 14% in Yorkshire and Humberside.

The pattern of alcohol consumption varies among the ethnic minority groups. A study by Cochrane and Ball (1990) found that, compared to white men, Muslim men drink the least amount of alcohol, followed by Hindu men. Sikh men reported approximately the same level of alcohol consumption as white men. It was also found that older Asian men (aged 40+) drink more alcohol than their young counterparts and older Sikh men drink more than white men in the same age category.

Use of health services

Studies indicate that patients with alcohol problems consult their GP nearly twice as often as the average patient (OPCS 1988). Heavy drinkers (50 units, men; 35 units, women) tend to be heavy users of hospital services. There is evidence to suggest that over 25% of British male in-patients have a current or previous alcohol problem (Lloyd *et al.* 1986). A significant proportion of patients admitted to general hospital wards (e.g. one in five men) have health problems which are either directly or indirectly related to their alcohol consumption (Barrison *et al.* 1982).

Alcohol consumption seems to be a significant factor for those presenting to casualty departments with accidental injuries (Department of Health 1993). In England, in 1986, there were 250 (172 men and 78 women) first admissions to psychiatric hospitals and units for alcoholic psychosis 3334 (2361 men and 973 women) admissions for alcohol dependence and 939 (610 men and 329 women), admissions for non dependent abuse of alcohol (Department of Health and Social Security (DHSS) 1987).

Although the numbers of women admitted to general hospitals with alcohol related health problems are proportionately lower than the figures for male admissions, it is likely that those women who do present to general hospitals do so when alcohol has caused a considerable degree of damage. About 15% of female admissions to general hospitals were found to be alcohol related (Northcote *et al.* 1983). Due to the apparent stigma still attached to women drinking, it is more difficult for women to come forward for advice or treatment at an early stage.

Chemical nature and production of alcohol

Ethyl alcohol or ethanol (C_2H_5OH) is a colourless, inflammable liquid with a characteristic smell and a burning taste. Alcohol is produced by fermenting a variety of organic materials, for example rye, wheat, corn, barley, various fruits or vegetables such as potatoes. Flowers, milk and honey can also be fermented to produce alcoholic beverages. Spirits or 'hard liquor', e.g. whisky, rum or gin, are produced through a process of distillation.

Metabolism of alcohol

Alcohol is a psychoactive substance that depresses the central nervous system and provides calories. Unlike other foods, alcohol does not have to be digested in order for absorption to occur. The rate that alcohol is absorbed varies widely among people, depending on individual differences in physiology and context or situational factors. Drinks with a higher concentration of alcohol, such as whisky or brandy, and carbonated drinks such as champagnes are absorbed more quickly.

After absorption, the blood distributes alcohol to all tissues. Most alcohol ingested is oxidised by the liver and only a small amount, about 5%, is excreted unchanged in the urine, sweat and breath. For the most part, absorption of alcohol takes place in the small intestine, but some strong alcohol is absorbed by the stomach. Once absorbed into the circulatory system it is carried to the liver for the process of oxidation by the portal system. The enzyme alcohol dehydrogenase is active in the oxidisation process. This produces acetaldehyde which is then changed to acetic acid by the enzyme acetaldehyde dehydrogenase. The acetic acid is rapidly converted to carbon dioxide and water with a major release of energy. It is worth pointing out that alcohol, although fattening, affects the body's ability to absorb and use food effectively. This adds to the problem of malnutrition or vitamin deficiencies in heavy drinkers.

Alcohol affects men and women in different ways. Women can become more intoxicated than men on the same amount of alcohol, even if they weigh the same. That is because women have less water in their bodies than men, so alcohol is less diluted and has a greater potency. Women are likely to combine their alcohol dependence with other psychoactive substances, particularly prescribed medications. Women do not metabolise alcohol as efficiently as men, which may make women more vulnerable to the consequences of drinking.

General effects of alcohol

Alcohol is the basis for all commonly used intoxicating beverages and acts as a cerebral depressant, although it is often associated with creating a 'high'. There appears to be a strong association between the degree to which an individual is dependent on alcohol and the severity of problems experienced by the individual. This is independent from the amount of alcohol consumed. It should be borne in mind that, for some people, even low or moderate levels of consumption can be damaging and that the health and social consequences of this type of drinking behaviour make a very significant impact on the nation's health status.

During acute intoxication with alcohol, the individual will show severe signs of behavioural dysfunction. Alcohol's effects include disinhibition, relaxation and feelings of euphoria. At a higher consumption, increasing intoxication occurs as do progressive levels of cognitive, perceptual and behavioural impairment. This may also include blackouts, insomnia and a hangover. For every individual, their lethal dose of alcohol is generally related to body size and physiology. Death can occur from high consumption of alcohol or from withdrawal of alcohol.

In women, menstrual disorders and fertility problems have been associated with chronic heavy drinking. women are more susceptible to the influence of alcohol just prior to or during their menstrual cycle than any other time during their cycle and they are more susceptible to physical damage than men (Department of Health & The Royal College of General Practitioners 1992). Babies of mothers who drink heavily can be born with fetal alcohol syndrome (FAS). This is a cause of birth defects and mental impairment and is prevented by not drinking during pregnancy (see Chapter 11). Ghodse (1990) suggests

> 'that there is a spectrum of severity of the effects of alcohol on the child, according to the level of daily alcohol consumption – although it is not clear whether binge drinking or sustained drinking is more harmful, or whether the use of other drugs in association with alcohol potentiates the teratogenic effects.'

The course of alcohol addiction progresses at a faster rate in men. Women are more likely to develop cirrhosis of the liver and other related diseases. Because heavy drinking is less socially accepted in women, they often hide their drinking and their problems related to alcohol are often mis-diagnosed. A summary of the problems associated with alcohol intoxication and with regular heavy drinking is found in Tables 5.1 and 5.2 respectively.

Table 5.1   Problems associated with alcohol intoxication.

Physical	Social	Psychological
Accidents	Absenteeism from work	Anger and fatigue
Acute alcohol poisoning	Accidents at work	Anxiety
Cardiac arrhythmia	Assault	Amnesia
Fetal damage	Burglary	Attempted suicide
Failure to take	Child neglect/abuse	Depression
prescribed medication	Criminal damage	Impaired interpersonal
Gout	Domestic violence	relationships
Gastritis	Domestic accidents	Insomnia
Hepatitis	Drinking and driving	Suicide
Impotence	Family arguments	
Pancreatitis	Football hooliganism	
Strokes	Homicide	
Trauma	Inefficient work	
	Public drunkeness	
	Public aggression	
	Road traffic accidents	
	Sexually deviant acts	
	Taking and driving away	
	Theft	
	Unwanted pregnancy	

Adapted From The Royal College of General Practitioners (1986) *Alcohol – A Balanced View. Reports from General Practice 24.* RCGP, London.

Table 5.2 Recognition of features which may indicate possible alcohol misuse.

Physical	❑ Gastrointestinal symptoms	Vomiting, diarrhoea, anorexia, abdominal pain, nausea
	❑ Trauma	Accidents, injuries, bruising
	❑ Collapse	Blackouts, fainting, fits
	❑ Smell	Smell of drink (may be camouflaged)
	❑ Obesity	
	❑ Hypertension	
Psychological	❑ Anxiety	
	❑ Depression	Suicide attempt
	❑ Sexual problems	Impotence or infertility
	❑ Polydrug use	Benzodiazepines, hypnosedatives
	❑ Behaviour (during consultation)	Inappropriate, emotionally labile, potentially aggressive
	❑ Behaviour at home	Spouse battering, child abuse
Social/familial	❑ Family disruption	Partnership problems, separation, divorce
	❑ Financial	Debts
	❑ Legal	Driving offences, civil or criminal charges
	❑ Work	History of frequent job changes, high absenteeism, loss of job
	❑ Homelessness	

Alcohol dependence and withdrawal

Alcohol dependence involves both psychological and physical dependence. In clinical practice, it is difficult to distinguish physical dependence from psychological dependence as the two components are mutually interrelated. However, the presence of physical dependence is shown when problem drinkers cease alcohol consumption abruptly or reduce the level of consumption. The alcohol withdrawal syndrome occurs when the concentration of alcohol in the body or the blood alcohol of a problem drinker drops below the level necessary for the individual to function. In order to avert withdrawal symptoms, the problem drinker may continue to ingest alcohol.

Some or all of the following signs and symptoms are noticeable in those who are physically dependent on alcohol:

❑ Tremors
❑ Sweating (night)
❑ Increase in heart rate and respiration
❑ Insomnia

❑ Headache
❑ Nausea and vomiting
❑ Anxiety
❑ Restlessness
❑ Irritability

For most problem drinkers, alcohol withdrawal will not progress to the severe stage of delirium tremens (DTs). When an individual has DTs, this can become a life-threatening condition. The problem drinker may exhibit the following signs and symptoms:

❑ Clouding of consciousness
❑ Disorientation of time and place
❑ Visual or tactile hallucinations
❑ Paranoid delusions
❑ Anxiety
❑ Fear, suspicion and anger
❑ Suicidal behaviour
❑ Withdrawal fits (approximately 12 hours after abstinence)

Table 5.3 lists various problems commonly associated with problem drinking.

Table 5.3 Problems associated with regular heavy drinking.

Physical	Social	Psychological
Brain damage	Debt	Attempted suicide
Cirrhosis	Divorce	Amnesia
Cancer of mouth, larynx,	Family problems	Anxiety
oesophagus	Fraud	Changes in personality
Cancer of breast(?)	Financial difficulties	Depression
Cardiomyopathy	Habitual conviction for	Delirium tremens
Diabetes	drunkeness	Dementia
Fatty liver	Unemployment	Gambling
Fetal damage	Vagrancy	Hallucinosis
Gastritis	Work difficulties	Misuse of other drugs
Hepatitis		Suicide
Haemopoietic toxicity		Withdrawal fits
Infertility		
Neuropathy		
Nutritional deficiencies		
Obesity		
Pancreatitis		
Raised blood pressure		
Reactions with other drugs		
Strokes		
Sexual dysfunction		

Adapted from The Royal College of General Practitioners (1986) *Alcohol – A Balanced View. Reports from General Practice 24.* RCGP, London.

Sensible and controlled drinking

The Royal College of Psychiatrists' guidelines for sensible drinking are less than 21 units per week for men and less than 14 units per week for women. A unit is equivalent to half a pint of normal strength beer or lager, a standard measure of spirits or a glass of wine. According to Waldron (1996) 'by their very nature, these divisions are arbitrary and could conceivably be set at higher or lower levels'. The Royal Colleges of Psychiatrists, Physicians and General Practitioners (The Royal Colleges Report 1995) jointly concluded that low to moderate alcohol consumption protected against coronary heart disease but confirmed that sensible limits of 21 and 14 units should continue because to increase them would be to do more harm than good.

In December 1996, the issue of a government report (Department of Health 1995b) aimed to redefine the benchmarks for sensible drinking and expanded the sensible limits of alcohol consumption from 21 to 28 for men, and from 14 to 21 units per week for women. They also supported the health benefits of drinking alcohol for certain groups in the population: those with coronary heart disease, ischaemic stroke and cholesterol gallstones, men older than 40 years and post-menopausal women. The report indicated the risks of long term heavy drinking and suggested that all causes of mortality of moderate drinkers, both men and women, are similar to those of non drinkers until the consumption rises above 14 units per week for women and 21 units for men. Women are considered more at risk compared to men on the basis of their physiological differences: weight, rate of alcohol metabolism, possible increased vulnerability to tissue damage, the possible link between alcohol consumption and breast cancer and risks to the fetus and early infant development. Guidelines of sensible drinking for men and women are shown in Table 5.4.

Marmot (1995) questioned the recommended safe limits of alcohol consumption per day as recommended by the government and suggested that a change in policy would lead to an increase in alcohol consumption and could damage the public health. He pointed to the conclusions of the government report on sensible drinking and suggested that there is conflicting information of what constitutes a safe level, although they were in full agreement with The Royal Colleges Report (1995) that over 4 units (men) and 3 units (women) daily are associated with progressive health

Table 5.4 Guidelines for sensible drinking.

	Men	Women
Group	Over 40 years of age	Post-menopausal
Health benefits	1–2 units/day	1–2 units/day
No significant health risks	3–4 units/day (all ages)	2–3 units/day (all ages)
Not sensible drinking	4 or more units/day	3 or more units/day

risks but that between 3 and 4 units a day for men and 2 to 3 units a day for women are safe. It is worth pointing out that alcohol consumption at home is more likely to be above the standard unit of consumption and this should be borne in mind when calculating the amount of alcohol consumed.

How much is moderate?

The idea that moderate alcohol consumption is associated with a lowered risk of cardiaovascular disease and mortality has some research support. It has been recommended that women who choose to drink should limit their consumption to no more than one alcoholic beverage per day. Men who choose to drink should limit their consumption to no more than two drinks per day. One drink means one glass of wine or one beer. The following example is a useful reference guide for making quick calculations (Association of Nurses in Substance Abuse 1997):

> One unit of alcohol = half a pint of ordinary strength lager/beer/cider (3.5% ABV) = one small glass of wine (9% ABV) = one single pub measure of spirit (40% ABV)

The exact number of units in a particular drink can be calculated by multiplying the volume of the drink (number of ml) by the % ABV (alcohol by volume) and dividing it by 1000. For example, the number of units in an alcoholic lemonade (e.g. Two Dogs) of 330 ml with a 4.0% ABV = 330 × 4.0 divided by 1000 = 1.5 units.

The Center for Substance Abuse Prevention (CSAP) recommends abstention from drinking for those who are:

- Under the age of 21
- Pregnant, breast feeding or trying to conceive
- Engaging in activities that require attention, judgement or psycho-motor skills
- Taking medication or prescribed drugs that interact with alcohol
- Recovering from drug dependence
- Likely to drink to intoxication
- Unable to drink moderately

Conclusions

Alcohol misuse clearly has a serious negative impact on individual and societal health. The negative health effects impinge on a wide range of personal and social life domains, ranging from the impact on physical well-being, to psychological and psychiatric disorders, to legal, family and work related problems. Currently there is much scope for improvement in the approaches to the management of alcohol related problems, especially in the areas of early identification and intervention.

As long ago as 1978 the Kessel report (Department of Health and Social Security and the Welsh Office 1978) recommended that the whole range of health care professionals should be involved with the identification and management of alcohol related problems. It stressed the need for non specialists and primary care workers to take a more active role, and that these workers should be trained in order to feel both confident and able to take on this responsibility. In practice little has really changed since the publication of the Kessel report, apart from a few initiatives. One of the major barriers to implementing the recommended changes in practice is the lack of adequate education and training. It is expected that in the future this deficit will be addressed in the nursing curricula and other training programmes.

Nurses clearly have an invaluable role to play in these particular areas and therefore must be ready and able to optimise opportunities which arise in the course of their everyday practice, in order to help those at risk. Telltale signs and symptoms or a history of accidental injury may provide a pointer to a hidden alcohol problem, which should then be followed through in a sensitive and non judgemental manner. Nurses should not regard alcohol problems as being the business of specialists only, as this attitude simply wastes precious opportunities to respond to the problem promptly and effectively. They should, however, not shy away from tapping into the resources of specialists in order to benefit from the information and skills which can and should be shared.

References

Anderson, P. (1988) Excess mortality associated with alcohol consumption. *British Medical Journal*, **297**, 824–6.

Association of Nurses in Substance Abuse (1977) *Substance Use: Guidance on Good Clinical Practice for Nurses, Midwives and Health Visitors. Working within Primary Health Care Teams.* ANSA, London.

Barrison, I.G., Mumford, J. & Murray, R.M. (1982) Detecting excessive drinking among admissions to a general hospital. *Health Trends*, **14**, 80–83.

Borg, S. (1978) Homeless men. A clinical and social study with special reference to alcohol abuse. *Acta Psychologica Scandinavia*, supplement 276.

Cochrane, R. & Ball, S. (1990) The drinking habits of Sikh, Hindu, Muslim and white men in the West Midlands: a community survey. *British Journal of Addiction*, **85**, 759–69.

Cole, D. (1990) Identifying the alcohol misuser. *Nursing Times*, **86**, 58–60.

Cooper, D.B. (1994) *Alcohol Home Detoxification and Assessment.* Radcliffe Medical Press, Oxford.

Creighton, S.J. (1984) *Trends in Child Abuse.* NSPCC, London.

Department of Health and Social Security and the Welsh Office (1978). *The Pattern and Range of Services for Problem Drinkers: Report by the Advisory Committee on Alcoholism.* HMSO, London.

Department of Health and Social Security (DHSS) (19870 *Mental Health Statistics for England 1986.* Government Statistical Service, London.

Department of Health and the Royal College of General Practitioners (1992) *Women and Alcohol.* HMSO, London.

Department of Health (1992) *The Health of the Nation. A Strategy for Health in England.* HMSO, London.

Department of Health (1993) *The Health of the Nation Key Area Handbook. Accidents.* HMSO, London.

Department of Health (1995a) *Fit for the Future: Second Progress Report on the Health of the Nation.* HMSO, London.

Department of Health (1995b) *Sensible Drinking. Report of an Inter-departmental Working Group.* HMSO, London.

Edwards, G. & Gross, M.M. (1976) Alcohol dependence: provisional description of a clinical syndrome. *British Medical Journal,* **1**, 1058–61.

Edwards, G., Anderson, G., Anderson, P., *et al.* (1994) *Alcohol Policy and the Public Good.* Oxford University Press, Oxford.

Fillmore, K.K. (1985) The social victims of drinking. *British Journal of Addiction,* **80**, 307–14.

Gayford, J.J. (1975) Wife battering. A preliminary survey of 100 cases. *British Medical Journal,* **1**, 194–7.

Ghodse, A.H. (1990) Problems of maternal substance abuse. In: *Substance Abuse and Dependence – an Introduction to the Caring Professions* (eds A.H. Ghodse & D. Maxwell), Chapter 10. Macmillan Press, London.

Goddard, E. & Ikin, C. (1991) Drinking in England and Wales. *Patient Education and Counselling in 1987,* **18**, 120–31.

Godfrey, C. (1992) *Alcohol in the Workplace – A Costly Problem.* Alcoholism. Centre for Health Economics, University of York, York.

Health Education Authority (1994) *Health Update: Alcohol.* Health Education Authority, London.

Jellinek, E.M. (1960) *The Disease Concept of Alcoholism.* Millhouse Press, New Brunswick.

Lloyd, G., Chick, J. Crombie, E. & Anderson, s. (1986) Problem drinkers in medical wards: consumption patterns and disabilities in newly identified male cases. *British Journal of Addiction,* **81**(6), 789–95.

Marmot, M. (1995) A not-so-sensible drinks policy. Letter. *Lancet,* **346**, 1643–4.

Northcote, R.J., Martin, B.J., Scallion, H. & Reilly, D.T. (1983) Changing patterns of alcohol abuse in female acute medical admissions. *British Medical Journal,* **286**, 1702.

Office of Population Censuses and Surveys (1988) *General Household Survey 1986.* HMSO, London.

Office of Population Censuses and Surveys (1992) *General Household Survey 1990.* Series GHS no 21. HMSO, London.

Office of Population Censuses and Surveys (1995) *Social Survey Division. Results from the General Household Survey 1994.* HMSO, London.

Platt, S. (1983) Parasuicide. Paper presented to the first Scottish School on Drug Problems. Cited in Health Education Authority (1993) *Health Update: Alcohol, 3.* HEA, London.

Priest, R. (1976) The homeless person and the psychiatric services. *British Journal of Psychiatry*, **128**, 128–36.

Royal College of Psychiatrists (1986) *Alcohol – Our Favourite Drug.* Tavistock, London.

Royal College of Physicians (1987) *A Great and Growing Evil – The Medical Consequences of Alcohol Abuse.* Tavistock, London.

The Royal Colleges Report (1995) *Alcohol and the Heart in Perspective: Sensible Limits Reaffirmed.* Royal Colleges of Physicians, Psychiatrists and General Practitioners, London.

Waldron, G. (1996) Estimating the prevalence of alcohol-related conditions. In: *Addictive Behaviour – Molecules to Mankind* (eds. A. Bonner & J. Waterhouse). Macmillan Press, London.

World Health Organization (1992) *The Tenth Revision of the International Classification of Diseases and Related Health Problems (ICD-10). WHO, Geneva.*

Chapter 6

It's Everybody's Business: The Responses of Health Care Professionals

G. Hussein Rassool

Introduction

Health care professionals in both primary health care and residential settings are usually the first point of contact for many substance misusers. The management of those with chronic dependency problems and those in the early stage of use is not the sole responsibility of specialist workers and addiction specialists. An active involvement of the different cadres of health workers in managing problems of substance misuse is necessary because of the sharp increase, in recent times, in the number of users of psychoactive substances with abuse potential (Rassool & Oyefeso 1993). This chapter will examine the role of health care professionals in hospital and primary health care settings in relation to intervention and management of substance use and misuse. It will also examine the attitudes of nurses and other health care professionals towards substance misuse. The rationale for working with substance misusers and the contributions that health care professionals may be able to provide are briefly described.

Rationale for working with substance misusers

In the UK, there has been a growing societal, professional and governmental interest in the prevention, treatment and rehabilitation of substance misusers (Rassool 1997). There is now an increased awareness by consumer interest groups, parents and society in general of the need to combat the complex challenges of substance misuse rather than find a way of 'living with drugs'. Society's expectations of the provision of accessible services to those in need have increased as a result of the recognition that substance misuse is preventable and that the associated harm can be reduced if proper intervention and treatment are offered.

One of the pivotal mandates for national policy in the promotion of good health and prevention of ill health is in the Department of Health's (1992) document on *The Health of the Nation*. This is a strategic plan aimed at achieving better health for all in England and sets out targets for the nation's health. Five major health goals are set, addressing health education, prevention and promotion activities. In the context of substance misuse, some of the particular areas identified as threats to the nation's health are smoking, alcohol related diseases and HIV disease. All the key areas for health education targets are invariably related to the misuse of psychoactive substances. In addition, the aim of the British government's strategy, as set out in the White Paper (Tackling Drugs Together 1995), is 'to take effective action by vigorous law enforcement, accessible treatment and a new emphasis on education and prevention'. Substance misuse education for all health and social care professionals is therefore needed (Advisory Council on the Misuse of Drugs (ACMD) 1994).

Primary health care team members, such as health visitors, district nurses, domiciliary midwives, practice nurses, community psychiatric nurses and others, are well placed to deal with substance misusers. The extent and nature of the substantial health problems associated with substance misuse highlight the pressing need for members of the primary health care team and nurses working in hospital and occupational settings to intervene effectively (Rassool & Oyefeso 1993). The need for the management and treatment of substance misuse problems is no longer confined to the specialist services. The ACMD (1982) report on treatment and rehabilitation stressed the need for a comprehensive approach to drug misuse with the emphasis and focus on a multi-disciplinary response from generic, voluntary and specialist agencies. However, only a minority of drug and alcohol misusers are likely to come into contact and seek treatment with specialist drug and alcohol agencies. Those early in their drug/drink taking career and those with a chronic dependency have the same rights as other patients to receive appropriate health care from the National Health Service. Every member of the health care profession has an important role to play in responding to substance misuse problems. Studies have shown that intervening in the lives of substance misusers at an early stage helps to limit the associated health damage. Prompt treatment from health care professionals can have a dramatic impact on preventing substance misuse becoming a long term problem (Babor *et al.* 1986; World Health Organization 1986; Anderson & Scott 1992).

Attitudes towards substance misusers

It is clear that, even when health care professionals do identify and recognise drug or alcohol related problems, they are reluctant to respond appropriately. Social prejudice, negative attitudes and stereotyped perceptions of problem drinkers and problem drug users are widely held amongst health care professionals, and this may lead to minimal care being accorded to this client group. In addition, the health related problems may go untreated and may potentially be exacerbated. These negative and ill informed beliefs about drugs can be expected to translate themselves into negative and ill judged reactions to users (Griffiths & Pearson 1988).

Several studies of nurses and health professionals have indicated negative attitudes towards substance misusers and a prevalent pessimistic outlook on successful treatment. Nurses tend to be moralistic towards alcoholics and perceive them as weak rather than ill (Starkey 1980). One study found that nurses with negative attitudes towards alcoholism not only overlooked symptoms of alcoholism but failed to refer for treatment those they did identify (Rosenbaum 1977). People with drinking problems are usually unpopular patients, and they are perceived as noisy and manipulative (Ferneau 1968; Cornish & Miller 1976; Kelly & May 1982; Manson & Ritson 1984). In general, past studies have shown that nurses were less tolerant to alcoholic than to non alcoholic clients (Schmid & Schmid, 1973; Rotheram 1980).

However, this negative attitude is not peculiar to nurses but applies across a whole spectrum of health care professionals. Negative attitudes have been found among medical practitioners (Potamianos *et al.* 1985), social workers (Cartwright 1980; Lightfoot & Orford 1986), drug counsellors and law enforcement agents (Sutker & O'Neil 1980). Carroll's (1995) study of the attitudes of nurses working within the prison health care service in Scotland found that both male and female prison nurses had negative attitudes towards substance misusers in custodial care. Farrell and Lewis (1990) demonstrated that patients with a history of alcohol problems were rated by psychiatrists to be less compliant, have a poorer prognosis, be less likely to need hospital admission and, significantly, to be less of a suicide risk. Such negative attitudes compromise the opportunities for potential preventive health education and minimal interventions. A report of the ACMD (1988) stated that 'a change in professional ... attitudes to drug misuse is necessary as attitudes and policies which lead to drug misusers remaining hidden will impair the effectiveness of measures to combat the spread of HIV'.

However, the negative perceptions of nurses and other health professionals toward substance misusers are changing. Sullivan and Hale (1987) found that nurses perceive alcoholism more as an illness than as a moral weakness and believe that alcoholic people should have medical treatment. This may suggest that attitudes about alcoholism are moving away from the moralistic model towards an increased acceptance of the medical model of intervention. Nevertheless, both physical and psychosocial interventions are required to meet the health needs of substance misusers. The development of a positive and non judgemental attitude towards substance misusers may be partly related to the provision of education and training. A study of the role of GPs in the identification and management of patients with alcohol related problems indicated that education about alcohol and alcohol problems was correlated with a number of positive attitudes (Clement 1986).

Health care professionals' roles

Health care professionals have considerable contact with individuals who are at high risk of health related problems as a result of misuse of psychoactive substances. Whether specialists or not, nurses must assume a multitude of roles which focus on the provision of effective care, prevention and education (Rassool 1993b). The roles of the nurse in relation to substance misuse have been highlighted in a document from the World Health Organisation and the International Council of Nurses (1991). These roles are:

- Provider of care
- Educator/resource
- Counsellor/therapist
- Advocate
- Promoter of health
- Researcher
- Supervisor/leader
- Consultant

A brief description of the roles is shown in Table 6.1.

In summary, these roles have the same commonalities to those subroles health care professionals embrace within the health care system (Hall 1980; Griffin 1983; Bottorf & D'Cruz 1984; Macleod Clark 1988; Burnard 1990). It

Table 6.1 Nursing roles in relation to substance misuse.

Provider of care	Caring for those who misuse or are affected by psychoactive substances
Counsellor/therapist	Focusing on the needs of the individuals, their families and colleagues
Educator/resource	Providing health information to community groups, schools, families, individuals and to professional and non-professional groups
Advocate	Lobbying for change and improved care
Health promoter	Campaigning for policy and legislation to reduce demands of abused drugs
Researcher	Determining the most effective method of helping, caring and preventing substance misuse
Supervisor/leader	Guiding professionals and non professionals
Consultant	Providing consultancy to professionals in this speciality

Source: World Health Organization and the International Council of Nurses (1991).

is recognised that these generic roles and skills of the health care professionals could be easily adapted to meet the needs of the problem drug user and problem drinker as well as the 'non using' population (Rassool & Oyefeso 1993a). It is fundamental that the central role of health care professionals, in hospital or community settings, should focus on early recognition and the provision of effective care, prevention and health education.

Generic interventions with substance misusers

The nature and extent of substance misuse in the community requires a multi-professional approach in working with substance misusers. Liaison with other health and social care agencies and specialist substance misuse services is part of the shared care approach which is currently in vogue. This section will provide a brief overview of the particular setting and speciality of health care professionals and some aspects of generic interventions.

Residential and occupational based nurses

Psychiatric nurse

Several studies have shown that substance misuse is a common problem in psychiatric patients where substance misuse co-exists with psychiatric disorders (Hall 1980; Glass & Jackson 1988). In addition, 14 000 patients are admitted each year to psychiatric hospitals for alcohol dependence and alcohol psychosis (Royal College of Psyhchiatrists 1986). Many psychiatric patients use psychoactive substances as a means of self-medication in order to relieve anxiety, depression and other psychopathological conditions (Gafoor & Rassool 1998). Some patients are admitted to acute psychiatric settings as a result of drug induced psychiatric reactions from stimulants and hallucinogens. Health-related problems include:

❏ Drug induced psychosis (stimulants and alcohol)
❏ Drug withdrawal psychosis (hypnosedatives and alcohol)
❏ Suicidal behaviour and depression as a result of substance misuse
❏ Withdrawal symptoms
❏ Dual diagnosis (mental illness co-existing with substance misuse)

The areas of interventions include screening, assessment of substance misuse and management of patients with dual diagnosis and drug induced psychotic reactions. Patient health education, smoking cessation and harm-minimisation or controlled drinking should be included in the intervention strategies.

General nurse

Patients who misuse psychoactive substances may be admitted to a general or surgical ward, but the health problems may or may not be associated with substance misuse. The Tomlinson report (1992) indicates that 30% of acute medical admissions to hospitals have alcohol problems. According to Maxwell (1990), the range of acute medical problems nurses are likely to encounter are as follows:

On medical wards

- Unexplained fever
- Acute or chronic infection of skin and joints
- Unexplained cardiac murmurs and endocarditis
- Venous or arterial thrombosis
- Jaundice, or abnormal liver function
- Lymphadenopathy or other features of immunosuppression
- Munchausen's syndrome

On surgical wards

- Abscess
- Acute abdomen
- Intestinal obstruction ('body packers')
- Vascular problems
- Trauma (such as road traffic accidents or burns)
- Rhinitis or rhinorrhoea

Aspects of interventions include the provision of total nursing care, assessment or taking a drug and alcohol history, minimal interventions and counselling, harm minimisation, dealing with withdrawal symptoms and referral to specialist agencies.

Accident and emergency nurses

Substance misusers may present to the Accident and Emergency department as a result of physical or psychological complications of substance misuse. It is recognised that the monitoring of drug related problems by hospital emergency departments is a good method of detecting changes in the prevalence and patterns of substance misuse (Ghodse *et al.* 1981) The health problems related to the misuse of alcohol or drugs include:

- Dealing with overdose or coma
- Management of intoxicated clients and disruptive behaviour
- Management of withdrawal behaviour
- Accidents

❏ Respiratory failure (common after opiate overdose)
❏ Drug induced psychosis or other mental health problems

Aspects of intervention include nursing care of unconscious or overdose patients, liaison with specialist nurse or services and the patient's GP, and the provision of health information.

Genito urinary nurse

Substance misusers will come into contact with genito-urinary medicine services as a result of concern relating to their HIV status or a sexually transmitted disease. Substance misuse by injecting is a high risk behaviour and may lead to unsafe sexual behaviour and practice while under the influence of drugs or alcohol. Substance misusers with HIV positive status will require care and management in relation to their substance use problems and HIV related disease. Close working relationships with substance misuse services are needed. Areas of intervention include taking a drug and alcohol history, pre-and post-test counselling, general counselling, health education and harm minimisation.

Midwife or obstetric nurse

It is common for health care professionals in these specialities to come into contact with and manage pregnant substance misusers. It is acknowledged that, for some women, this may be their only contact with the statutory health services. Health related problems include:

❏ Disorders of fetal growth and development
❏ Risk of transmission of infection
❏ Withdrawal effects in the newborn (irritability and convulsions)

Aspects of intervention include screening, promotion of harm minimisation, encouragement of screening for cervical cytology (antenatal care) and the observation of babies undergoing withdrawal symptoms for those born with a high degree of dependence on opiates. Health education related to maternal health is indicated, as well as antenatal counselling and, as appropriate, education on the use of tobacco, drugs and alcohol and management of the abstinence syndrome. After care and support to the mother and child will be necessary, and liaison with specialist services.

Prison health care nurse

Prison health care services deal with the health needs of the prison population. These include the provision of general medical services and psychiatric treatment. The priority issues for the health care services for prisoners (Department of Health 1992b) are the management of alcohol and drug withdrawal, harm minimisation and HIV infection and AIDS. Since 1996, prison health care staff have responsibility for random drug screening. Health related problems include:

- ❑ Accidental overdose
- ❑ Withdrawal problems from drug or alcohol
- ❑ HIV or AIDS
- ❑ Hepatitis
- ❑ Psychiatric related problems, suicide

Aspects of intervention include the taking of a drug and alcohol history, assessment, initiation of a detoxification programme, harm minimisation, dealing with accidental overdose arising from loss of tolerance during custodial care, liaison with substance misuse services and other self-help groups, health information and counselling.

Primary Health Care Team

Community mental health nurses

Community mental health nurses are exposed to a wide range of patients with varying degrees of psychiatric disorders. Part of their case load will include individuals with substance use problems, involving both illicit and prescribed medications. In 1990, 134 specialist community mental health nurses were identified as working in the field of substance misuse (Butterworth & Rushforth 1995). This figure is probably underrepresented as more community mental health nurses are taking the opportunity to follow courses in substance misuse and addictive behaviour. These community nurses face the ethical dilemma of encouraging their clients to adhere to medication compliance, while at the same time discouraging and rationalising their alcohol or other drug use. This may play a part in the ambivalence that nurses experience, resulting in the resistance to use specialist services in a consultative capacity, preferring to refer the client to them for 'treatment and management' (Kennedy & Faugier 1989). Health related problems include:

- ❑ Dual diagnosis
- ❑ Problems related to withdrawal from alcohol, benzodiazepines, opiates, etc.
- ❑ HIV and AIDS; hepatitis
- ❑ Amphetaine or cocaine psychosis
- ❑ Dementia
- ❑ Smoking related problems

Aspects of intervention include screening, the assessment of mental health/substance misuse problems, counselling, harm minimisation, health education, alternative therapies in the rational use of psychoactive substances, alternatives to drug prescribing, home detoxification and the prevention of substance misuse.

School nurse

The use of tobacco, alcohol and illicit drugs by young people and school children is the source of much public concern. One of the key areas of the government's report (*Tackling Drugs Together* 1995) is to reduce the acceptability and availability of drugs to young people in schools. Solvents, cannabis, amphetamines, LSD and Ecstasy are the drugs most commonly used by young people. Experimental use of drugs or alcohol is common during adolescence. An account of the prevalence of substance misuse in young people is inappropriate here but is documented in Chapter 22. Aspects of intervention include the provision of advice, information and health counselling to parents and children, health promotion and referral to other specialist or non specialist agencies if appropriate. The school nurse should be among the core personnel who contribute to the school policy on substance use.

Practice nurse

Practice nursing has expanded and developed rapidly since the implementation of a cost effective health service based on the principles of market economy and consumer choices. It is stated that a future role of the nurse practitioner should be in the areas of health promotion and the diagnosis and treatment of disease in the setting of a neighbourhood clinic (Cumberledge 1986). The nurse practitioner has a valuable role to play in the prevention of substance misuse. Aspects of intervention include the early identification and recognition of substance misuse, screening for drugs and alcohol, brief interventions with clients with early drinking or drug taking problems, health education and counselling.

Health visitor

The health visitor will encounter a large client group – the family and significant others – misusing alcohol, tobacco and prescribed and illicit drugs. Although health visitors are responsible for child health, they are mainly concerned with preventative health education. Aspects of intervention include advice, counselling, health education, health promotion and harm minimisation.

District nurse

District nurses usually encounter patients at different stages in their illness and are responsible for the provision of total nursing care. They too have a role to play in prevention and harm minimisation in relation to substance misuse. Aspects of intervention include the early identification and recognition of substance misuse, health education and the generic assessment of health problems related to substance use.

Occupational health nurse

The misuse of psychoactive substances in the work place is one of the major concerns of management, professional organisations and occupational health staff. The use and misuse of psychoactive substances such as tobacco and alcohol by workers have resulted in absenteeism, accidents and loss of efficiency. There is evidence to suggest that a policy on tobacco smoking or alcohol use can lead to reduced absenteeism, improved safety performance, lower maintenance costs, lower air-conditioning and ventilation costs, increased productivity, improved morale among non smokers, fewer accidents and a lower risk of losing skilled employees through premature retirement or death (McEwen 1991). The occupational health nurses have a major role to play in health education and promotion regarding the use of psychoactive substances and in meeting the health and safety needs of the employees. Aspects of intervention include screening, health promotion, detoxification harm minimisation and controlled drinking and smoking cessation clinics.

Nurses working in family planning and well men and women clinics

There is ample opportunity for screening and early recognition of substance use and misuse for those attending family planning and well men or women clinics. During the process of health monitoring, time must also be used for the provision of health counselling, risk reduction advice and harm minimisation for alcohol use, tobacco smoking and drug use and misuse.

Conclusions

Health care professionals share many commonalities with their addiction specialist counterparts. Their skills in assessment, counselling and health education are quite legitimately applicable in working with the public – non-users, experimental, recreational and dependent or chronic substance misusers and their families. The recognition and early identification of problem or alcohol drug use is an important aspect of the health care professional's role, as this is a significant means to prevent the widespread misuse of psychoactive substances and to limit the damage done to the individual and society.

References

Advisory Council on the Misuse of Drugs (1982) *Treatment and Rehabilitation.* HMSO, London.

Advisory Council on the Misuse of Drugs (1988) *Aids and Drug Misuse. Part 1.* HMSO, London.

Advisory Council on the Misuse of Drugs (1994) *Aids and Drug Misuse. Update.* HMSO, London.

Anderson, P. & Scott, E. (1992) The effect of general practitioners' advice to heavy-drinking men. *British Journal of Addiction,* **87**, 891–900.

Babor, T.F., Hodgson, R.J. & Ritson, E.B. (1986) Alcohol-related problems in primary health care settings: a review of early intervention strategies. *British Journal of Addiction,* **81**, 23–46.

Bottorf, J.L. & D'Cruz, J.V. (1984) Towards inclusive notions of 'patient' and 'nurse'. *Journal of Advanced Nursing,* **9**, 549–53.

Burnard, P. (1990) Recording counselling skills in nursing. *Senior Nurse,* **10**, 26–7.

Butterworth, T. & Rushforth, D. (1995) Issues in the development of community mental health nursing services. In: *Stress and Coping in Mental Health Nursing* (eds J. Carson, L. Fagin & S. Ritter). Chapman & Hall, London.

Carroll, J. (1995) Attitudes and perceptions of prison nurse officers to drug misusers. Paper presented at the *ANSA Conference,* March 1995.

Cartwright, A. (1980) The attitude of helping agents towards the alcoholic client: the influence of experience, support, training and self-esteem. *British Journal of Addiction,* **75**, 413–31.

Clement, S. (1986) The identification of alcohol related problems by general practitioners. *British Journal of Addiction,* **81**, 257–64.

Cornish, R.D. & Miller, M.V. (1976) Attitudes of registered nurses towards the alcoholic. *Journal of Psychiatric Nursing,* **14**, 19–22.

Cumberledge, J. (1986) *Neighbourhood Nursing – A Focus for Care.* HMSO, London.

Department of Health (1992) *Health of the Nation: A Strategy for Health in England.* HMSO, London.

Department of Health and the Home Office (1992) *Review of Health and Social Services for Mentally Disordered Offenders and Others Requiring Similar Services.* Cmnd 2088. HMSO, London.

Farrell, M. & Lewis, G. (1990) Discrimination on the grounds of diagnosis. *British Journal of Addiction,* **85**, 883–90.

Ferneau, E.W. (1968) What student nurses think about alcoholic patients and alcoholism. *Nursing Research,* **17**, 41–57.

Gafoor, M. & Rassool, G.H. (1998) The co-existence of psychiatric disorders and substance misuse: working with dual diagnosis patients. *Journal of Advanced Nursing,* **27**, 497–502.

Ghodse, A.H., Edwards, G., Stapleton, J., *et al.* (1981) Drug-related problems in London accident and emergency departments. *Lancet,* **2**, 859–62.

Glass, I. & Jackson, P. (1988) Maudsley Hospital survey: prevalence of alcohol problems and other psychiatric disorders in a hospital population. *British Journal of Addiction,* **83**, 1108–11.

Griffin, A.P. (1983) A philosophical analysis of caring in nursing. *Journal of Advanced Nursing,* **5**, 149–59.

Griffiths, R. & Pearson, B. (1988) *Working with Drug Users.* Wildwood House, Hants.

Hall, D.C. (1980) The nature of nursing and the education of the nurse. *Journal of Advanced Nursing,* **5**, 149–59.

Kelly, M.P. & May, D. (1982) Good and bad patients: a review of the literature and a theoretical critique. *Journal of Advanced Nursing,* **7**, 147–56.

Kennedy, J. & Faugier, J. (1989) *Drug and Alcohol Dependency Nursing.* Heinemann, London.

Lightfoot, P.J.C. & Orford, J. (1986) Helping agents' attitudes towards the alcoholic client: the influence of experience, support, training and self-esteem. *British Journal of Addiction,* **75**, 413–31.

Macleod Clark, J. (1988) Communication: the continuing challenge. *Nursing Times,* **84**, 24–7.

McEwen, J. (1991) Interventions in the workplace. In: *The International Handbook of Addiction Behaviour* (ed. I. Glass). Routledge, London.

Manson, L. & Ritson, B. (1984) *Alcohol and Health. A Handbook for Nurses, Midwives and Health Visitors.* Medical Council on Alcoholism, London.

Maxwell, D. (1990) Medical complications of substance abuse. In: *Substance Abuse and Dependence* (eds A.H. Ghodse & D. Maxwell). Macmillan Press, London.

Potamianos, G., Winter, D. Duffy, S., *et al.* (1985) The perception of problem drinkers by general hospital staff, general practitioner and alcoholic patients. *Alcohol,* **2**, 563–6.

Rassool, G.H. (1993a) Nursing and substance misuse: responding to the challenge. *Journal of Advanced Nursing,* **18**, 1401–7.

Rassool, G.H. (1993b) Prime movers. *Nursing Times,* **89**, 40–42.

Rassool, G.H. (1997) Addiction nursing – towards a new paradigm: the UK experience. In: *Addiction Nursing: Perspectives on Professional and Clinical Practice* (eds G. Rassool & M. Gafoor). Stanley Thornes, Cheltenham.

Rassool, G.H. & Oyefeso, N. (1993) The need for substance misuse education in health studies curriculum: a case for nursing education. *Nurse Education Today,* **13**, 107–10.

Rosenbaum, P.D. (1977) Public health nurses in the treatment of alcoholic abusers. *Canadian Journal of Public Health,* **68**, 503–8.

Rotheram, F. (1980) Nurses and alcohol problems. *Nursing Times,* **76**, 2197–8.

Royal College of Psychiatrists (1986) *Alcohol: Our Favourite Drug.* Tavistock, London.

Schmid, N. & Schmid, D. (1973) Nursing students' attitudes towards alcoholics. *Nursing Research,* **22**, 246–8.

Starkey, P.J. (1980) Nurses' attitudes towards alcoholism. *AORN,* **31**, 822.

Sullivan, E.J. & Hale, R.E. (1987) Nurses' beliefs about the etiology and treatment of alcohol abuse: a national study. *Journal of Studies on Alcohol,* **48**, 456–60.

Sutker, P.B. & O'Neill, P.M. (1980) Evaluation of a drug abuse education course for law enforcement and treatment specialists. *International Journal of the Addictions,* **15**, 125–35.

Tackling Drugs Together (1995) *A Strategy for England 1995–1998.* HMSO, London.

Tomlison, B. (1992) Report of the inquiry into London's health service. *Medical Education and Research,* **17**.

World Health Organization (1986) *Drug Dependence and Alcohol-Related Problems: A Manual for Community Health Workers with Guidelines for Trainers.* WHO, Geneva.

World Health Organization and the International Council of Nurses (1991) *Roles of the Nurse in Relation to Substance Misuse.* ICN, Geneva.

Part 2
Prevention, Recognition and Intervention

Chapter 7

Prevention and Health Education

G. Hussein Rassool

Introduction

In the current climate of the changing nature of alcohol drinking and drug taking behaviours, health education and prevention increasingly form part of the role of the health care professionals and the central part of public health policy. In the UK, there is a recognition that substance use and misuse cut across every aspect of health which requires the conception and delivery of a prevention and health education strategy that is not simply confined to the specialist services but to professional disciplines and organizations. Every encounter with a patient affords an opportunity for health care professionals to transmit knowledge about health care and harm minimisation in relation to tobacco smoking, alcohol, psychoactive drugs and sexual health. Health promotion has emerged over the last few years as a significant entity within the health movement and now forms an important part of the health services of most developed countries (Bracher *et al.* 1995).

The aims of this chapter are to examine the relationships of health education and nursing and the concept of prevention in the context of substance misuse. A brief overview of health promoting hospitals, schools and workplaces and the personal health education of health care professionals is given.

Nursing and health education

Health education and health promotion can be identified throughout nursing practice. Together they represent an integral part of the nurse's role and a component of nursing care (Rassool 1984; United Kingdom Central Council 1986; Maben & Macleod Clark 1995). Health education and health promotion have been widely used in the nursing literature but confusion still exists in the clarification and operational definitions of both concepts. According to Tones (1990) health education is 'any planned activity which promotes health or illness related learning, that is, some relatively permanent change in an individual's competence or disposition.' This is an acceptable definition but it is too vague to be used in the context of substance misuse. Some writers have incorporated the concept of health education within the aegis of health promotion.

Maben and Macleod Clark (1995) proposed a definition of health promotion which incorporates the concept of health education. Health promotion is seen as

> 'an attempt to improve the health status of an individual or community, and is also concerned with the prevention of disease ... At its broadest level it is concerned with the wider influences on health and therefore with the policy and legislative implications of these. Health education through information-giving, advice, support and skills training as part of, and a necessary prerequisite to, health promotion.'

That is, health education is a component of health promotion activities where the goal is to enhance and promote health through the implementation of effective educational and training programmes, taking into account the socio-political influences. It is not within the scope of this chapter to provide a fuller exposition of health promotion and health education. For a more comprehensive examination of the concepts of health promotion and health education the reader is referred to Naidoo and Willis (1994) and Maben and Macleod Clark (1995).

Part of the goal of health education includes the process of enabling an individual to change his life-style and behaviour. In the context of substance use and misuse, the goal of health education is to promote the health of the general population and prevent the use of psychoactive substances and minimise the harm. Helping people to make informed choices about the use of tobacco, alcohol and drugs is part of that process. Accordingly, nurses should utilise health education materials to assist in reducing the demand for substances through the promotion of healthy life-styles and suitable alternatives (World Health Organization/International Council of Nurses (WHO/ICN) 1991). Interventions to prevent substance misuse may be implemented both formally and informally, during one-to-one interactions and in groups. However, there is an urgent need to shift substance use education from its narrow focus of simply providing health information or leaflets, to those at risks of substance misuse, to the provision of advice and brief interventions. Table 7.1 summarises the models, goals and interventions of health education in relation to drugs and alcohol.

Health education and prevention

A variety of models and approaches have been used in an attempt to prevent and reduce substance misuse (Ewles & Simnett 1992). Traditionally health education activities have been viewed as existing on three levels: primary, secondary and tertiary prevention. This three-stage model

Table 7.1 Health education approaches to substance misuse.

Approach	Goals	Health education intervention	Examples
Medical/public health problems	Reduction of morbidity and mortality	Prevention of ill health. Clinical interventions	Early recognition, care, treatment and rehabilitation
Behaviour change	Change of life-style and behaviour	Media campaign. Health information: controlled drinking, safer drug use and safer sex	Prevent non smokers from starting to smoke. Persuade smokers to stop. Counselling. Reducing or minimising ill effects or harm from alcohol and drugs
Educational	Change attitudes. Increase knowledge and awareness. Develop skills in decision making	Health information on smoking, drinking and drug taking. Learning coping skills and stress management	Information about effects of substance misuse and health related problems. Provision of resources. Referral to specialist services
Consumer empowerment	Enabling individuals to identify their health concerns	Advocacy. Meeting specific health and socio-economic needs	Clients identify health needs, types and access to services. Community anti-drug campaign
Social change	Enabling changes to health and social policies. Bringing changes to the social environment. Improvement in health and social equality in access to services and treatment interventions	Lobbying. Political and social actions	Alcohol and drug policy in work place. Limit the marketing and advertising of psychoactive substances. Labelling on alcoholic beverages

Source: Rassool & Gafoor (1997).

was modified by the Advisory Council on the Misuse of Drugs (ACMD) (1984) on the grounds that it was not comprehensive enough to cover all the elements of prevention policies. The ACMD's approach to prevention is based on meeting two basic criteria:

(1) Reducing the risk of an individual engaging in substance misuse and
(2) Reducing the harm associated with substance misuse

Primary prevention

Primary prevention is a process that includes efforts to reduce the demand for and stop illegal drug use, drinking alcohol or tobacco smoking. for example, primary prevention campaigns would seek to discourage any alcohol drinking among children and adolescents and those in high risk groups. Prevention has been defined as 'a process to inhibit or reduce physical, mental, emotional or social impairment which results in or from the abuse of chemical substances' (National Institute on Drug Abuse 1989). Thus, primary prevention involves the provision of health information/teaching and media campaigns and mobilisation of the community.

The focus of primary prevention should not only be the non using population, but also experimental, recreational and dependent users. Certain groups are more vulnerable in regard to high risk behaviour, such as young people, pregnant women, prisoners, prostitutes and the homeless. The implications for nursing in the area of primary prevention include information and education, formally and informally, about substance misuse with the emphasis on reducing risk factors associated with these substances.

Secondary prevention

This is the prevention of the sequelae of the misuse of psychoactive substances and the limitation of disability or dysfunction. Secondary prevention seeks to reduce and limit further health and social harm done by the use and misuse of psychoactive substances through early recognition, intervention or rehabilitation. Examples include the rational use of prescribed medication (see below), health information on safer alcohol and drug use and safer sexual practices. The harm minimisation approach, as part of secondary preventive strategies, has been widely implemented in the drug and alcohol field as a response to the threat presented by HIV and hepatitis.

Harm minimisation approach

This approach focuses on reducing the harm that substance misusers do to themselves and to their families. This may involve drawing attention to technique specific hazards (related to injecting and the sharing of equipment) and/or the dangers of specific risks in the misuse of particular psychoactive substances. It has been pointed out that more benefits would be achieved from everyone drinking somewhat less rather than persuading the chronic problem drinker to become abstinent (Kreitman 1986). Similarly in the case of drug taking, some individuals may be unwilling to contemplate stopping their drug life-style but can still benefit from interventions intended to reduce harm.

Harm minimisation techniques are relevant to health education and preventive strategies for the misuse of psychoactive substances. Advising people about the dangers of intoxication, drinking and driving, and the ways to minimise harm all come under harm minimisation and form part of the health education role of the nurse (Kennedy & Faugier 1989). Harm minimisation strategies are also applicable to those who continue to use illicit drugs. The advent of HIV makes it essential for generic services in contact with drug misusers to provide health care information and advice on the risks of HIV and how to reduce risks in both sexual health and injecting behaviour.

Tertiary level

The tertiary level of prevention seeks to limit and reduce further complications or dysfunctions through effective care, treatment and rehabilitation services. The aim of the tertiary level is to restore the individual to an optimal level of functioning and prevent relapse. In particular, tertiary prevention includes the engagement of residential and community facilities for those who are seeking help for their alcohol or drug related problems. Services available for those with substance use problems are examined in Chapter 10.

It has been pointed out that all three levels of prevention can be incorporated in the work of health care professionals in an approach combining assessment, intervention and evaluation (Tether & Robinson 1986). The focuses of preventive interventions for generic health professionals are based on primary and secondary interventions. It is worth pointing out that the notion of completely 'stopping' the whole population from using a variety of mind altering psychoactive substances is extremely idealistic and, of course, is unachieveable in reality. Nurses need to acknowledge this limitation and address the areas where health education can reduce the harm caused as a result of continuing use and misuse of prescribed, over-the-counter and illicit drugs.

General interventions

There are grounds for optimism that if information, advice and health education on sexual health and the dangers relating to the misuse of drugs, alcohol and tobacco smoking are provided by nurses and others, that this may reduce the casualties in terms of harm and dependency. Early recognition and minimal intervention are also part of the process of preventive health education (Babor *et al.*, 1986; WHO 1986). Advice given to patients to help change their drinking habits has produced demonstrable benefits to their health in the ensuing year (Chick *et al.* 1985). There is evidence that patients in both hospitals and in primary health care would welcome clearer guidance concerning a healthier life-style, including information about sensible drinking practices and smoking (Hartz *et al* 1991; Faulkner & Ward, 1983). Early recognition and minimal interventions can be simultaneously achieved during a brief assessment which includes taking a drug/alcohol/tobacco history, risk assessment and counselling. (Chapters 8 and 9 deal with screening and brief interventions.)

Community approach

Nurses in primary health care teams and other health care professionals are more likely to be involved with preventive health behaviour at the community level. Helping people to change their life-style and behaviour is not only about targeting individuals, but also about helping the community to change. An element of this approach is mobilising the community, and suggestions on mobilising the community for the nurse as a primary health care worker has been documented elsewhere (WHO 1986). However, the strategy of preventive health education cannot be operated by nurses in isolation. A workable strategy for nudging the community towards healthier life-styles and behaviour requires positive partnerships with key agents of change within the community. This community partnership involves community leaders, members of the public, social services, education services, non statutory and voluntary agencies, police services and the media.

It has been suggested that, to be effective, any drugs campaign or production of safer sex strategies needs to be 'ground roots' based and use credible trained peers (Kelly & Murphy 1991). Within the framework of this approach, the individual is also encouraged to maintain a healthier life-style, for example by taking up physical and recreational activities or using stress reduction techniques and other coping skills. Helping people to make informed choices about the rational use of legal psychoactive substances is part of that process.

Rational use of psychoactive substances

In the context of this chapter the term rational use means that the right drug is taken by the right patient, in the right dose and for the right duration of therapy, and that the risks of therapy are acceptable (WHO 1989). Many of the prescribed psychoactive drugs such as hypnotics, sedatives and tranquillisers are frequently the subject of widespread misuse and can result in health related problems and dependence. Health care professionals have a responsibility to ensure the rational use of psychoactive drugs. The importance of promoting the rational use of psychoactive drugs and the need to educate health care professionals in this area have been recognised (Ghodse & Khan 1988; WHO 1989; WHO–ICN 1991; Rassool & Winnington 1993).

The knowledge and clinical skills of health care professionals in relation to a wide range of medications and to the sequelae of their misuse can form a basis for effective nursing interventions (Rassool & Winnington 1993). Nursing interventions and non pharmacological therapies such as counselling and relaxation may be used instead of psychoactive substances. Several studies have shown that educating patients in the art of relaxation reduces the need to use hypnosedatives and tranquillisers (Temez *et al.* 1978; Tilly & Weighillk 1986; Gournay 1988). It is stressed that while the focus is on the misuse of psychoactive drugs, consideration must also be given to the proper use of therapeutic medications (Rassool & Winnington 1993).

Health promoting institutions

Health and safety aspects of the working environment have had a long history in the UK, but health promotion in the work place is a relatively new concept and practice. In the next sections the concept and practice of health promotion in hospitals and other work places will be examined briefly in relation to health care professionals.

Health promoting hospitals

In recent years the idea of 'health promoting hospitals' has been slowly emerging in Europe, with the emphasis on health gain through health promotion and disease prevention. The Budapest Declaration on Health Promoting Hospitals (WHO 1991) stated that

> 'Beyond the assurance of good quality medical services and health care, the health promoting hospital encourages and supports health promoting perspectives and activities among staff, patients, relatives and the wider community.'

In England the report on *The Health of the Nation* (Department of Health 1992) reinforced the same theme and stated that

> 'hospitals exist to provide treatment and care but they also offer unique opportunities for more general health promotion for staff, patients and all who come into contact with them.'

The principle behind this movement is to use hospitals to promote positive health within its own environs and to the wider local community.

The shifting focus from illness to health oriented and public concerns within the hospital environments should enable organisations to implement health education and health promotion activities for both staff and patients. A number of initiatives in the creation of health promoting hospitals are under way and the key principles are derived from the Ottawa Charter for Health Promoting Hospitals (HPHs) (World Health Organization 1992; Asvall 1993). The implementation of health promoting programmes in the work place has benefited organisations in terms of reductions in staff stress, absenteeism, sickness and turnover and increases in organisational efficiency (Health Education Authority 1992; Audit Commission 1993). Information on tobacco smoking and the case of alcohol and other psychoactive substances should be incorporated in health education and health promotion activities. The personal health education of the staff in relation to substance use and misuse should also be on the health policy agenda.

Health promoting schools

Young people constitute one of the high risk groups who experiment with or recreationally use legal and illicit psychoactive substances. Within this age group, primary prevention initiatives are the most appropriate in motivating young people to avoid drug experimentation. The aim of preventive health education in schools is to raise young people's awareness of the facts about drug misuse and associated risks, emphasise the benefits of life-styles and develop skills needed to make informed and responsible decisions to resist drug misuse (Department of Health 1995).

The Tackling Drugs Together (1995) report on *A Strategy for England 1995–1998* has been introduced by the government to tackle drug misuse. One of the aims of the strategy is to reduce the accessibility (demand) and availability (supply) of drugs to young people. The objectives of the strategy are:

❑ To discourage young people from using drugs
❑ To raise awareness among staff, governors and parents of issues related to drug misuse
❑ To ensure that schools offer effective programmes of drug education and the availability and accessibility of a range of services: advice, counselling, treatment, rehabilitation and after care services

The plan of action in relation to young people and substance misuse includes the training of teachers, the support of innovative projects in drug education and prevention, the development of school policies on managing drug related incidents and drug education. Other initiatives focus on new interdepartmental publicity campaigns with advertising and media expertise, and role models aimed at helping young people to resist drugs.

School nurses (see Chapter 14) are more likely to be involved in primary and secondary prevention in the provision of information on health and the risk factors of psychoactive substances, in offering advice and counselling to parents and young people about drugs and by taking an active part in health education projects aimed at reducing the experimentation in tobacco smoking and the use of drugs (Ecstasy, amphetamines, cannabis) and alcohol by young people. It is acknowledged that it is important to adopt a school policy that recognises a variety of responses to tackle substance misuse. Prevention of substance use and misuse is the primary target for schools but, for those few who become entangled with psychoactive substances beyond experimentation, treatment and rehabilitation (if appropriate) should be made available rather than a punitive sanction imposed.

Health promotion: substance misuse and the work place

The work place is an ideal environment for the capture of sizeable numbers of adults as recipients for promotional information on health and prevention of the use and misuse of tobacco smoking, alcohol and drugs. In a review of current approaches to health promotion in the work place and their effectiveness in preventing and controlling alcohol and drug related problems, the WHO (1993) drew attention to the need for workers' participation in programme development and implementation, and for the needs of specific occupational groups and the diversity of cultural settings to be taken into account. Compared to other countries, the UK has a low rate of work place health promotion practice (Fhilo *et al.*, 1993) and only 40% of the work places studied were involved in health promotion (Health Education Authority 1993).

Health promotion activities are slowly being introduced in the work setting. For instance, the occupational health service of British Rail developed an advisory unit for those with an alcohol or drug problem in 1992 (McHugh 1995), and a new and updated drug and alcohol policy was introduced in 1993 with the full support of the trade unions.

Gossop and Grant (1990) identified three principal concerns in the drug education of employees: impersonal information, employee participation and health promotion activities. It is anticipated that organisations will encourage the participation of all staff, management, trade unions or professional organisations in decision making related to health care policy. Health care professionals have an important contribution to make in the development of occupational health services and policy regarding health in the work place, including substance misuse educational programmes.

Personal health education of nurses

Health promotion activities within hospital and community settings represent a significant change for the personal health education of nurses and others. Besides the general health related programmes and activities, there is a need to focus on health education and prevention programmes in the use and misuse of tobacco, alcohol and other drugs. The personal health education of health care professionals has been somehow neglected on the health agenda in both policy development and practice.

There is a dearth of nursing literature on the incidence and prevalence of substance misuse among nurses and other health care professionals. A recent study of student nurses, medical students, qualified nurses and junior and qualified doctors in London, by Koffman and Hudson (1995), found that a small but significant proportion of health care professionals and an even larger proportion of health care trainees are drinking above the recommended safe alcohol limits. Furthermore, the findings suggest that health care professionals and students may be more prone to drinking alcohol excessively than the general public.

Research on smoking shows that nurses smoke more than doctors and that nurses in particularly stressful situations, such as psychiatric units and casualty wards, smoke more than nurses in community settings (Hawkins *et al.* 1982). Among community psychiatric nurses, the findings of a study on stress and mental health suggested that alcohol drinking and smoking habits are related to stress experiences at work (Leary & Brown 1995). There is also evidence to suggest, from the same study, that ward based psychiatric nurses who have high levels of involvement and decision making in their practice demonstrate a significantly lower intake of tobacco and alcohol. In a Scottish study by Plant *et al.* (1992) the findings showed that men who showed higher levels of work related stress were more likely to be heavy drinkers and that women mental health nurses were generally more likely to be heavy drinkers, smokers and users of illicit drugs than women in other nursing fields. The use of alcohol, tobacco or illicit psychoactive substances has been demonstrated to be a common coping strategy among nurses when dealing with emotional situations and stress. Studies by Plant *et al.* (1992) and Lees and Ellis (1990) showed that smoking, alcohol or drug use are often cited by nurses as their method of coping with stress.

Conclusions

The role of nurses and other health care professionals in relation to substance misuse is to support, educate, prevent and provide care, all of which refer to the general term of 'nursing intervention'. Both primary and secondary health prevention initiatives in substance use and misuse are within the realm of most nurses. Prevention, health education and health promotion in the use and misuse of psychoactive substances should be part of the agenda for health and educational policy development. The national policy on substance use and misuse (*Tackling Drugs Together* 1995), currently encourages substance misuse education and health promotion activities that can be widely supported in all arenas. A review of models of health education and health promotion suggests that the best form of drug education makes no reference to drugs *per se* and is not substance focused. A better approach, according to Tones (1987) is to

'focus on the general personal and social development of people within the context of general health promotion strategies which seek to make healthy choices, easy choices by removing the social concomitants of drug abuse – poverty and deprivation, disadvantage and lack of self fulfilment.'

The success of any health promoting activity depends upon a co-ordinated approach using existing prevention strategies. Health care professionals, schools, families and other interested parties should combine their efforts to prevent and reduce the casualties from substance misuse. Above all, we should not forget the health education of caring practitioners.

References

Advisory Council on the Misuse of Drugs (1984) *Prevention*. HMSO, London.

Asvall, J.E. (1993) *Message from the Regional Director of WHO-Europe. Health Promoting Hospitals Newsletter*. World Health Organization Regional Council of Europe, Geneva.

Audit Commission (1993) *What Seems to be the Matter: Communication between Hospitals and Patients*. HMSO, London.

Babor, T.F., Ritson, E.B. & Hodgson, R.J. (1986). Alcohol-related problems in the primary health care setting: a review of early intervention strategies. *British Journal of Addiction*, **81**, 23–46.

Bracher, E., Burns, I. & Cantrell, J. (1995) Module for change. *Nursing Standard*, **28**, 22.

Chick, J., Lloyd, G. & Crombie, E. (1985). Counselling problem drinkers in medical wards. *British Medical Journal*, **290**, 965–7.

Department of Health (1992) *The Health of the Nation*. HMSO, London.

Ewles, L. & Simnett, I. (1992) *Promoting Health*. Wiley, Chichester.

Faulkner, W. & Ward, L. (1983). Nurses as health educators in relation to smoking. *Nursing Times*, **79**, 47–58.

Fhilo, J., Russell, J., Pettersson, G., *et al.* (1993) *Health at Work: A Needs Assessment in South West Thames Regional Health Authority*. SWTRHA, London.

Ghodse, A.H. & Khan, I. (eds) (1988) *Psychoactive drugs: improving prescribing practices*. WHO, Geneva.

Gossop, M. & Grant, M. (eds) (1990) *Preventing and Controlling Drug Abuse*, pp. 76–7. WHO, Geneva.

Gournay, K. (1988) Sleeping without drugs. *Nursing Times*, 16–22 March, 46–9.

Hartz, C., Plant, M. & Watts, M. (1991). *Alcohol and Health*. Medical Council on Alcoholism, London.

Hawkins, L., White, M. & Morris, L. (1982) Smoking – stress and nurses. *Nursing Mirror*, **10**, 19–22.

Health Education Authority (1992) *Health at Work in the NHS: Action Pack*. HEA, London.

Health Education Authority (1993) *Health Promotion in the Workplace: A Summary*. HEA, London.

Kelly, J.A. & Murphy, D.A. (1991) Some lessons learned about risk reduction after ten years of the HIV/Aids epidemic. *Aids Care*, **3**, 8.

Kennedy, J. & Faugier, J. (1989) *Drug & Alcohol Dependency Nursing*. Heinemann Nursing, London.

Koffman, J. & Hudson, M. (1995) Purely medicinal. *Nursing Standard*, **9** 18–19.

Kreitman, N. (1986) Alcohol consumption and the preventive paradox. *British Journal of Addiction*, **81**, 353.

Leary, J. & Brown, D. (1995) Findings from the Claybury study for ward based psychiatric nurses and comparisons with community psychiatric nurses. In: *Stress and Coping in Mental Health Nursing* (J. Carson, L. Fagin & S. Ritter) Chapman & Hall, London.

Lees, S. & Ellis, N. (1990) The design of a stress-management programme for nursing personnel. *Journal of Advanced Nursing*, **15**, 946–61.

Maben, J. & Macleod Clarke J. (1995) Health promotion: a conceptual analysis. *Journal of Advanced Nursing*, **22**, 1158–65.

McHugh, K. (1995) How British Rail guards its greatest asset: 'people'. *Addiction Counselling World*, May/June, 17–19.

Naidoo, J. & Willis, J. (1994) *Health Promotion: Foundations for Practice*. Balliere Tindall, London.

National Institute on Drug Abuse (1989) *Prevention*. NIDA, Rockville, MD.

Plant, M.L., Plant, M.A. & Foster, J. (1992) Stress, alcohol, tobacco and illicit drug use amongst nurses: a Scottish study. *Journal of Advanced Nursing*, **17**, 1057–67.

Rassool, G.H. (1984) Mental health: the role of the community psychiatric nurse as health educator. MSc dissertation, University of London (unpublished).

Rassool, G.H. & Gafoor, M. (1997) *Addiction Nursing: Perspectives on Professional and Clinical Practice*. Stanley Thornes, Cheltenham.

Rassool, G.H. & Winnington, J. (1993) Using psychoactive drugs. *Nursing Times*, **89**, 38–40.

Tackling Drugs Together (1995) *A Strategy for England 1995–1998*. HMSO, London.

Tether, P. & Robinson, D. (1986). *Preventing Alcohol Problems: A Guide to Local Action*. Tavistock, London.

Tilly, S. & Weighillk, V.E. (1986) How nurse therapists assess and contribute to the management of alcohol and sedative drug use among anxious patients. *Journal of Advanced Nursing*, **11**, 499–503.

Temez, E.G., Moore, M.J. & Brown, P.L. (1978) Relaxation training as a nursing intervention versus pro rata medication. *Nursing Research*, **27**, 160–65.

Tones, K. (1987) Devising strategies for preventing drugs misuse: the role of the health action model. *Health Education Research*, **2**, 4.

Tones, K. (1990) Why theorise: ideology in health education. *Health Education Journal*, **49**, 1.

United Kingdom Central Council (1986) *Project 2000: A New Preparation for Practice*. UKCC, London.

World Health Organization (1986) *Drug Dependence and Alcohol Related Problems – A Manual for Community Health Workers with Guidelines for Trainers*. WHO, Geneva.

World Health Organization (1989) *Report of the WHO meeting on nursing/midwifery education in the rational use of psychoactive drugs*. DMP/PND/89.5. WHO, Geneva.

World Health Organization (1991) *Europe. Budapest Declaration on Health Promoting Hospitals. HPH Networking Documents.* WHO Regional Office for Europe, Geneva.

World Health Organization (1992) *Europe. Health Promoting Hospitals. Networking Documents.* WHO Regional Office for Europe, Geneva.

World Health Organization Expert Committee (1993) *Health Promotion in the Workplace: Alcohol and Drug Abuse.* Technical Report Series, No 883, iii–33. WHO, Geneva.

World Health Organization/International Council of Nurses (1991) *Roles of the Nurse in Relation to Substance Misuse.* ICN, Geneva.

Chapter 8

Screening and Generic Assessment

G. Hussein Rassool

Introduction

Screening and drug and alcohol history taking are components of the assessment process and form part of the stages within the framework of the systematic approach to nursing care and interventions. In most settings, assessment takes the form of interviewing and taking and recording a medical/nursing and psychosocial history. It is through the process of screening and history taking that patients are given the opportunity to understand their 'addiction', and they are enabled through counselling and other interventions to modify or change their life-style and behaviour.

There are three types of assessment (Association of Nurses in Substance Abuse (ANSA) 1997): triage for emergencies screening and initial/specialist assessment. The purpose of screening and assessment is to determine the degree and patterns of substance use and misuse, the consequences of the sequelae and to develop a plan of effective nursing and health interventions appropriate to meet the needs of the patients. In addition, both screening and substance use history serve to identify the appropriate professional help for the patients and significant others and to monitor care and treatment. In emergency situations a triage assessment may be essential, for those presenting within the primary health care settings with overdose, lost prescriptions, withdrawal seizures, delirium tremens and deliberate self-harm (ANSA 1997).

The aims of this chapter are to provide an overview of the use of screening and history taking for substance use behaviour. An outline of screening for high risk behaviours in relation to substance use is presented. The different types of screening instruments that non specialist health care professionals may incorporate within their general assessment procedure are described. An assessment of current prescribed medication of psychoactive drugs is also included.

Context and setting for screening substance use history

There is a host of physical, psychological and social problems related to substance misuse that are present covertly in almost every nursing encounter. Within the primary health care setting there is ample opportunity for health care professionals to use screening tools and for taking substance use history (drugs, alcohol and tobacco). The context and settings when opportunities for screening and history taking can be undertaken include:

❑ New patient registration
❑ Well woman clinics/family planning clinics
❑ Well men clinics
❑ Pre-birth checks
❑ Under 5 and 16 year old checks
❑ Specialist clinics, e.g. asthma/diabetic/blood pressure/travel
❑ Accessing primary care for other health related problems

According ANSA (1997) in the case of patients with problematic or dependent substance use:

❑ The GP surgery/health centre is more accessible.
❑ Some patients are reluctant to attend specialist services because of the fear of being labelled an 'addict', stigma, etc.
❑ Some patients do not consider themselves 'addicts' and do not wish to attend a specialist service.
❑ The specialist clinics may not have such flexible opening hours as the GP's surgery/health centre/clinic.
❑ They may lack knowledge about available specialist services.

Screening for high risk behaviour

In view of the diversity of individuals considered at risk of developing alcohol or drug related problems, and the assumptions about the aetiology and nature of substance misuse, a broad based screening approach is preferable. It is argued that this approach would detect more people consuming harmful levels of alcohol and avoid negative stereotyping (Gafoor 1994). There is considerable debate between researchers and clinicians on the question of selective or mass screening. Murray (1977) has suggested that selective screening for alcohol related problems is more efficient and cost effective than mass screening of the population. The following groups of individuals should be targeted for screening:

❑ Hospital patients suffering from conditions such as pancreatitis, gastritis, tuberculosis and cardiomyopathy
❑ Patients attending Accident and Emergency services (see Chapter 15)
❑ Patients who have attempted suicide
❑ Individuals arrested for drink driving and public intoxication offences

Other groups considered to have high risks of developing alcohol problems are middle aged males, migrant workers and certain occupational groups such as business executives, bar workers, chefs, publicans and seamen.

Screening methods for alcohol and drugs

A number of methods can be used to identify use of drugs or alcohol. These include questionnaires, 'drinking diaries', biological markers and physical examinations which may be used alone or in combination. These methods of screening may help to confirm and support the history taking. The instruments or assessment tools used to screen for drug and alcohol problems are used also for the following reasons:

❑ The early identification of substance use behaviour
❑ To discover the extent of misuse and its health effects
❑ To examine the social context of substance use in both the patient and significant others
❑ To determine a care plan and appropriate nursing interventions

It is stated that in identifying the existence of problematic drug/alcohol use, a screening assessment may be an enabling process that can motivate the problem drug user or dependent drug user to move from a pre-contemplative to a contemplative stage and take action in changing their substance use behaviours (Prochaska & DiClemente 1986). The outcome of screening will enable the nurse to determine the degree of interventions appropriate to this particular client in terms of the provision of health information and advice and brief interventions or counselling by the primary health care professionals. If substance misuse is problematic, referral to the GP or specialist drug and alcohol services is recommended.

In both residential and primary health care settings, the use of screening questionnaires has been gaining popularity in the identification of alcohol and drug related problems. Instruments that may be used include CAGE (Mayfield *et al.* 1974), the Short Michigan Alcoholism Screening Test (SMAST) (Selzer *et al.* 1975) and the Problem Drinking Scale (Valliant 1983). However, many of the screening questionnaires have a limited ability to detect problem drinkers accurately. Over half of the patients who screen positive on either CAGE or MAST do not have a current alcohol problem (Barry & Fleming 1993). Some tend to pick up rather late and chronic cases (Von Knorring *et al.* 1987). The CAGE questionnaire has a tendency to miss patients or patients whose consumption is over the level of safe drinking or problem-free drinking. It should be emphasised that these instruments should not replace vigilant and sympathetic questioning (Edwards 1982).

The Alcohol Use Disorder Identification Test (AUDIT) is a screening instrument developed for primary health care settings (Babor *et al.* 1986). It has ten items covering alcohol consumption and symptoms and consequences of alcohol use. The mean daily alcohol intake detected by AUDIT was reported to be 66% of that indicated by the drinking diary (Anderson 1985). This questionnaire is easy to administer and can be included in life-style and health behaviour questionnaires. It can also be used opportunistically when patients consult their GP or practice nurse for routine health check ups.

The CAGE questionnaire is the simplest and its four questions could easily be incorporated in the routine assessment process. Two or more positive responses are said to identify the problem drinker. The questionnaire concentrates on the consequences rather than on the quantity or frequency of alcohol use. It includes the following four questions:

(1) Have you ever felt you should *cut* down your drinking?
(2) Have people *annoyed* you by criticizing your drinking?
(3) Have you ever felt bad or *guilty* about your drinking?
(4) Have you ever had a drink first thing in the morning to steady your nerves, or get rid of a hangover (*eye-opener*)?

The Addiction Prevention in Primary Care Programme has developed a screening questionnaire (Ghodse *et al.* 1994) which may also be may be incorporated within the assessment framework of any nursing specialties, see Table 8.1.

Table 8.1 Addiction Prevention in Primary Care Programme

1. Do you smoke or have you ever smoked?	YES/NO
2. How much do you smoke? (Per day or week)	
❏ All smokers should receive further assessment and advice	
3. Do you drink or have you ever drunk alcohol?	YES/NO
4. In an average week, how much alcohol do you drink?	
❏ If greater than 21 units (male) or 14 units (female) a more detailed assessment of the patient's drinking history is necessary	
5. Do you use any pills, medicines, drugs or tablets other than those prescribed for medical reasons?	YES/NO
e.g. to help you – relax, sleep, cope with stress	YES/NO
– feel good	YES/NO
– have fun or excitement	YES/NO
6. Do you ever need to use more of your medicines than prescribed?	YES/NO
7. Do you regularly use non prescription medicines from the chemist?	YES/NO

Source: Addiction Prevention in Primary Care Programme, Centre for Addiction Studies, Department of Addictive Behaviour, St George's Hospital Medical School, University of London.

Special investigations

If the screening instrument indicates that the patient or client misuses drugs or alcohol, laboratory investigations may be undertaken to aid early identification and diagnosis. These investigations are also helpful in contributing objective information to the assessment of the health status of the patient. Drugs can be measured directly in serum, urine, exhaled air and hair. Essential investigations include gamma glutamyltransferase (GTT), appartate aminotransminase (AST), mean corpuscles volume (MCV) and blood alcohol concentration (BAC). Screening of patients attending Accident and Emergency departments involves blood ethanol levels, the mere smell of alcohol on a patient's breath and the use of a breathalyser test. This is simple and has many advantages over other biochemical measures.

Skinner *et al.* (1984) have shown the value of a brief enquiry about a history of trauma, supported by chest X-ray investigations. A history of trauma or injury may signal the misuse of drugs or alcohol, or addiction. A combination of a brief questionnaire such as CAGE with biological investigations such as GGT and MCV with ethanol estimates would be an appropriate screening battery or may be combined with other relevant measures (e.g. the trauma scale).

Nursing assessment

Nursing assessment is a comprehensive analysis of the patient's needs and related problems which is based on the collection of data of the physical/ medical, psychosocial and spiritual needs of the individual. It is to facilitate the identification and recognition of substance using/abusing behaviour and its resultant health related problems. In the context of this chapter, assessment is concerned with the taking of an accurate substance misuse history, along with a history of associated health problems and the utilization of screening tools and questionnaires in the identification and recognition of substance misuse. A specialist or full assessment is carried out if more information regarding the substance use status and health status of the patient is required for clinical care, and this kind of assessment is usually performed by addiction nurses. For a framework for an in-depth assessment, the reader is referred to Clancy and Coyne (1997).

Assessment and history taking

Each professional discipline has their own established method of making their own detailed assessment of the patient's health needs. Documentation varies according to the setting and context where health and social care are provided. The nurse or member of the primary health care team uses various frameworks or models of care on which to base their clinical practice and interventions. Incorporation of the substance use history within a particular model of assessment would cause few problems, if any, and would certainly help with accurate and relevant information gathering.

Generally, assessment is based on a brief health check and a full medical and psychosocial history. The generic worker (e.g. a nurse in a general hospital setting or an occupational nurse) is primarily concerned with the interim, brief history taking of drug, alcohol and tobacco use and misuse rather than a full or specialist assessment. The latter is usually carried out by an addiction nurse specialist or other health care professional as part of a multi-disciplinary assessment of needs and subsequent specialist interventions.

A specialist assessment tool is the Substance Abuse Assessment Questionnaire (SAAQ) (Ghodse 1995) which incorporates the following assessments: medical and psychological, alcohol use, drug use, forensic, psychosocial and family, profile of the substance misuser and treatment programme. For a framework for an in-depth assessment the reader is referred to ANSA (1997). The characteristics which may suggest possible drug and alcohol misuse are summarised in Table 8.2.

The taking of a substance use history includes the process of identifying

Table 8.2   Characteristics which may suggest potential drug and alcohol misuse.

	Drug	Alcohol
How the patient presents for help	❑ with a specific request for drugs of misuse ❑ outside normal GP surgery hours ❑ repeated attempts for repeat/lost prescriptions ❑ as a temporary resident	❑ alcohol misusers are frequent attenders, however alcohol use may be disguised by other physical or psychological problems
Signs and symptoms	❑ injection marks, scars and pigmentation over injection sites ❑ pupils markedly constricted or dilated ❑ unexplained constipation or diarrhoea	❑ smell of drink at interview ❑ withdrawal symptoms ❑ obesity, gastrointestinal symptoms, hypertension ❑ unexplained injury, bruising, memory blackouts ❑ anxiety and depression
Behaviour during consultation	❑ unaccountably drowsy, elated or restless ❑ loss of interest in appearance	❑ inappropriate behaviour in the surgery ❑ emotionally labile ❑ aggressive
Social behaviour	❑ family disruption ❑ frequent changes of GP ❑ history of offences to obtain money	❑ family disruption ❑ frequent changes of GP ❑ history of offences to obtain money

Source: ANSA (1997).

with the client whether alcohol, drug or tobacco use is problematic or could potentially result in health related problems. That is, the problem drinker or problem drug taker has the opportunity to assess accurately the impact that alcohol and other psychoactive substances have on their health, relationships and employment and on other socio-economic domains of their life. If a substance use history is taken in a non judgemental, skillful way, it can be a potent factor in motivating the patient to change problem drinking behaviour (Miller 1983). Most of the professionals are well placed and already possess the necessary basic skills to undertake a drink/drug history. The patient or client may already be in their care in hospitals, health centres or community agencies, or may have been referred because of particular physical or psychological/psychiatric problems.

A drug or alcohol history is a detailed assessment of the current presentation of an individual's drug or alcohol taking pattern. One of the initial tasks of the history taking is to discern the client's views of their drug or alcohol consumption. The history taking should then focus on the current pattern of drug taking, the type of drug used and the quantity, frequency and route of administration of psychoactive substances.

In order to ascertain the presence and level of dependency, it is important to ask about experience of withdrawal symptoms or any medical problems. The history should also include details of the use of tobacco and other psychoactive substances. An outline of taking a drug and alcohol history is shown in Table 8.3. This schedule can also be adapted to include tobacco smoking.

Assessment of current prescribed medication of psychoactive drugs

The assessment of a patient's use of psychoactive medication is an essential part of the nursing process (Rassool & Winnington 1993). In addition to the taking of a drug and alcohol history, information gathered in the assessment model should include:

- ❏ Current prescribed medication being taken
- ❏ The patient's potential for self-medication
- ❏ The need for health information concerning particular medications to be provided to the patient
- ❏ The need for prescribed drugs to be given where necessary
- ❏ The current appropriateness of the medication for the patient
- ❏ A history of self-harm/self-poisoning

Conclusions

The focus of this chapter is on the process of screening and the taking of a drug and alcohol history. Nurses or other health care professionals could

Table 8.3 Taking a drug and alcohol history.

Current drug or alcohol use	Type, quantity, frequency and route of administration (drug)
Pattern of drug or alcohol use	Details of drug/alcohol taking for the past week/month Drugs of choice
Current use of other substances	Prescribed, illicit or over-the-counter drugs
Level of dependence	Any withdrawal symptoms Evidence of increasing tolerance
Associated problems	Any medical, psychiatric, social or legal problems
Risk behaviours	Source of injecting equipment Sharing of equipment/knowledge about sterilisation Sexual behaviour when intoxicated
Periods of abstinence/relapse	Duration; periods of abstinence – voluntary or enforced; reasons for relapse
Sources of help	Statutory agencies. Local authorities, voluntary agencies or self-help groups

easily incorporate the substance use history into their assessment model. The uses of screening measures and brief intervention methods in primary care settings have been demonstrated to lead to a reduction in alcohol use of between 10 and 30% (Babor *et al.* 1986). It must be acknowledged that most patients with a drink or drug problem will be reluctant to provide an accurate history of their use of psychoactive substances. A patient may be offended by a health care worker making unsympathetic enquiries about his drinking or drug taking habits.

Furthermore, if the patient is, for example, drinking to excess or above the recommended limits, he or she may not take too lightly any suggestion of change in the drink behaviour pattern. Individuals may feel guilt or remorse as well as an understandable fear of withdrawing from the effects of drugs or alcohol, and this may be expressed in hostile or aggressive behaviour. Patients may be ambivalent and reluctant to accept help and support. Even if a drinking or drug problem is suspected, many patients are more likely to deny or minimise the extent of their misuse of psychoactive substances.

Health care professionals need to be non judgemental and accepting in order to establish a positive therapeutic alliance with the patient or client. Through one to one nursing interventions or counselling, where a degree of trust may be established, the patient may gain insight into his or her drinking or drug taking (or both) behaviour. Members of the primary health care team and nurses in hospital are well situated for the early identification of patients with potential addictive problems. In addition, these professionals can help motivate the individual to modify his or her life-style and behaviour or to seek specialist assistance where appropriate.

References

Anderson, P. (1985) Managing alcohol problems in general practice. *British Medical Journal*, **290**, 1873–75.

Association of Nurses in Substance Abuse (1997) *Substance Use: Guidance on Good Clinical Practice for Nurses, Midwives and Health Visitors. Working within Primary Health Care Teams.* ANSA, London.

Babor, T.F., Ritson, E.B. & Hodgson, R.J. (1986). Alcohol related problems in the primary health care setting: a review of early intervention strategies. *British Journal of Addiction*, **81**, 23–46.

Barry, K.L. & Fleming, M.F. (1993) The Alcohol Use Disorders Identification Test (AUDIT) and the SAMSF-13: predictive validity in a rural primary care sample. *Alcohol and Alcoholism*, **28**, 33–42.

Clancy, C. & Coyne, P. (1997) Specialist assessment in addiction. In: *Addiction Nursing: Perspectives on Professional and Clinical Practice* (eds G.H. Rassool & M. Gafoor), Stanley Thornes, Cheltenham.

Edwards, G. (1982) Alcohol education. *British Journal of Addiction*, **77**, 337–9.

Gafoor, M. (1994) Early intervention in primary care setting (Personal communication).

Ghodse, A.H. (1995) *Drugs and Addictive Behaviours: A Guide to Treatment*, 2nd edn. Blackwell Science, Oxford.

Ghodse, A.H., McShane, E., Priestley, J.S. & Saunders, V.J. (1995) *Addiction Prevention in Primary Care Programme Review 1993/1994.* Centre for Addiction Studies, Department of Psychiatry of Addictive Behaviour, St George's Hospital Medical School, London.

Mayfield, D., McLeod, G. & Hall, P. (1974) The Cage Questionnaire: validation of a new alcoholism screening instrument. *American Journal of Psychiatry*, **131**, 1121–3.

Miller, W.R. (1983) Motivational interviewing with problem drinkers. *Behavioural Psychology*, **11**, 147–72.

Murray, R.M. (1977) Screening and early detection instruments for disabilities related to alcohol consumption. In: *Alcohol Related Disabilities* (G. Edwards, M.M. Gross, M. Keller *et al.* pp. 89–105.), World Health Organization, Geneva.

Prochaska, J. & DiClemente, C. (1986) Toward a comprehensive model of change. In: *Treating Addictive Behaviours* (eds W. Miller & N. Heather), pp. 3–27. Plenum, New York.

Rassool, G.H. & Winnington, J. (1993) Using psychoactive drugs. *Nursing Times*, **89**, 38–40.

Selzer, M.S., Vinokur, A. & Rooijien, E.V. (1975) A self-administered Short Michigan Alcoholism Screening Test (SMAST). *Journal of Studies on Alcohol*, **36**, 117–26.

Skinner, H.A., Holt, A., Schuller, R., *et al* (1984) Identification of alcohol abuse using laboratory tests and a history of trauma. *Annals of Internal Medicine*, **101**, 847–51.

Valliant, G.E. (1983) *The National History of Alcoholism.* Harvard University Press, Cambridge, Mass.

Von Knorring, L., Oreland, L. & Von Knorring, A.L. (1987) Platelet MAO activity as a biological marker in subgroups of alcoholism. *Acta Psychiatrica Scandinavia*, **75**, 307–14.

Chapter 9
An Overview of Intervention Strategies

G. Hussein Rassool and Bridget Kilpatrick

Introduction

The underlying aim of intervening with substance misusers with health related problems is essentially a straightforward one. That is, to restore an individual to an improved state of health and independent function through a hierarchy of goals and a sequential process of change. The first contact between the health care professional and the substance misuser is vital, and during this initial phase of seeking help the likelihood of drop-out is high. Additionally, the longer a patient has been involved in substance misuse, the greater the prospect of a range of problems experienced by the user. To change any established pattern of behaviour is difficult, and hence to transform a complex addiction successfully at the first attempt is unrealistic. Supporting a patient usually involves dealing with a person who can be unwilling, ambivalent, uncertain, despondent, anxious or unrealistic about their ability to change. The interventions are appropriate for those who have acknowledged their problems and want to change.

Substance misuse problems can occur at any point along an imaginary line stretching from minimal use or experimentation at one end through to regular use and onto established dependence at the other. Thus, health problems can vary to reflect the pattern, frequency and method of use. Intoxication is a direct consequence of excessive consumption, but can be found both at the experimental stage of use as well at the other extreme of persistent and dependent use. Once drinking or drug taking becomes more regular, habitual and greater in quantity, then the likelihood increases that health and other problems will also increase in their nature, effect and severity. Patients may be admitted to general hospital wards with reasons not associated with or attributed to their drinking or drug taking. Whilst intervention does occur within the specialist addiction setting, it can be undertaken or started in other non specialist settings where nurses and other health care professionals are likely to encounter such patients. These settings include medical, surgical, orthopaedic, ante-and post-natal wards and out-patient clinics, health care settings in prison and other custodial institutions and through to primary care. Although specialist interventions are provided by designated addiction services, nurses in other settings can initiate and contribute to the early recognition and management of substance misusers who are in the early stages of their substance use career.

This chapter aims to examine the principles of intervention and provide an overview of the intervention strategies used in the management and treatment of substance misusers in generic and specialist agencies.

Principles of clinical interventions

Treatment programmes should have clear and cogent policies, procedures, goals and objectives that are familiar to staff and patients and should be flexible in order to provide individualised treatment planning and implementation. Nursing interventions will depend upon the needs and health related problems of the substance misuser. It is through the screening process and the taking of a drug and alcohol history that a decision is made whether the patient may be treated in a non specialist setting or referred to a specialist addiction service.

In the hospital and primary settings, suitable interventions can be directed to those groups of patients who are beginning their drug taking career, or consume low levels of alcohol, or who are recreational users of psychoactive substances, and have no mental health problems or co-existing medical problems. An explicit treatment alliance, such as a contract and review(s), will measure the expected outcome and overall progress, but this may be more applicable to specialist addiction settings. Local policy will dictate whether a review is undertaken informally or carried out on a more formal basis.

Intervention strategies

A number of interventions exist, and all involve behavioural changes to a greater or lesser extent. The intervention strategies used in the care, management and treatment of substance misuse or addictive behaviours incorporate a range of nursing, pharmacological, psychosocial and behavioural treatments. Nursing recognition of a substance misuse problem will not necessarily mean that intervention will have a positive outcome. The appropriateness of the intervention and the willingness of the patient to accept the need to change voluntarily are vital components.

The types of interventions that generic nurses are capable of providing include health information and awareness, health and preventive education and brief or minimal interventions. In some generic settings, such as primary care health centres, occupational centres, etc., counselling, family support and complementary therapies may also be provided. More specialist interventions are required for those who are multiple-drug users, dependent or addicted patients, those who have a history of poor compliance to treatment or numerous attempts at detoxification and those who have child care problems or are pregnant. A brief overview of selected treatments for substance misusers is given below. Further details about specific interventions can be found in Davidson *et al.* (1991), Ghodse (1995) and Jarvis *et al.* (1995).

Brief intervention

The term brief or minimal intervention generally refers to screening and health education techniques designed to raise problem awareness and provide advice on changing substance use behaviour. It is cost effective and can reach a wide population within the health care delivery systems (Bien *et al.* 1993). In brief interventions, the number of sessions may vary from one to eight and their length may vary from 10 to 20 minutes each. This type of intervention has been found to be particularly effective in influencing a change in drinking behaviour (Watson 1992; Freemantle *et al.* 1993).

The elements that have been incorporated in brief interventions are summarised under the acronym FRAMES (Bien *et al.* 1993):

- ❑ **Feedback** about risks of substance use and misuse
- ❑ **Responsibility**
- ❑ **Advice** to cut down or abstain
- ❑ **Menu** of options and choices to change the substance use pattern
- ❑ **Empathic** interviewing
- ❑ **Self-efficacy** – using a counselling style which encourages and reinforces strength within a patient

A framework of brief or minimal interventions for alcohol misuse has been suggested by Anderson (1987). These intervention strategies include:

- ❑ Ask patients if their alcohol consumption is affecting their health.
- ❑ Stimulate a discussion of recording their drinking behaviour: weekly consumption, types of drinks, regular heavy drinking days, etc.
- ❑ Encourage completion of a drink diary to record and monitor consumption for the previous week.
- ❑ Compare the patient's health status to the general population.
- ❑ Raise awareness of the current or likely risks or negative effects.
- ❑ State the benefits of reduced drinking or abstinence.
- ❑ Give sound, but friendly advice.
- ❑ Give health education literature, e.g. booklet on alcohol and a self-help manual.
- ❑ Try and arrange a follow-up appointment within 2 to 4 weeks to review alcohol consumption and monitor behaviour change.

This type of intervention can easily be adapted within the therapeutic framework of settings such as Accident and Emergency departments, general acute wards and the primary health services. Brief interventions are likely to be highly effective with drinkers with moderate dependence rather than those with severe alcohol-related problems. It may also be extended to the misuse of prescribed, over-the-counter or illicit drugs. Jarvis *et al.* (1995) stated that there is no reason why early and brief forms of intervention should not be extended to opiates or stimulants, especially in settings which have embraced a harm minimisation approach to drug use.

Individual counselling

Counselling is a major component of the intervention strategies in working with substance misusers and those with addictive behaviours. The principles and processes of counselling remain the same whether the patient is a substance user or not. The same skills used in general counselling are also effective for counselling patients with substance misuse problems.

The counselling process embraces general psychological support, review and monitoring and offers specific client-centred, cognitive-behavioural, psychodynamic and other therapeutic approaches. For example, individual counselling may be offered to support and retain a patient waiting for admission into a residential or in-patient unit, or it may be part of an ongoing assessment process or it may be used to monitor the progress of a planned alcohol or drug reduction programme. Counselling does not undermine or suggest that the patient does not have the ability to succeed, but recognises that addressing an addiction can involve several, if not many, attempts. Counselling is useful in getting patients to assess their own situation and get help before a deterioration or 'slip' becomes a full-blown drinking or drug relapse.

Counselling may be offered on a time-limited basis of minimal intervention in one to two sessions or it may be part of a longer term contract. Frequency of contact can vary, from weekly to monthly or longer. For some, the continued offering of regular or sporadic appointments, often many months in advance, may be preferable to ceasing formal contact altogether. Other patients may function without maintaining such frequent support but it is important to stress to the patient that help may be sought at any time in the future, should they feel the need. Such action is viewed as a positive step.

There is a variety of reasons why people misuse psychoactive substances and an implicit aim of counselling is to attempt to address some of the underlying problems and conflicts which have contributed to, exacerbated or derived from the substance misuse. The empathic process of counselling may enable patients to recognise, acknowledge, reveal, disclose and address sensitive or distressing information. Thus, counselling a substance misuser can range from alcohol and drug specific tasks such as refusal skills, dealing with high risk situations and relapse prevention through to dealing with losses, past trauma, generalised anxieties or specific psychological problems, relationship difficulties and ill health, both physical and mental.

Group therapy

There are many orientations to group therapy; they may be supportive, cognitive behavioural, educative and for growth and development. Providing intervention on a group basis is well established in addiction treatment. However, while some patients may be apprehensive and refuse to talk in front of others, it can be an effective therapeutic tool, if initial reluctance or anxiety can be overcome, in dealing with both general and specific aspects of substance misuse. A long term abstinence-based open support group run by an addiction service may attract someone who would not feel otherwise that he or she could walk into an unfamiliar group of people. Groups can constructively assert that their members assume greater responsibility for their behaviour and utilise peer support and confrontation as a part of this process of change.

Other groups may be run for specific reasons or according to designated principles. A short term group may offer assertive training, social skills training, relapse prevention and drink refusal skills, while another group will include them as part of a longer term 'staying stopped' group. Attracting women into treatment is difficult for most addiction services and providing easy access and setting aside a time for women only, either on a drop-in or group basis, may help. Education on safe and sensible drinking skills can be offered on a short term basis and may be particularly attractive for patients in employment. Groups can meet in a variety of community and institutional settings such as church halls, hospitals, prisons and clinics.

Couples therapy

Substance misuse and addictive behaviour not only cause harm to the individual but also to the spouse, partner and family. People who are emotionally close to the family can exert a strong influence on the substance misuser to seek help and receive treatment, and may also become the primary carer in the management of a home or community detoxification programme. Couples therapy can be offered either with an individual couple or in a specific family or in a group setting. The style of intervention strategies may encompass supportive, behavioural and psychodynamic orientations and a systems approach. Couples therapy is only appropriate when there is agreement that the involvement of others would be beneficial (Jarvis *et al.* 1995). The overall aim is to support, educate and strengthen the relationship patterns of the couple to enable the substance misuser or both (if both partners are substance misusers) to attain, within their capacity, a change in their drinking or drug taking behaviour. For a comprehensive exposition of working with couples and families see O'Farrell and Cowles (1989) and O'Farrell (1989).

Motivational interviewing

Motivational interviewing is a counselling approach which aims to influence and enable patients to change. It is a technique which has been widely adopted in the addiction field to enhance retention (Miller 1983). It involves a style of behaviour adopted by the counsellor and demands a non judgemental approach, open-ended questioning and reflective listening. It aims to raise the patient's self-esteem, self-efficacy and increase awareness of their problems. It elicits self-motivational statements from the patient and highlights their motivated behaviour whilst underlining that responsibility for change lies with patient. Jarvis *et al.* (1995) equate motivational interviewing to the patient 'talking themselves into change'. As with most forms of intervention, it is only going to be successful if the patient remains in, and actively participates in the process.

Motivational interviewing has offered both a way of approaching the initial interview or, later on during counselling with a patient, of assessing their perception of the situation, in order to suggest or target a specific intervention. It is also a particularly useful technique for nurses working in a non specialist setting, such as in a liaison function in GP surgeries or general hospital departments, when patients are more likely to have little or no awareness of the effects of their substance use and misuse.

Relapse prevention

Relapse prevention is based on social learning theory of behaviour change (Bandura 1977; Marlatt 1979). The framework of relapse prevention relies on a variety of cognitive behavioural approaches in the treatment of addictive behaviours and implies

❑ That the person is capable of change and self-control and
❑ That alternative coping strategies are needed to achieve either abstinence or controlled use (Salazar 1997)

The self-efficacy model (Annis 1986; Annis & Davis 1987) enables patients to identify their particular high risk situations so as to cope with them. High risk situations are the context that encourage the use of a substance which may sometimes lead to maladaptive behaviour and heavy or uncontrolled use. A programme of the relapse prevention model stresses the learning and practice of coping skills to enable the patient to prevent relapse and maintain drug or alcohol free behaviour. It also enhances the self-care approach whereby the patients take responsibility for their own health and make active decisions to adapt coping skills in risky situations. Relapse prevention is targeted to individuals in the action, maintenance and relapse stages as described in the process of change model (see Prochaska & DiClemente 1982; Wanigaratne *et al.* 1990).

Pharmacological therapy

Pharmacological therapy involves the clinical management of withdrawal and detoxification from alcohol or drugs. Many patients stop dependent drinking or drug taking without taking any medication provided for withdrawal symptoms. This does not mean that abrupt withdrawal should be or can be achieved by every patient. Some substance misusers feel unable to tolerate the distress, anticipated and real, that would occur in the withdrawal stage as well as deal with any specific dangers involved in withdrawal from high dose and regular use of some substances: for example, delirium tremens and grand mal convulsions from alcohol, and convulsions in withdrawal from benzodiazepines, chlormethiazole and barbiturates. If it is agreed to prescribe substitute drugs for withdrawal, is this to be done in an out-patient or in-patient setting?

Withdrawal from alcohol and drugs, often referred to as detoxification, is swifter in hospital and follows a standard regime of stopping use of the abused substance, substitution with a cross-tolerant drug by stabilisation and then gradual withdrawal to zero. In out-patient, community and home settings a similar approach is used, but the reduction process is often slower and varies between drugs. for detoxification with alcohol problems, the most popular and widely used drug is a benzodiazepine, such as chlordiazepoxide (Librium) or diazepam (Valium). Withdrawal using medications, regular psychological support and monitoring is similar in ward, out-patient or community settings and is generally accomplished in 7 to 10 days.

Opiate dependent patients can be withdrawn using a non opioid or less addictive drug, such as lofexidine (Britlofex) or dihydrocodeine tartrate, particularly if the addiction is short. Where it is decided to use a substitute opioid for withdrawal, the drug of choice is methadone mixture. It may be decided to undertake a more gradual withdrawal from heroin, over many months (Department of Health *et al.* 1991). Once withdrawal has been completed or stabilisation achieved, in the case of opiate dependence, the patient is in a more comfortable state for further intervention to continue. Although not a drug withdrawal procedure, methadone maintenance treatment merits a brief mention; this involves prescribing for an indefinite period. A review of this treatment has been carried out and has suggested there are benefits to this approach for patients (Farrell *et al.*, 1994). For a comprehensive overview of specific methods of pharmacological therapies for substance dependence see Ghodse (1995).

Complementary therapies

People are increasingly seeking help and treatment from complementary therapies. The use of complementary therapies in the addiction field has been the product of a paradigm shift from a medical-oriented model to the development of a bio-psychosocial model. While there may be a pharmacological or prescribing component to a patient's care, individuals are now seeking a non pharmacological adjunct or alternative to conventional addiction treatment. There has been a growing interest by addiction nurses and others to introduce complementary therapies as part of the treatment regimes offered by addiction services, and those include acupuncture, aromatherapy, reflexology, shiatsu, etc (McDonald & Rassool 1997).

Since the early 1970s, auricular acupuncture has been used to treat most forms of substance misuse and addictive behaviours, for example alcoholism (Smith 1979), methadone detoxification (Gomez & Mikhail 1974), detoxification of opiate, cocaine, crack cocaine, alcohol and tobacco addiction (Low 1977; Chen 1979; Smith & Khan 1988) and in the prevention of relapse (Katims *et al.* 1992). Complementary therapies are mainly used for the purposes of detoxification, massage, relaxation, stress reduction and pain relief. In the clinical management of HIV/AIDS, patients are offered therapies such as massage, reflexology, acupuncture and aromatherapy (The London Lighthouse 1990).

The integration of complementary therapies with conventional treatment for substance misuse remains a valuable option in providing choices for patients, depending on their individual needs and problems. It is stated that in order for therapies to become part of the professional nursing practice we must also be prepared to undertake research in order to ensure that our actions are based upon knowledge rather than belief (Rankin-Box, 1987). Addiction nurses should examine their scope, nature and benefits so that these therapies may be appropriately offered in the management of substance misusers (McDonald & Rassool 1997).

Conclusions

There are a number of interventions that can be used for patients at any stage in their drug taking career. The utilisation of new or the adaptation of existing medical, psycho-social and spiritual approaches has broadened the range of interventions that can be offered to patients, from simple advice and health information to more specialised counselling techniques such as motivational interviewing.

The nature and form of the problems associated with substance misuse have led addiction nurses to incorporate these approaches and techniques within their clinical nursing practice. The papers by Winship & Unwin (1997) and McDonald & Rassool (1997) contain further references to the use of the psychodynamic approach, relapse prevention and complementary therapies. Generic nurses and other health care professionals can develop their repertoire of skills to respond effectively to those who use and misuse psychoactive substances.

References

Anderson, P. (1987) Early intervention in general practice. In: *Helping the Problem Drinker* (eds T. Stockwell & S. Clement), pp. 61–2. Croom Helm, London.

Annis, H.M. (1986) A relapse prevention model for treatment of alcoholics. In: *Treating Addictive Behaviours: Process of Change* (eds W.R. Miller & N. Heather). Plenum, New York.

Annis, H.M. & Davis, C.S. (1987) Self-efficacy and the prevention of alcoholic relapse: initial findings from a treatment trial. In: *Addictive Disorders: Psychological Research on Assessment and Treatment* (eds T.B. Baker & T. Cannon). Praeger, New York.

Bandura, A. (1977) Self-efficacy: toward a unifying theory of behaviour change. *Psychological Review*, **84**, 191–215.

Bien, T.H., Miller, W.R. & Tonigan, J.S. (1993) Brief interventions for alcohol problems: a review. *Addiction*, **88**, 315–36.

Chen, J.Y.P. (1979) Treatment of cigarette smoking by auricular acupuncture: a report of 184 cases. Presented at the *National Symposia of Acupuncture and Moxibustion and Acupuncture Anaesthesia*, Beijing, China, 1–5 January.

Davidson, R., Rollnick, S. & MacEwan, I. (eds) (1991) *Counselling Problem Drinkers*. Routledge: London.

Department of Health, Scottish Office Home and Health Department and Welsh Office (1991) *Drug Misuse and Dependence: Guidelines on Clinical Management*. HMSO, London.

Farrell, M., Ward, J., Mattick, R., *et al.* (1994) Methadone maintenance treatment in opiate dependence: a review. *British Medical Journal*, **309**, 997–1001.

Freemantle, N., Gill, P., Godfrey, C., *et al.* (1993) Brief interventions and alcohol use – are brief interventions effective in reducing harm associated with alcohol consumption? *Effective Health Care*, no 7.

Ghodse, A.H. (1995) *Drugs and Addictive Behaviour*, 2nd edn. Blackwell Science, Oxford.

Gomez, E. & Mikhail, A. (1974) Treatment of methadone withdrawal, with cerebral electrotherapy (electrosleep). Presented at the *Annual Meeting of the American Psychiatric Association*, Detroit, MI, 6–10 May.

Jarvis, T.J., Tebutt, J. & Mattick, R.P. (1995) *Treatment Approaches for Alcohol and Drug Dependence: An Introductory Guide*. John Wiley & Sons, Chichester.

Katims, J.J., Ng, L.K.Y. & Lowinson, J.H. (1992) Acupuncture and transcutaneous electrical nerve stimulation: afferent nerve stimulation (ANS). In: *Treatment of Addiction in Substance Abuse: A Comprehensive Textbook* (eds J.K. Lowinson, P. Ruiz, R.B. Millman & J.G. Langrod), 2nd edn, pp. 574–83. Williams and Wilkins, Baltimore.

Low, S.A. (1977) Acupuncture and nicotine withdrawal. *Medical Journal of Australia*, **2**, 687.

McDonald, J. & Rassool, G.H. (1997) Complementary therapies. In: *Addiction Nursing: Perspectives on Professional and Clinical Practice* (eds G.H. Rassool & M. Gafoor). Stanley Thornes, Cheltenham.

Marlatt, G.A. (1979) A cognitive-behavioural model of relapse process. *NIDA Research Monograph*, **25**, 191–200.

Miller, W.R. (1983) Motivational interviewing with problem drinkers. *Behavioural Psychotherapy*, **1**, 147–72.

O'Farrell T.J. (1989) Marital and family therapy in alcoholism treatment. *Journal of Substance Abuse Treatment*, **6**, 23–9.

O'Farrell, T.J. & Cowles, K.S. (1989) Marital and family therapy. In: *Handbook of Alcoholism Treatment Approaches: Effective Alternatives* (eds R.K. Hester & W.R. Miller), pp. 183–205. Pergamon, New York.

Prochaska, J.O. & DiClemente, C.C. (1982) Transtheoretical therapy: toward a more integrative model of change. *Psychotherapy: Theory, Research and Practice*, **19**, 276–88.

Rankin-Box, D. (1987) (ed.) *Complementary Health Therapies. A Guide for Nurses and the Caring Professions*. Chapman and Hall, London.

Salazar, C. (1997) Relapse prevention and nursing interventions. In: *Addiction Nursing: Perspectives on Professional and Clinical Practice* (eds G.H. Rassool & M. Gafoor). Stanley Thornes, Cheltenham.

Smith, M.O. (1979) Acupuncture and natural healing in drug detoxification. *American Journal of Acupuncture*, **7**, 97.

Smith, M.O. & Khan, I. (1988) An acupuncture program for the treatment of drug addicted persons. *Bulletin of Narcotics*, **15**(1), 35–41.

The London Lighthouse (1990) *Groups, Creative & Complementary Therapies, Activities & Classes for People living with HIV & AIDS*. The London Lighthouse, London.

Wanigaratne, S., Wallace, W., Pullin, J., *et al.* (1990) *Relapse Prevention for Addictive Behaviours: A Manual for Therapists*. Blackwell Scientific Publications, Oxford.

Watson, H.E. (1992) *A study of the effectiveness of brief intervention for problem drinkers in acute hospital setting*. Unpublished dissertation, University of Strathclyde, Glasgow.

Winship, G. & Unwin, C. (1997) Psychotherapeutic approaches and nursing interventions. In: *Addiction Nursing: Perspectives on Professional and Clinical Practice* (eds G.H. Rassool & M. Gafoor). Stanley Thornes, Cheltenham.

Chapter 10

Service Provision For Substance Misusers

G. Hussein Rassool

Introduction

There are wide variations in the provision of services for substance misusers in the UK. They range from the National Health Service (NHS) (drug dependence unit, community substance misuse team, etc.) the social services and the Probation Service (hostels or half-way houses) to the non statutory and voluntary sectors (street agencies, advice and counselling centres, telephone help-lines etc.). Services for alcohol have been in existence in the NHS since the late 1950s, when the first specialised NHS alcohol treatment unit (ATU) was established in the UK (Kennedy & Faugier 1989). As a result of health policy changes in the 1970s, it was recommended that community services should be developed and integrated with existing hospital services (DHSS 1978). A number of community alcohol teams (CATs) came into existence to provide consultancies to generic health care professionals in the management and treatment interventions of problem drinkers.

In the case of services for drug users, the report of the Brain Committee recommended that treatment units should be set up to provide appropriate treatment for problem drug users and addicts and to maintain opiate addicts on heroin (Ministry of Health and Scottish Home and Health Department 1965). In 1968, drug dependency units (DDUs) were established throughout the country to treat individuals with opiate, especially heroin, problems. In the 1980s due to the rising trends in the misuse of psychoactive substances, community drug teams (CDTs) were set up to provide consultancies to generic workers and to have an input into clinical work. Nowadays, a number of CDTs and CATs have been combined to form community substance misuse teams. There is a wide variety of approaches to services for drug and alcohol clients and there is also a variation in the availability of these services throughout the country. It is acknowledged that generic professionals and services are more likely to encounter patients or clients with alcohol and other drug related problems than specialist substance misuse services.

This chapter aims to describe the statutory, non statutory and voluntary services for drug and alcohol clients in the UK. These include specialist services such as in-patient units, community based teams, residential rehabilitation and self-help groups. Although substance misuse problems can effectively be managed by non specialist workers, it is essential that health care professionals should get to know the sources of help and resources available in their particular areas.

Non specialist services

General practitioners

Nowadays, GPs are likely to encounter patients who misuse drugs and alcohol. They have a role in the provision of basic health care to substance misusers and their clinical management. A study of GPs (Glanz & Taylor 1986) found that one in five doctors attended an opiate user during a 4-week period. A report of the Medical Working Group (Department of Health 1991) stated that doctors have a role in both the primary prevention of substance misuse and its clinical management. Doctors should also seek to ensure that patients understand the dangers of drug misuse, particularly high risk groups such as young people and those patients receiving pre-scribed tranquillisers such as the benzodiazepines or who have a drink problem.

GPs have a legal duty to notify the Addicts Index, at the Home Office, of contact with opioid and cocaine addicts and should report details of patients with any recent drug problem to the Regional Drug Misuse Database. The involvement of GPs not only provides general health care needs to substance misusers, within the context of their general practice, but can also provide an effective response to patients with substance use problems or drug related problems. Services that can be provided by GPs include smoking cessation clinics, health education regarding the use of alcohol, tobacco and other psychoactive substances, substitute prescribing, harm minimisation and abstinence programmes.

Accident and Emergency departments

Accident and Emergency (A&E) departments are considered to be the 'shop door' of the health service (Sbaith 1993) and function on an open house policy. These departments are important health care providers for substance misusers suffering from the effects of overdose, acute toxic reactions such as hyperactivity, aggression or even violence, panic attacks, withdrawal symptoms, deliberate self-harm or the physical com-plications of injecting drugs such as abscesses or septicaemia. Appro-priate referral to local substance misuse teams is sometimes the gateway for patients to come into contact with specialist drug and alcohol agencies.

Occupational health departments

In addition to intervening when workers have stress related, health or family problems, occupational health departments have a crucial role in both prevention and minimal interventions with workers who have a problem with alcohol or psychoactive substances. Many institutions and companies have incorporated alcohol and drug policies in the work place. The services provided to employees include screening, counselling and work site health information on the use and misuse of psychoactive substances.

Child guidance service

The child guidance service provides help with children and families in all aspects of health care. The family GP may refer children with drug related problems and their families to the clinic.

Youth counselling

Support and help are also made available by the youth counselling centres. Counselling regarding drug and alcohol misuse in young children is offered in some youth centres.

Specialist services

Drug Dependence Units

Drug dependence units (DDUs) are specialist units which in the past have dealt primarily with opiate addiction. Currently, many units see a variety of clients with cocaine, heroin and hypno-sedative dependence as many of the patients attending treatment or rehabilitation centres are poly-drug users. The source of referral to the local DDU may be the patient's GP or other medical personnel, social worker, probation officer or statutory and voluntary agencies. DDUs are usually staffed by doctors, nurses, social workers, psychologists, occupational therapists and other supportive staff. The intervention strategies include detoxification, individual and group psychotherapy, health education, social skills training, stress management and relapse prevention.

Community Drug Teams

Community Drug Teams (CDTs) have been in existence since the mid 1980s and are usually attached to hospital based units. The Advisory Council on the Misuse of Drugs recommended the establishment of drug teams. CDTs offer a number of services to the local population by providing health information, advice, counselling and home detoxification family therapy and relapse prevention. CDTs are more likely to encounter patients with a variety of substance misuse problems, for whom community based approaches are likely to be more appropriate. CDTs are staffed by nurse specialists, medical practitioners and social workers and/or psychologists.

Community Alcohol Team

Community Alcohol Teams (CATs) have been in existence since 1968. During recent years there have been the new developments in the services provided to the local population by CAT. A London based CAT will serve a population of approximately 600 000 where there are 48 000 alcohol misusers, 6000 being severely alcohol dependent. During 1994, one CAT received 505 referrals (T. Hartnett, personal communication). CATs accept referrals from all professionals and most do not accept self-referrals from patients. Services provided include assessment, community detoxification, home detoxification, counselling, group programmes and relapse prevention.

Crisis intervention

Crisis intervention centres provide emergency care for those dependent users who require medical and nursing management as a result of withdrawal from drugs. The centres provide detoxification from psychoactive substances or, where immediate prescribing may be necessary, complementary therapies for symptoms alleviation, counselling and support. They also act as a short term residency for dependent or chaotic poly-drug users and are often followed by referral to other specialist services.

Addiction prevention services

The addiction prevention project was established in September 1991 in South London. The aims are to educate primary health care staff in the early recognition of, and intervention in, the problems associated with substance use and misuse (Ghodse *et al.*, 1997). The project deals with alcohol and tobacco, prescribed drugs and illicit drugs. The counsellors offer screening, a surgery based counselling service to patients with an early stage of hazardous substance use and also a smoking cessation programme.

Drug and alcohol liaison team

The drug and alcohol liaison team (DALT) service is available to all in-patients of St George's Hospital, London and to those attending A & E department who have a drug and/or alcohol problem. The services that are offered include assessment, advice on detoxification regimes, guidance on the management of patients with substance use problems and possible interactions with other treatments, and liaison work with other specialist agencies.

Street agencies

Street agencies or advice and counselling services are especially found in large urban areas and are accessible to individuals and their families. They provide a 'user-friendly' link for those with substance use problems who are unwilling to attend statutory services for help or treatment. Street agencies have drop-in centres offering advice and help with practical problems, counselling and sometimes medical help. Some of them offer a needle and syringe scheme. No referral or appointment is necessary.

Self-help groups

Various self-help groups exist for those with drug, alcohol and non pharmacological addictions, their families and significant others. Within the substance misuse field, the self-help groups include Alcoholics Anonymous (AA), Tranx (for problems with tranquilliser use), Narcotics Anonymous (NA), Families Anonymous (FA) and Gamblers Anonymous (GA).

Residential rehabilitation services

There are a number of centres throughout the UK who offer residential rehabilitation for those who cannot sustain a drug-free lifestyle. Most require that substance misusers are drug-free on admission and the length of stay varies between one and two years. However, the length of stay has been reduced considerably as a result of changes in community care and finance policies. The therapeutic approaches of the rehabilitation services include group work, social skills training, counselling and health maintenance. Some of the residential services are abstinence orientated and base their approach on the 'twelve steps' model of the AA's programme of recovery. Other facilities focus on the spiritual dimension of substance misuse and are based on the Judeo-Christian tradition. The community based facilities offer services which primarily focus on alcohol or drugs.

Private sector facilities

There has been a growth in the development of treatment and rehabilitation services for substance misusers in the private sector during the last few years. Private clinics offer a range of services and these facilities charge fees to the residents or their families. The treatment and rehabilitation programmes offered vary in length from a few weeks to several months. The therapeutic approaches are mainly based on the 'Minnesota model' (Wells 1987) and incorporate strict adherence to the principles of Narcotics Anonymous.

Resources: national organisations

There are a number of resources in the UK that may be helpful to health and social work professionals, patients and their families. Release, which runs a 24-hour help line, provides information and advice on the legal aspects of drugs. Alcohol Concern provides information on services offering advice, information and support to those experiencing alcohol related problems. A directory of alcohol services is published annually. The Standing Conference on Drug Abuse (SCODA) publishes a comprehensive national directory of drug services. A useful address list is provided in the Appendix of this book.

Conclusions

This chapter summaries the main services provided by statutory, non statutory, voluntary and private sectors in the treatment and rehabilitation of substance misusers. The services or facilities operate upon different philosophical approaches to the treatment of substance misusers and their families. The variety of the residential and community based services provides a rich menu for individual clients or patients to select the particular services that will accommodate their specific needs. The need to make services more economically viable in relation to the provider/purchaser climate of the NHS must also be balanced against the need to maintain good clinical standards and practice in all settings.

References

Department of Health (1991) *Drug Misuse and Dependence. Guidelines on Clinical Management.* HMSO, London.

DHSS (1978) *The Pattern and Range of Services for Problem Drinkers. Report of the Advisory Committee on Alcoholism.* HMSO, London.

Ghodse, A.H., McShane, E., Priestley, J. & Saunders, V. (1997) *Addiction Prevention in Primary Care Project Review (1996/1997).* Department of Psychiatry of Addictive Behaviour, St George's Hospital Medical School, London.

Glanz, A. & Taylor, C. (1986) Findings of a national survey of the role of general practitioners in the treatment of opiate misuse. *British Medical Journal,* **293,** 427–30.

Kennedy, J. & Faugier, J. (1989) *Drug and Alcohol Dependency Nursing.* Heinemann, London.

Ministry of Health and Scottish Home and Health Department (1965) *The Brain Committee.* HMSO, London.

Sbaith, L. (1993) Accident & Emergency work. *Journal of Advanced Nursing,* **18**, 957–62.

Wells, B. (1987) NA and the Minnesota Method in Britain: time to build bridges. *Druglink,* **2**, 1.

Part 3

Generic Responses: Different Contexts and Settings

Chapter 11

Drug Use, Pregnancy and Care of the New-Born

Faye Macrory

Introduction

Pregnancy, childbirth and motherhood are an intrinsic part of women's experience whether or not they become mothers themselves (Ussher 1989; Phoenix *et al.*, 1991). Society today continues to gear females up for the occupation of maternity and the idea that only women with children are real women is pervasive in spite of public commitment to sexual equality. As Ussher (1989) reminds us, society continues to define motherhood, and particularly childbearing as the supreme route to physical and emotional fulfilment and as essential to all women. But while motherhood is socially constructed as valued and important, the circumstances and age at which women are supposed to become mothers outlaw motherhood for women who are too young, too old, too poor, although never too rich, too uneducated or too unsuitable because they use illicit drugs. Women who are seen to be in the wrong group are therefore in the contradictory position of being immediately devalued, although they have entered a status that is, in theory, valued (Phoenix *et al.* 1991).

The unspoken and spoken assumption is that drug using women have not planned their pregnancies, do not want their babies and will not be able to love and care for them as other mothers will. It should therefore come as no surprise that drug using women who have children are then stigmatised because they have contravened dominant ideological notions about what are supposed to be the normal circumstances in which to have children. It is important at this point to look at what 'drug use and misuse' actually does.

For some it meets the need for stimulation or pleasure, or conversely acts as a need for a chemical crutch when there is an overwhelming desire to obliterate the reality of a miserable existence. The use and misuse of any substance can be of a legal, illegal or prescribed nature and many over-the-counter medications can have the potential for harm.

The aims of this chapter are to examine the relationship of drug use in pregnancy and the antenatal care provided for drug-using mothers.

Treatment protocol for the management of drug users and both intra-partum and postpartum care are discussed. Issues such as contraception and sexual health and aspects of child protection are examined.

Women, drug use and pregnancy

Every woman, both drug user and non-drug user alike, may experience ambivalent feelings about their pregnancy, especially if it is their first. While many women experience happiness and fulfilment, some may also experience great anxiety and fear surrounding their change of role, their ability to parent and the changes a new baby may bring to existing relationships and children. Many women may also suffer low self-esteem, depression, anxiety states and extreme guilt. Poverty and financial diffi-culties, domestic violence, legal issues and homelessness and housing difficulties can add further to these very real anxieties. For the woman who is dependent on drugs, all these potential problems are aggravated by her dependence and, where illegal drugs are concerned, the risky life-style that goes with it. Drug use and procuring money for drugs are also very time consuming and stressful. Contraception may be of little concern when obtaining funds to buy drugs is the predominant daily activity. Many drug users consider contraception to be unnecessary or of low priority in relation to their drug habit, and hence first contact with family planning services is either post delivery or post termination. Reasons for the low rate of contraception among female drug users include the belief that they are infertile as a result of drug use, confusion between amenor-rhoea and infertility and experience of menstrual abnormalities, with a consequent underestimate of the risks of pregnancies (Miller 1996). Therefore it is often a shock for some women users to find that they have conceived.

For a proportion of these women, this can cause such emotional turmoil that it is unrealistic to expect immediate and lasting abstinence from sources of coping, such as drugs or alcohol. However, for many women pregnancy can serve as a catalyst, prompting them to try to address their drug use and lifestyle and making them keen to accept help. As Hepburn (1993) suggests, there should be a pragmatic approach to appropriate individual management, with control of drug use and subsequent stabili-sation of life-style being the objective. Many of the women are reluctant to contact health care agencies or reveal their drug use, fearing that the child or existing children may be taken from them should their drug use become known to health or social work staff. A woman may withdraw from contact with the caring agencies or suspect the motives of those workers she does come in contact with because of previous experiences with unsympathetic or hostile health or social workers.

Antenatal care

Ex-users may also require support as well as any woman whose partner is a drug user. Illicit drug use includes both experimental and recreational drug use, and users may request or need information and advice, as may those women who drink alcohol. Misuse of amphetamine, cocaine and benzo-diazepines may be more harmful than opiate use. Continuing antenatal care should be undertaken monthly or as regularly as possible in a venue acceptable to the woman. It should be remembered that an early morning appointment is not usually a realistic option for women taking methadone or other 'street drugs'.

Long waiting periods in clinics can be very distressing for women suf-fering from drug withdrawal; therefore the appointment clerks should notify the midwifery staff when such women book in. Having blood taken may cause distress to women who are trying to discontinue their intra-venous drug use and a sensitive approach should be used. If drugs have been recently injected, blood may have to be taken at a later date. In certain circumstances, for example antibody screening, it may be appropriate for the woman to take her own blood if she prefers. Tests on blood samples should include hepatitis B screening. Hepatitis C screening should not be done routinely but must be preceded by pre-test counselling as for HIV. Urine testing for the presence of illicit substances is not indicated; this is only appropriate as part of a treatment programme planned by the drug service. Should HIV testing be requested, and a trained counsellor is not available, the client should be referred to the genito-urinary medicine (GUM) clinic or back to their drug agency for confidential testing.

An early ultrasound scan is beneficial in determining gestation and, if appropriate, should be done at the booking appointment. More scans may be useful if growth is not maintained, but for some women the suggestion of serial growth scans can reinforce a fear that their drug use is adversely affecting their baby's well-being, and may greatly increase anxiety and existing feelings of guilt. Conversely, some women may request frequent scanning for reassurance. In either case, any advantages or disadvantages should be explained sensitively, while taking the above into account. Should a home birth or domino delivery be requested this should be dis-cussed and assessed on an individual basis. The woman's drug use should not be seen as an automatic contraindication.

Treatment protocol for the management of drug users on the ward area

Illicit drug use is a chronic relapsing condition. Clients presenting for treatment will invariably have been using drugs on a dependent basis for several years. The treatment of drug misuse is therefore a planned exercise and not a medical emergency. The rationale for prescribing methadone in pregnancy includes the following:

❑ Methadone replaces illicit opiates of uncertain composition and dose and thereby reduces the risk of infection from injecting.
❑ There will be less or no need to engage in drug related crime or prostitution to finance their habit and the woman will be relieved of the burden of drug seeking.
❑ Regular medication allows for the stability of the fetus *in utero*, avoiding the potentially harmful effects of the peaks and troughs of illicit drug taking often determined by both the availability of the drug and the money to pay for it.
❑ Nutritional intake is also usually improved as the opportunities to stabilise a previously chaotic life-style are increased (McEvilly 1991).

Should a woman request admission to the maternity services for reduction or detoxification the specialist drug service must be contacted, as in-patient treatment within the maternity services is not usually appropriate for this client group. Emergency treatment of drug misuse problems should never be initiated without obtaining specialist advice. An admission to the maternity or gynaecology services may occur in the case of an associated condition and advice should also be sought for the drug dependence from the drug services at the earliest opportunity. Close liaison between the drug services and any hospital wards is very helpful to patient management.

Treatment is usually only necessary for those who take opiates and, more rarely, tranquillisers – usually benzodiazepines – on a regular basis. Persons who use stimulants, i.e. amphetamines or cocaine, will not usually show a true withdrawal syndrome, although they may exhibit intense drug craving behaviour and can become quite depressed. Specialist advice should be sought if either of these behaviours poses a problem for management.

A person using opiates on a daily basis will start to have opiate withdrawal symptoms when their opiate intake ceases. For heroin, symptoms start at about 6 hours and peak at about 48 hours. For methadone, the symptoms may not start for 12 hours or more and will not peak until 72 to 96 hours. Features of withdrawal include craving, irritability, restlessness and later vomiting and diarrhoea. Heroin users not in a treatment programme should be offered methadone during their stay in hospital and contact with the drug services should be offered. Treatment already being prescribed should be continued during admission. Some patients may prefer to take their medication in one dose, others in divided doses. Methadone prevents the physical discomforts of withdrawal, and does not achieve the 'high' heroin does; therefore, staff need not feel that they are condoning or colluding in the women's drug use, an anxiety that has been expressed on several occasions. Flexibility in prescribing should be taken into account according to each individual's needs. It is important however, that independent checks are made to confirm the treatment regime to avoid under or over prescribing.

For those not already in treatment, or where it is not possible to confirm that they are in fact in treatment, for example weekend or statutory holidays, the following regime should be prescribed for opiate withdrawal until advice from the drug services can be obtained. A methadone mixture, 1 mg in 1 ml, should be given, 10 mg 4 hourly prn (as necessary). The dose should be given every 4 hours provided that the woman requests it and that she is not at all drowsy or intoxicated. After 24 hours the dose required can then be given on a twice daily basis. A person requiring 10 mg every 4 hours will then be stabilised on 60 mg a day, or 30 mg bd (twice a day). Any woman apparently requiring larger doses than this will need expert advice. Women who are definitely in receipt of prescribed benzodiazepines outside hospital should have their prescription continued, but those who are not in receipt of such drugs should not be prescribed them at all during admission unless under specialist advice. This includes the prescribing of temazepam for night sedation.

Methadone should be given in the privacy of the office or the treatment room, and not carried on to the ward in view of the other women. Should the woman be confined to bed, confidentiality can be preserved by placing the medicine pot inside a cup/saucer. Family members and friends may not be aware of the woman's drug use and it should be remembered that relationships can be irrevocably damaged if confidentiality is breached. The woman's drug use should not be discussed on the ward round under any circumstances. Persons receiving prescriptions for methadone or similar drugs outside hospital, and who are admitted to hospital, will have outpatient prescriptions which are continuing to run and other persons may continue to collect these drugs while the patient receives their supplies in hospital. To avoid this the patient's prescriber should therefore be contacted as soon as possible after admission so that out-patient supplies can be stopped. Liaison will also need to take place at an early stage so that clients can pick up their out-patient prescription again on discharge. It should usually be possible for the drug services, or the GP if one is prescribing, to take up treatment immediately on discharge, so that no take home methadone has to be supplied by the hospital.

Should discharge occur unexpectedly over the weekend period, no more than 3 days' supply of medication should be issued to be taken home. Again, close liaison is necessary so that a patient does not simultaneously receive take home supplies from the hospital and their normal out-patient prescription at the same time. In the case of new patients, early liaison with the drug service is vital if they are to be taken into ongoing treatment after they leave hospital – should they wish to avail themselves of this. Any woman suspected of using illicit substances should be asked not to do so while on hospital premises. Conflict should be avoided and security involved only if absolutely unavoidable.

Intrapartum care

For opiate dependent women receiving antenatal care, the management and duration of labour and the incidence of caesarean section are no different from those of a matched population (Fraser 1976 1983). If the woman is maintained on methadone, this should be continued during labour. Standard analgesia is indicated during labour as a daily dose of methadone will not provide pain relief. There is also little evidence to suggest that pain relieving opiates are harmful to the fetus already sensitised to opiates during pregnancy (Fraser 1976). It should be remembered that, for everyone, pain is a subjective experience which is influenced by several factors. Siney *et al.* (1995) found that opiate dependent women who have their methadone levels maintained do not usually require any more analgesia in labour or post-delivery. However, some opiate users may require larger amounts for pain relief as normal doses may be ineffective if tolerance has developed. Drug misuse is not a contraindication to having a patient controlled analgesia (PCA) pump following caesarean section and post-delivery pain control and relief should be available as for every woman.

Withdrawal from opiates in labour may be shown by fetal distress on the cardio tocograph (CTG) monitor, e.g. tachycardia, bradycardia, increased fetal movements, meconium stained liquor. Therefore it is helpful to ensure that a woman has an adequate amount of opiate throughout labour, so that opiate withdrawal induced fetal distress can be excluded from other obstetric emergencies. Maternal signs include:

❑ Restlessness
❑ Tremors
❑ Sweating
❑ Abdominal pain
❑ Cramps
❑ Anxiety and
❑ Vomiting

Routine care in labour should be carried out with careful observation of the mother and fetus for withdrawal. The paediatricians and special care baby unit should be informed of the woman's admission and delivery.

The woman's drug problem may be recognised or disclosed for the first time during labour. The woman may be extremely anxious about an unaware partner or relatives noticing injecting sites, therefore discreet clothing should be an available option. Any drug user who goes into opiate withdrawal during labour should be treated by a small dose of opiate. Fetal distress will dramatically improve, thus reducing the risk of asphyxia and meconium aspiration due to withdrawal. A paediatrician should be present if fetal distress or meconium liquor is present.

Naloxone, an opiate antagonist, must not be given as it may precipitate abrupt withdrawal symptoms in both fetus and mother. Senior medical/paediatric advice should be sought if necessary. Depending on the particular hospital's policy, the baby is either transferred to the postnatal area with its mother, or routinely admitted to the special care baby unit. The latter often causes great distress to mothers and may be their reason for non-disclosure. Again, confidentiality is paramount as partners and relatives may be unaware of the woman's drug use, and will understandably want an explanation as to why an apparently healthy baby is being transferred to the special care baby unit. If, for legal reasons, the baby must be cared for separately, transfer to the unit usually takes place following delivery.

Postpartum care

If possible, and hospital policy allows, the mother and baby should go to any bed in the postnatal area. The neonatal abstinence score chart is used for assessing the onset, progression and lessening of symptoms of abstinence. Research in Liverpool (Shaw & McIvor 1994) has shown that neonatal withdrawal symptoms from methadone, which has a longer half-life than heroin, generally occur, if at all, after 24 hours and within 72 hours. The mother should therefore be encouraged to remain in hospital for a minimum of 72 hours so that any major symptoms of opiate withdrawal in her baby can be monitored and treated as per protocol. Antenatally, the score system and chart will have, when possible, been explained to the mother and she should be involved in the scoring process. However, the score chart should not be seen as a prescriptive tool, but as a guide to overall observation. Babies are often fractious even if they do not require treatment and the mother should be supported in comforting her baby – use of dummies, swaddling etc. The score chart should be kept in the office area, not on the end of the cot, to maintain confidentiality. Most drug using women are also very anxious that other women in the ward remain unaware of their drug use.

Apart from all the well documented benefits, breast feeding will certainly support the mother in feeling that she is positively comforting her baby, should it be harder to settle. Most psychoactive drugs of misuse do not pass into the breast milk in quantities which are sufficient to have a major effect on the new-born baby. There may be some effect on the baby, such as drowsiness with opiates or tranquillisers. However, the important point is that women should be given all the information they need to make an informed choice about breast feeding, and having made that decision, they should be fully supported by all the professionals involved. (Institute for the Study of Drug Dependence 1995).

When contraception and sexual health are discussed, the only consistent advice usually given to drug users is about the effect of drugs on their pregnancy, not about the effects of drugs on menstruation and fertility or the appropriateness of different types of contraception. The provision of information and education empowers drug users to take responsibility and make informed choices, therefore maternity services need to emphasise the important role of the GP, as well as the roles of GUM and family planning services in encouraging women to address their sexual health. The importance of cervical screening must be stressed (Miller 1996). Ideally, discussion should be instigated in the antenatal period, rather than when the woman is about to be discharged post-delivery. Factors that need to be considered when discussing contraception with drug using women include the following:

❑ Personal choice
❑ Availability and accessibility of contraception
❑ Medical status or contraindications and
❑ Compliance.

Also for those women who work as prostitutes, condoms may not be an option in their personal relationships, because of the association with their work.

Discharge

Mother and baby should be notified to the community midwifery service as per protocol. Some babies may go home on medication. The health visitor will, when possible, have been informed during the antenatal period so early contact can be instigated. The drug service should also be informed of impending discharge as soon as possible, so that arrangements for the methadone script to be re-issued can be made. Methadone or other pre-scribed drugs, such as Diazepam or temazepam, should be given TTO (to take out) without prior consultation with the drug services. Should discharge occur over a weekend or bank holiday period and no liaison with the drug services is possible, no more than 3 days supply of medication should be given to take home.

Social services and child protection issues

It is now increasingly recognised that drug use does not in itself cause poor parenting. Drug using parents tend to share a spectrum of characteristics which predominate among social services clients, rather than there being a direct correlation between drug use and child neglect or abuse. Drug misuse goes along with a chaotic lifestyle, poverty and bad housing and many drug users have a personal history of neglect and abuse. However, many people, both drug users and non drug users, need support from time to time with their child care. This need should not necessarily or automatically invoke child protection services. Disclosure of drug use should not immediately warrant social worker involvement, unless there are other causes for concern – as per procedure for any client of the maternity services. Any discussion of social worker involvement should be handled in as sensitive a manner as possible.

Some women will already be involved with social services and this should be recorded in the notes with any contact numbers. When indicated, the relevant worker should be notified. If a case conference is required it should ideally be held several weeks before the estimated date of delivery. This is a social services decision. This system enables the parent/s concerned to have time to accept any decisions made and also for hospital staff to be aware if child protection action is to be taken or, more importantly, not. Documentation of any case conference decisions should be placed in the appropriate confidential file.

The following SCODA (Standing Conference on Drug Abuse 1989) guidelines should be borne in mind when referral is being considered.

'Drug use by parents does not automatically indicate child neglect or abuse. Automatic child abuse registration will deter parents from approaching drug dependence clinics or other professionals for help and should be avoided. In families where drug use is a factor, a comprehensive assessment of the relationship between parental drug use and child care is indicated. Each family should be assessed individually.'

Case vignette

Sally was stable on methadone and 16 weeks pregnant with her second child when her drug worker referred her to me. In her first pregnancy she had been too scared to disclose her heroin use to the maternity services as she believed her baby would be taken into care if the staff found out. Her family was also unaware of her drug use and she was extremely anxious whether staff would breach confidentiality if her baby had to go to the special care baby unit. Sally had very negative memories of her whole experience of pregnancy and her first few months of motherhood. She was delighted when she knew that her next baby would remain with her on the ward area, that staff were very supportive and aware of the need for confidentiality to be respected and that there would not be an automatic referral to the social services. Sally was then able to continue to address her drug use realistically, rather than desperately and unsuccessfully try to be drug free by the birth to avoid being separated from her baby.

Conclusions

While it is recognised that there may be difficulties in attempting to provide a specialised service that at the same time does not appear to stigmatise, it is hoped that the women involved will ultimately feel empowered to address other difficulties in their lives by knowing that there is non judgemental and sympathetic support available to assist them. The importance of training in the many areas related to drug use is that it gives the staff the understanding and confidence to care for the babies in the ward area following delivery. Once the women know that their babies will not be separated from them automatically, they then have the chance to address their drug use during pregnancy realistically, rather than try desperately, and usually unsuccessfully, to be drug free by the time of the birth.

Although drug using women certainly need special services, projects may run several risks in concentrating help to women during this time of their life. By focusing all their resources and attention on pregnant women, they may simply be reinforcing the already strong societal message women receive – and internalise – that their only value is in producing offspring, and that the only attention they will get is in their role as potential mothers (Weissmann 1991). For women whose sense of self and self-esteem is already precarious, the feeling that they are only valued when pregnant may increase their suspicion of or, conversely, their reliance on statutory services. It must always be remembered that the pregnant woman is a whole person and that pregnancy is only one part of her life.

References

Fraser, A.C. (1976) Drug addiction in pregnancy. *The Lancet,* **8**, 96–9.

Fraser, A.C. (1983) The pregnant drug addict. *The Journal of Maternal and Child Health,* November, 461–3.

Gossop, M. (1993) *Living With Drugs,* 3rd edn. Avebury, Aldershot.

Hepburn, M. (1993) Drug misuse in pregnancy. *Current Obstetrics and Gynaecology,* **3**, 54–8.

Institute for the Study of Drug Dependence (1995) *Drugs, Pregnancy, and Childcare: A Guide for Professionals.* ISDD, London.

McEvilly, S. (1991) *Factors to consider when working with the pregnant opiate user.* Rochdale Drug Advice and Information Centre, Rochdale.

Miller, J. (1996) Addressing the issues of contraception in substance misuse services: is it a concern? *Psychiatric Care: ANSA,.* **3** (Suppl. 1).

Phoenix, A., Woolett A. & Lloyd E. (1991) *Motherhood. Meaning, Practices and Ideologies.* Sage Publications, London.

Shaw, N.J. & McIvor, L. (1994) Neonatal abstinence syndrome after maternal methadone treatment. *Archives of Disease in Childhood,* **71**, 203–20.

Standing Conference on Drug Abuse (SCODA) (1989). *Drug using parents and their children: the second report of the National Local Authority Forum on Drug Abuse in conjunction with SCODA.* Association of Metropolitan Authorities, London.

Siney, C., Kidd, M., Walkinshaw, S., *et al.* (1995) Opiate dependence in pregnancy. *British Journal of Midwifery*, **3**, 69–73.

Ussher, J. (1989) *The Psychology of the Female Body*. Routledge, London.

Weissmann, G. (1991) *Working with pregnant women at high risk for HIV infection: Outreach intervention*. National Institute On Drug Abuse, Rockville, Maryland.

Chapter 12

Health Visiting and Substance Misuse

Julie Gafoor

Introduction

The health, social and economic costs incurred on society through the widespread use and misuse of drugs and alcohol have become a matter of national concern in recent years. Statistics from the Office of Population Censuses and Surveys (1992) showed 28% of women smoked during their pregnancy. Substance misuse during pregnancy is known to be linked with higher rates of prematurity, low birth weight and retarded intrauterine growth (Chasnoff 1988). Furthermore, research has shown substance misuse to be a major factor in 80% of all cases of child abuse and neglect (Children's Defense Fund 1992). In recent years several policy documents (Department of Health 1992; Advisory Council for the Misuse of Drugs 1994; Tackling Drugs Together 1995) have highlighted the need for greater involvement by health care professionals in responding to the health needs of substance misusers. Reducing smoking and alcohol consumption are both targets set in *The Health of the Nation* documents. The emphasis on the importance of non specialists in working with substance misusers followed research demonstrating the effectiveness of brief and opportunistic interventions in primary care settings (Russell *et al.*, 1979; Babor *et al.*, 1986).

Health visitors are community nurses who have a responsibility for health promotion and preventive care for all children under the age of 5 years and their families. They provide an accessible and non stigmatising home visiting service to clients and facilitate access to health and social services. The principles of health visiting allow a framework for health visiting practice based on a philosophy of promoting health, health assessment, primary prevention, public health and human development. As a member of one of the main health professional groups who are in regular contact with pre-school children and their families, the health visitor is well placed to develop interventions in the prevention and treatment of substance misuse. This chapter will examine the main problems associated with parental substance use and misuse and outline the interventions and treatment strategies which can be adopted by health visitors in working with this group of patients. A case vignette is used to illustrate the work of the health visitor.

Nature of problems in parents who are substance misusers

Substance misuse during pregnancy is associated with increased medical risks to both mother and baby and there is a direct relationship between perinatal mortality and antenatal care (Tylden 1983). The use of opiates during pregnancy may be associated with premature delivery and low birth weights (Riley 1987) and withdrawal effects can lead to miscarriage. Injecting drug users who use unsterile injecting equipment are a high risk group for medical complications such as HIV, hepatitis, abscesses, gangrene and septicaemia. Other complications such as anaemia, chest infections, malnutrition and vitamin deficiencies may occur as a result of smoking, poor diet and inadequate housing and medical care.

Both the intoxicating and withdrawal effects of substances and chaotic life-styles of some illicit drug users may impair their parenting abilities and adversely affect the safety, health and development of young children. Money for food, clothing and heating may be spent on drugs, and young children might be at risk of drugs and injecting equipment left lying around the house. It has been shown that children from economically deprived families have higher rates of chronic illness, respiratory infections, hearing loss, nutritional and growth problems and accidents (Kurtz & Stanley 1995).

Feelings of depression and low self-esteem are common among substance misusers and these may lead to ambivalent and hostile feelings towards a new-born baby (Griffith 1988). Some drug dependent mothers may harbour feelings of guilt concerning possible harm their drug use during pregnancy may have caused the infant. Such feelings may be especially strong if the baby had suffered from withdrawal symptoms at birth. Babies born to mothers who are addicted to drugs such as opiates, benzodiazepines, barbiturates and alcohol can develop withdrawal symptoms – for example irritability, twitching, diarrhoea, dehydration and in some instances convulsions during the first few days of life. The onset may sometimes be delayed for days or weeks if the mother was addicted to methadone (Robson 1992) and the baby may have difficulties feeding and sleeping.

The use of social drugs during pregnancy can also have a detrimental effect on child development. Alcohol misuse during pregnancy can cause fetal alcohol syndrome with growth retardation, irritability and hyperactivity (US Department of Health and Human Services, 1990); and infants born to smokers have a lower birth weight than those born to non smokers (Royal College of Physicians 1992). Infants with parents who smoke are also likely to suffer from chest infections, increased asthmatic attacks, 'glue ear' and irritations to the eyes, throat and respiratory tract (Chappell & Lilley 1994).

Summary of problems

❏ Medical complications such as HIV, hepatitis B and C, thrombophlebitis, gangrene and septicaemia can result from injecting drugs with unsterile injecting equipment.
❏ Anaemia, chest infections, malnutrition and vitamin deficiencies may occur due to smoking, poor diet, inadequate housing and medical care.
❏ Substance misusing parents often suffer from feelings of guilt, low self-esteem and depression.
❏ Babies born to mothers addicted to opiates, alcohol, benzodiazepines and barbiturates can develop withdrawal symptoms at birth.

Role of the health visitor in substance use and misuse

Most health visitors are attached to primary health care teams and every client who is registered with a general practitioner (GP) has access to a health visitor. They provide an accessible and non stigmatising service to the practice population and see patients in a variety of community settings such as their homes, GP surgeries, health centres, etc. The health visitor can make statutory home visits at any time during pregnancy, birth and pre-school years and this provides a unique opportunity to access patients who may not otherwise come into contact with health professionals. The health visitor is therefore ideally placed to identify and work with the substance misuser.

For the majority of clients their first contact with the health visitor will be during pregnancy or shortly after birth. At this stage the health visitor will aim to develop a therapeutic relationship with the client by explaining her role, policies on confidentiality of information provided and clarifying any concerns that the client may have regarding the well-being of the child. It is widely acknowledged that pregnant substance misusers are unwilling to admit to their substance misuse and are reluctant to present for antenatal care for fear that their baby may be removed at birth. On the other hand expecting a baby may give some parents an incentive to stabilise their drug use or give up altogether.

Health visiting interventions

Assessment

Although, as outlined earlier, children whose parents are substance misusers are more susceptible to neglect and abuse. It should be borne in mind that substance misuse does not automatically indicate child neglect or abuse. As part of the health visitor's role, he/she is able to assess proactively for health needs within the family and to prepare and support parents in child care. Most health visitors will routinely ask clients about their use of tobacco and alcohol but may lack the confidence and knowledge to enquire about illicit substances. The child protection remit of the health visitor's role could act as a barrier in getting patients to admit to substance use. However, in a study carried out by Pearson (1991) on patients' perceptions of the health visitor's role, it was found that parents valued the health visitor in having a role in identifying family stress and worries. If the health visitor establishes a warm and friendly rapport and listens carefully to the client's concerns, it will make it easier for the client to disclose details of substance use. Clients are more likely to be open about the use of substances if they feel confident that their concerns will be adequately addressed and that the health visitor will act in their best interests.

In cases where substance misuse is identified, it is important for the health visitor to assess the degree of risk to both the parent and child. Information on the type of drugs, amounts, costs, duration of use, route of administration, extent of HIV risk-taking behaviour and presence of withdrawal symptoms are necessary to determine the nature and severity of the client's substance misuse. Other factors such as partner's use of substances, parenting abilities and relationship with the child, availability of family resources and support networks are important when making a comprehensive assessment.

Health education/harm minimisation

Health education may be defined as

> 'any communication activity aimed at enhancing positive health and preventing or diminishing ill health in individuals and groups, through influencing the beliefs, attitudes and behaviour of those with power and of the community at large' (Tones & Tilford 1994).

Thus health visitors should provide their clients with accurate and up to date information on the effects and consequences of their use of drugs and alcohol. Such information can enable patients to make informed choices and decisions regarding their use of substances. As a result, it may be possible to help a client to stabilise or cease their use of substances by providing them with health education regarding the adverse effects of various drugs together with the possible risks of HIV infection through needle sharing and unsafe sexual practices. Pregnant clients should be informed at the earliest opportunity of the possible harmful effects their use of substances might have on the developing fetus, particularly during the first trimester. They should also be told that the withdrawal effects from drugs such as opiates, alcohol and other sedatives may cause miscarriage.

However, for some clients, information by itself will not be enough for them to avoid harmful use of substances and health visitors will need to adopt harm minimisation principles for working with this group. This means helping the client to choose the safest possible way of using substances and providing her with the necessary support and means in order to achieve the best possible outcome. For example, a client may not be able to give up injecting drug use but may stop sharing injecting equipment if provided with sterile needles and syringes. Likewise some patients may be encouraged to change from injecting to oral drug use. In both cases, the client remains at risk but the likelihood of harm is reduced.

Psycho-social support

Parents who are substance misusers often experience feelings of guilt and shame relating to the consequences their use of substances might have on their children. Women in particular may feel inadequate as mothers, given the negative views that are held in society regarding female substance users. Some may be involved in violent or exploitative relationships with men and may feel hopeless in their ability to make positive changes. Individual counselling and a non judgmental attitude by the health visitor can help to increase patients' self esteem and allay feelings of guilt and inadequacy. Skills in assertiveness, stress management and positive parenting can be taught at antenatal or postnatal classes. Some clients may need practical support to deal with issues such as housing, benefits and child care. Attendance at a family centre can also be useful in learning parenting skills and reducing social isolation.

Interagency liaison and treatment

Health visitors throughout the course of their work liaise with a number of health and welfare agencies on behalf of their patients. With the pregnant substance misuser, there should be regular liaison between the health visitor, midwife, GP and paediatrician and substance misuse service. However, it is important to recognise that the client may have concerns about confidentiality of information. Failure to address these concerns could lead to denial of substance misuse or non compliance by patients in responding to help. Clients should be informed clearly of the roles of any professional who is involved in their care and should be invited to attend any planning meetings to review child care. In some instances, it might be more appropriate for the health visitor to become the key worker and to ensure that other professionals involved are working closely together and towards the same goal.

Clients who are physically dependent on substances such as opiates, alcohol and benzodiazepines may require detoxification either in hospital or in the community. This should be carried out during the second trimester to reduce the risk of miscarriage in the first trimester and fetal distress in the third trimester (National Institute on Drug Abuse 1985). Substitute prescribing of drugs such as methadone and benzodiazepines may help to stabilise drug use and drug-seeking behaviours in some patients. Clearly the health visitor is not expected to be an expert in substance misuse and should seek clinical support and advice from specialist staff where necessary. The involvement of a community addiction nurse (with the client's permission) should be considered in some cases for a joint assessment. He/she can also advise on prescribing issues and play an important therapeutic role in relapse prevention and ongoing toxicology.

Case vignette

The following case history briefly outlines the health visitor's role in assessment, health education and support of a young family affected by substance misuse. Linda was 17 years old and expecting her first child. Her partner, Paul, was 27 and had a long-standing history of drug misuse. They met while staying at a local hostel for young homeless people. Linda claimed to have been sexually abused by her brother and subsequent arguments with her parents resulted in her leaving home at the age of 13 and living rough for a while. Her relationship with Paul had been an 'on and off' one. He saw other girlfriends and had a history of violent behaviour. Linda initially denied illicit drug use to the midwife during antenatal visits, although she admitted to smoking around 20 cigarettes a day.

Linda was introduced to the health visitor by the midwife and a home visit was arranged. She had been reconciled with her parents and had returned home to live. At the first visit the health visitor explained her role and responsibility towards the unborn child. She discussed with Linda the likely harmful effects of her smoking on the baby *in utero* and after it was born, and the importance of healthy eating and sleeping habits. Linda showed concern for the baby's health and later admitted to the health visitor an intermittent use of intravenous heroin and amphetamines. She was provided with information regarding the risks of infection: for example, HIV and hepatitis associated with sharing injecting equipment and unsafe sexual practices. The possible risks of miscarriage due to opiate withdrawal were also discussed, although Linda did not show any signs of being physically dependent on opiates.

The health visitor explored with Linda the factors relating to her use of illicit drugs and she was able to identify certain situations in which drug use occurred. These were mainly confined to arguments with Paul and being in the company of other drug users. A joint meeting with Paul and Linda was arranged and he agreed to attend the substance misuse treatment centre where he was stabilised on a methadone prescription. He attended an anger management group and was persuaded to accompany Linda at antenatal classes. Shortly after the birth of their baby son, Linda and Paul moved into a flat offered by the housing association following a letter of request by the health visitor. They both agreed to attend the well-baby clinic fortnightly in order for the baby's growth and development to be monitored. In addition, they were encouraged to attend a postnatal support group where they met other new parents and shared information on aspects of child care such as feeding, sleep, safety and play.

The health visitor managed to develop a trusting and caring relationship with Linda who then felt safe enough to admit to illicit drug use and was willing to make changes in her use of substances during her pregnancy. Higgins *et al.* (1995) found that over 50% of pregnant women reported positive changes in their drug taking behaviour because they wanted a healthy baby. Linda was provided with health education and helped by the health visitor to avoid the use of street drugs by identifying the high risk situations and developing alternative coping strategies. Her partner was also encouraged to seek treatment since his use of drugs had a direct effect on Linda and the baby's well being. The couple were also supported socially with help in finding suitable accommodation and developing new relationships away from a drug-using subculture.

Conclusions

The physical, social and psychological problems experienced by families who are substance misusers are a matter of concern for all health care professionals. Most female substance misusers are of a child bearing age and the use/misuse of substances during and after pregnancy can have harmful effects for the woman, fetus and newborn child. Health visitors as community nurses are ideally placed to address the needs of parents who are substance misusers. The government's *Health of the Nation* documents (Department of Health 1992, 1993) have identified health targets for health care professionals in relation to alcohol, HIV and sexual behaviour. These and other health policy directives have all highlighted the need for health care professionals to receive appropriate training and education in substance misuse in order for them to intervene effectively with this group of patients.

It is clear, however, that many generic workers including health visitors still regard substance misuse as something to be dealt with by specialists and tend to view their role largely as a referral agent. An education and training programme for health visitors should include the effects and health sequelae associated with the range of commonly used psychoactive substances along with the different kinds of interventions that are required. This would complement the existing core skills already practised by health visitors in assessment, counselling and health promotion and help them to fulfil their role in the prevention, recognition and management of substance misuse. It is also important for issues on substance misuse to be incorporated into the health visitor's training curriculum.

The diversity of their role in health promotion, prevention, treatment and as referral agents provides health visitors with a unique opportunity to identify and develop intervention strategies for the substance misuser. A background knowledge on the effects and complications of the range of commonly misused substances along with assessment, counselling and stress management skills would enable the health visitor to make an effective contribution in dealing with substance misusers. In some cases clinical support, advice and training from specialist substance misuse workers will be required. The changing patterns of drug taking and widespread use of substances in the community make it necessary for all health visitors to develop their role in working with patients who use and misuse psychoactive substances.

References

Advisory Council for the Misuse of Drugs (ACMD) (1994) *Aids and Drug Misuse: Update*. HMSO, London.

Babor, T.F., Ritson, E.B. & Hodgson, R.J. (1986) Alcohol related problems in the primary health care settings: a review of early intervention strategies. *British Journal of Addiction*, **81**, 23–46.

Chappell, C. & Lilley G. (1994) Effects of smoking on the fetus and young children. *British Journal of Midwifery*, **2**, 587.

Chasnoff, I.J. (1988) Drug use in pregnancy: parameters of risk. *Pediatric Clinics in North America*, **35**, 1403–12.

Children's Defense Fund (1992) *The State of America's Children, 1992*. Children's Defense Fund, Washington, DC.

Department of Health (1992) *The Health of the Nation: A strategy for England*. HMSO, London.

Department of Health (1993) *The Health of the Nation: Key Area Handbook on HIV/AIDS and Sexual Health*. HMSO, London.

Griffith, D.R. (1988) The effects of prenatal cocaine exposure on infant neurobehaviour and early maternal–infant interactions. In: *Drugs, Alcohol, Pregnancy and Parenting* (ed. I.J. Chasnoff), pp.105–13. Kluwer Academic Publishers, Boston.

Higgins, P.G., Clough, D.H., Frank, B. & Wallerstedt, C. (1995) Changes in health behaviours made by pregnant substance abusers. *The International Journal of the Addictions*, **30**, 1323–33.

Kurtz, Z. & Stanley, F (1995) Epidemiology. In: *Community Child Health and Paediatrics* (eds D. Harvey, M. Miles & D. Smyth). Butterworth-Heinemann, London.

National Institute on Drug Abuse (NIDA) (1985) *Drug Dependency in Pregnancy: Clinical Management of Mother and Child*. National Institute on Drug Abuse, Rockville, MD.

Office of Population Censuses and Surveys (1992) *Infant Feeding in 1990*. OPCS, London.

Pearson, P. (1991) Patients' perceptions: the use of case studies in developing theory. *Journal of Advanced Nursing*, **16**, 521–8.

Robson, P. (1992) Opiate misusers: are treatments effective? In: *Practical Problems in Clinical Psychiatry* (eds K. Hawton & P. Cohen), pp.152–7. Oxford Medical Publications, Oxford.

Royal College of Physicians (1992) *Smoking and the Young*. Royal College of Physicians, London.

Riley, D. (1987) The management of the pregnant drug addict. *Bulletin of the Royal College of Psychiatrists*, **11**, 362–5.

Russell, M.A.H, Wilson, C., Taylor, C. & Baker, C.D. (1979) Effect of general practitioners' advice against smoking. *British Medical Journal*, **6184**, 231–5.

Tackling Drugs Together (1995) *A Strategy for England 1995–1998*. HMSO, London.

Tones, K. & Tilford, S. (1994) *Health Education, Effectiveness, Efficiency and Equity*, 2nd edn. Chapman & Hall, London.

Tylden, E. (1983) Care of the pregnant drug addict. *MIMS*, June.

US Department of Health and Human Services (1990) *Alcohol and Birth Defects: The Fetal Alcohol Syndrome and Related Disorders*. Department of Health and Social Services Publication No. ADM 87-1531, Rockville, Maryland.

Chapter 13
Practice Nurse: Recognition and Early Interventions

Clare Cowan

Introduction

Health care strategies implemented by the Government (Department of Health 1987, 1992) over the past decade, together with simultaneous reorganisation of the National Health Service affecting primary health care provision (Department of Health 1990), have resulted in general practice being recognised as a key contributor to health promotion and disease prevention in the UK. In addition, general practice has been identified as providing a frequent point of contact for those seeking help for substance misuse (Tackling Drugs Together 1995). It is estimated that 98% of the UK population is registered with a GP (Anderson 1992); 90% of patients present to their GP at least once in a 5 year period and 78% present at least once annually. It is this frequency of patient contact which potentially allows a proactive approach by health care professionals working within the general practice setting to identify and offer intervention strategies to patients regarding substance use.

However, accurate statistics regarding attendance at general practices as a result of substance use and misuse are difficult to calculate due to lack of agreement over definitions, difficulties in establishing harmful levels of intake and problems with carrying out the necessary surveys (Paton 1994). In terms of alcohol use it has been estimated that the average GP with 2000 adult patients would be expected to have 186 'heavy drinkers', of whom 37 are likely to be 'problem drinkers' and 19 to be dependent on alcohol (Paton 1994). Yet, recent morbidity statistics indicate that only 13 per 10 000 general practice consultations are for an alcohol dependent problem (Office of Population Censuses and Surveys 1995). Moreover, it is believed that doctors recognise only half the 'problem drinkers' they see (Kitchens 1994), and most fail to include alcohol misuse as a differential diagnosis (Wenrich *et al.* 1995).

In terms of drug use, morbidity statistics indicate that 19 consultations per 10 000 are for drug dependence, and 17 consultations per 10 000 are for non dependent drug misuse. The ratio between consultation rates and prevalence is reported as high, thus indicating that those drug misusers who do consult their GP do so on a frequent basis (Office of Population Censuses and Surveys 1995). Furthermore, the figures highlight the fact that many patients with a problem do not consult their general practice at all.

Previous studies indicate that alcohol and nicotine related disorders and their management and interventions have been dealt with in general practice for many years with varying degrees of success (Russell *et al.* 1978; Babor *et al.* 1986; Anderson 1987), yet drug misuse problems have, to a great extent, been ignored and under diagnosed. The government White Paper (Tackling Drugs Together 1995) hopes to redress this balance by promoting 'shared care' arrangements for drug users between GPs (and other agencies as appropriate) and the specialist substance misuse services.

This chapter argues that the practice nurse is well placed to fulfil a crucial role in the recognition and early intervention of substance misuse in the general practice setting. It will explore the rationale for practice nurse involvement and present a brief outline of the role. Guidelines for the assessment of patients will be considered, and early intervention techniques described. Professional and educational issues will be discussed in relation to the expanding role of the practice nurse.

General practice versus specialist services

Although some substance misusers will require specialist support and counselling, many others could be managed either exclusively by their GP and his team or in collaboration with the specialist services using various models of 'shared care' (Tackling Drugs Together 1995). The potential benefits for the patient from these types of arrangements include easier and more flexible access to care in a familiar, non stigmatised setting (Anderson 1992). The notion is thought to be particularly important for those who do not consider themselves 'addicts' or who lack knowledge of the specialist services. It is also envisaged that more substance misusers will register permanently with a GP, thus ensuring equitable access to NHS services. In relation to substance misuse patients, GPs have a dual role:

❑ The provision of general medical services;
❑ The provision of care and treatment appropriate to the degree and type of substance misuse (DHSS 1984).

Both facets of care are considered to be interrelated and of equal importance. However, GP attitudes to substance misusers vary widely (Parker & Gay 1987; Abed & Neira-Munoz 1990) and it is not unknown for a patient to be faced with an unsympathetic response. This may occur because

(1) The GP lacks the necessary skills required to deal effectively with the situation;
(2) The GP has an inherent mistrust of substance misusers resulting in a negative attitude of care; and
(3) There is a time constraint.

Whatever the reason, it is important that the patient does not risk deterioration of his/her problem as a result of not being offered advice, support or access to services.

Why the practice nurse?

Some patients find it less threatening to discuss potentially embarrassing or awkward problems with a member of the practice team other than the GP, for example the practice nurse. The nurse may be seen as a means of 'demedicalising' or trivialising the problem, and is perceived as having more time and being more approachable for informal discussion. While each practice nurse's role varies considerably depending on skills, work environment and the needs of the practice population (Royal College of Nursing 1991), a unique function of the role, and perhaps the most important one for patients, is 'the permanence and stability of her presence on the practice premises for direct access by the practice population' (Hyde 1995).

Practice nursing occupies a gatekeeping, sifting and sorting role which because of its specific approach to health promotion through screening and chronic disease management (English National Board 1990), lends itself to recognition and early intervention strategies. In the context of substance misuse, the practice nurse is therefore ideally placed to offer care focused towards affected patients. Due to increasing involvement with anticipatory and preventative care (Tettersell & Luft 1994) many opportunities exist for the practice nurse to screen and assess patients, enabling recognition and identification of problematic/non problematic substance use.

Working within the framework of her role and *The Scope of Professional Practice* (United Kingdom Central Council 1992), the practice nurse may then offer interventions appropriate to the level of substance use. These may include interventions aimed at preventing or minimising harm associated with initial problematic or dependent substance use, interventions linked with treatment regimes, e.g. urine testing, or, realising the limitations of her own role, onward referral to an appropriate colleague, voluntary or statutory service. Having discussed the rationale behind the use of general practice as a key contributor for substance misuse disorders, and having justified the importance of the practice nurse role, the next section will deal specifically with the practical and problematic nature of assessing patients. However, first it would be beneficial to look at how patients may present to the practice nurse.

Patient presentation

In her everyday contact with the practice population, the practice nurse can expect to encounter numerous patients who have, or have had, a substance misuse problem. Important groups of patients who should not be over-looked are those who have been taking prescribed medications over long periods and patients with the phenomenon of polypharmacy. Patients may present with problems which do not initially indicate a substance misuse related problem, e.g. minor injuries, obesity, dizziness, while others will present with a direct request for help. Some may have been referred from a colleague or present as an emergency. Whatever the presentation, the nurse will be expected to assess the situation and intervene appropriately. Assessment may take the form of

❏ Screening
❏ In-depth assessment
❏ Triage for emergency (Association of Nurses in Substance Abuse 1997)

Assessment

The three forms of assessment will be considered in detail, together with the outcomes arising from each assessment process.

Screening

The underlying principle of screening is the early identification of sub-stance misusers or substance misuse related disease, so that some form of intervention can be offered before the patient presents with the serious medical and psychosocial consequences resulting from his/her behaviour and life-style. Every contact with a patient provides a potential opportunity to conduct a brief screening assessment to identify whether a substance misuse problem exists or not. This could be performed as part of general life-style questioning:

❏ Either opportunistically during a routine consultation;
❏ As part of a new patient check; or
❏ During attendance at a special clinic, e.g. well person, travel, chronic disease management.

A comprehensive, simple questionnaire format should be used, such as CAGE (Mayfield *et al.* 1974). Short questions, which avoid jargon and progress from non-threatening to more sensitive issues may be beneficial. Specificity and precision of answers can be encouraged through clarification of points, especially when initial responses are equivocal or vague. Care should be taken to use non judgmental questioning techniques (Carroll 1995) which take into account the particular needs of the individual and practice community with regards to race, religion, culture, gender, sexuality and age.

Outcomes arising from screening

If the screening interview elicits no cause for concern the opportunity may be taken:

- ❑ To reassure the patient that everything appears normal;
- ❑ To reaffirm positive health messages, e.g. sensible drinking limits;
- ❑ To highlight information about services and support systems which may be of benefit in the future;
- ❑ To increase awareness of potentially harmful situations, e.g. alcohol and water sports, drink driving, alcohol and diabetes, polypharmacy.

If problems are identified following initial screening then consideration needs to be given to the need for an in-depth assessment. It may be necessary to discuss the patient with, or refer them to, a colleague or other agency, e.g. GP, Substance Misuse Services or Alcoholics Anonymous (Association of Nurses in Substance Abuse 1997).

In-depth assessment

The in-depth assessment will require time, co-operation, trust and tact. The practice nurse will need to be proficient in both asking open ended questions and reflective listening in an effort to gain insight and elicit detailed information regarding

- ❑ Past and present substance use and treatments;
- ❑ Physical, psychological and social consequences of use;
- ❑ Patient perception and self-awareness of problem.

Outcomes arising from in-depth assessment

Once collected the information will give the practice nurse a clearer notion of the extent of the problem. Depending upon the assessment outcomes, practice policy, availability of resources, the nurse's confidence and competence and the patient's preference, a decision will need to be made as to the most appropriate intervention of care. In cases which appear to require minimal intervention this decision may be made by the practice nurse herself. Other more complex cases may require discussion with practice colleagues and/or local substance misuse services, and a full medical examination by the GP. Clearly not all patients will be suitable for management within the general practice setting, and certain factors may influence the decision making process regarding treatment venue (Association of Nurses in Substance Abuse 1997).

Triage for emergency

Due to the direct accessibility of the practice nurse by the practice population, and the reception staff, she is often the first practitioner that the substance misuser will come into contact with in the event of an emergency. As the practice nurse has little opportunity to prepare herself in advance of the consultation (Hyde 1995), it is vital that prior consideration be given to the formation of policy procedure and agreements. This is particularly important in general practices where the practice nurse may be the only trained health care professional available, at certain times of the day, to respond to a patient's needs.

Life threatening emergencies may range from

❑ Overdose with intoxication or coma
❑ Attempted suicide
❑ Epileptic fits due to alcohol or drug withdrawal
❑ Delirium tremors
❑ Aggravated psychiatric symptoms
❑ Violence and aggression
❑ Abuse
❑ Needle stick injury

Managerial emergencies may include

❑ Lost prescriptions
❑ Non collection of medication
❑ Patients presenting out of hours
❑ Substance misusers presenting as temporary residents
❑ Patients presenting with atypical or unusual pain requesting analgesics

All emergencies will demand competent, safe and appropriate clinical management, as well as diplomatic and tactful handling. Phoning for the emergency services and giving acute care may be the most important response in some cases. Other situations can be managed solely by the GP or in conjunction with other agencies, e.g. Accident and Emergency Department, psychiatric liaison team, child protection staff. All patients undergoing care interventions within the practice should be advised of all relevant policies before commencement of treatment.

Planning care and interventions

Following the in-depth assessment it is necessary to establish the patient's willingness to accept help and to explore his/her readiness to change. By getting the patient to articulate his/her needs, desired goals and outcomes, the practice nurse will have a clearer understanding about what the patient is motivated to consider and/or do. At this preparatory stage of work with the patient it is important to set the boundaries of the working relationship.

Issues which need to be considered include aspects of confidentiality, the use of written contracts regarding the professional's expectations of the patient's behaviour during the treatment stage, methods and duration of review policies and non compliance with negotiated treatment goals, for example lack of attendance.

The practice nurse is well placed to become involved in a number of patient centred interventions, ranging from minimum to maximum involvement, depending upon her level of confidence and competence. These may include

- Raising health awareness
- Health education and provision of information
- Effecting change in patient behaviour
- Support
- Clinical management
- 'Shared care'

Interventions are not mutually exclusive. An experienced practice nurse may find she uses a combination of the above interventions when dealing with individual patients at any given time.

Raising health awareness

The aim of this type of intervention is the prevention of, and/or minimisation of, substance misuse related harm in all patients. Using visual aids and verbal and non verbal cues from patients, the practice nurse can draw attention to health issues relating to substance misuse, forming a possible focus for discussion. By maximising potential opportunities to increase patient knowledge and understanding, the nurse can raise issues relevant to patients particular needs. These may include:

- Prevention of overdose by non mixing of alcohol and drugs;
- Prevention of overdose due to reduced tolerance following abstinence;
- Prevention of infection, HIV/AIDS by advising patients of syringe exchange centres and safe injection techniques;
- Prevention of unwanted side effects due to polypharmacy by providing clear instructions on how to take prescribed medication and checking simultaneous use of over-the-counter medicines and alcohol intake.

Health education and provision of information

The practice nurse may provide verbal and written health education materials on a number of directly and indirectly related substance misuse issues to patients, family and concerned or interested others. A variety of culturally and intellectually sensitive literature should be available including information regarding local self-help groups, free syringe exchange centres and alternative therapy treatments, for example aromatherapy, massage, traditional Chinese medicine, which may be culturally more acceptable to ethnic minority groups (Carins 1997).

Written information to support advice given during consultation should be provided, and could include information about broad based issues, such as dietary advice and healthy eating plans to help avoid accidental overdose in patients suffering from malnourishment (Carins 1997). Opportunities should be harnessed which allow health education activities to be linked with local or national promotions, for example a 'no smoking day', in an effort to reinforce positive health messages.

Effecting changes of behaviour

Everyone finds it difficult to change an established habit and substance misusers are no exception. Simply giving information and advice to a patient will not effect a change in that person's behaviour, although it might do (Wanigaratne *et al.* 1990). The practice nurse may therefore wish to use the Prochaska and DiClemente (1986) model to identify the patient's readiness, in terms of motivation and commitment, to change, thus enabling the choice of a suitable approach to achieve change.

Support

Individual patients will require varying degrees of support over different time scales. This is usually dependent on the patient's overall condition, its severity and their individual responses to support intervention. The practice nurse may also find herself in the situation of supporting members of a patient's family or friends who approach her with a request for advice on how to deal with a specific situation, e.g. strained relationships. While the patient's confidentiality is paramount (Cooper 1994), the nurse may be able to help dispel some negative attitudes, fears and anxieties by increasing knowledge and skills, in the context of specific substances. Where possible the nurse, in conjunction with the patient, should encourage family involvement during the intervention stages in an effort to provide additional support and encouragement towards a more sensible way of life (Wells 1990). The nurse may also find herself in the position of providing support for colleagues, e.g. clinical supervision.

Clinical management

Specific clinical interventions may occur during any consultation with a patient. They may form part of the initial screening process, the on-going treatment stage of a substance misuse disorder or the provision of general medical services. The practice nurse may therefore find herself involved with

❏ The collection and testing of samples, e.g. measurements of liver function and haematological parameters for alcohol misusers or urine toxicology for drug misusers;
❏ Screening for hepatitis B and C and the provision of hepatitis B vaccination;
❏ Supervision of prescribed medication during detoxification programmes;
❏ BMI measurements.

Shared care

Finally, practice nurses may become involved in a number of models providing shared care for patients in the GP setting. These may entail:

❏ Practice nurse clinics – the practice nurse provides care and onward referral to the specialist services when necessary;
❏ Transferred care – the patient is initially assessed by the specialist services and transferred to the GP setting for continued care and treatment;
❏ Specialist nurse led clinics – a named specialist nurse runs a clinic within the GP setting;
❏ GP/practice nurse attachment – the GP/practice nurse works on a sessional basis with the specialist services, thereby increasing their knowledge base and experience with substances misusers;
❏ Part care – the patient receives part of his/her care from the GP setting and part from the specialist services.

The practice nurse may be responsible for the co-ordination and continuity of care for the patient, using agreed treatment policies and protocols set up in collaboration with the GP, the local specialist services and the local medical advisor. This may entail attendance at multi-disciplinary and multi-agency reviews requiring good liaison skills and careful record keeping.

Evaluation

Evaluation and monitoring of intervention strategies should take place at regular intervals in an effort to provide optimum individual, and communal, health care to the practice population. Nurses with the potential for maximum involvement may also provide input for contractual policies and agreements with the various statutory and non statutory services available for substance misuse problems. In an effort to relate theory to practice it would be useful to view the role of the practice nurse in the following two cases.

Case vignette 1

Elsie, a 70 year old widow, was discharged from hospital following surgery for a wrist injury after a recent fall. She also sustained abrasions to her legs and has arrived at the surgery to see the practise nurse for change of dressings. Elsie complains of feeling drowsy and 'showing my age'.

Assessment and interventions

- ❏ Assess injuries.
- ❏ Elicit detailed history of all prescribed medications and self administration of OTC medications and other drugs not indicated from the GP.
- ❏ Check dosage, compliance and efficacy.
- ❏ Enquire about alcohol intake.

Elsie reveals that she has been prescribed night sedation and analgesics from the hospital. She takes her analgesia three times daily, the last dose at bed time with her sleeping tablet. She also admits to taking a 'night cap or two' of whisky to help her relax, 'something I missed in hospital'.

Plan care

- ❏ Discuss with GP, who is to make a detailed assessment/examination of the patient's physical and mental state. Review her medication regime and alcohol intake leading to alternative drugs/alteration of dosages/ cessation of some drugs and/or alcohol for present time.

Intervention

- ❏ Change dressings.
- ❏ Establish Elsie's willingness and motivation to change.
- ❏ Provide clear verbal and written instructions on how to take medications using pre-filled containers, with all drugs to be taken at a specific time.
- ❏ Provide explanations for all actions.

Evaluation

- ❏ Arrange follow up appointments and observe for improvement in overall condition.

Case vignette 2

Richard is 38 years old and attends the surgery for travel advice before going to India on a business trip. He has not attended the surgery for over 4 years.

Assessment

❑ Assess travel health care needs.
❑ Take the opportunity to update the patient's life-style details using the agreed practice screening questionnaire.

Richard admits that his alcohol intake has increased in recent months, since separating from his wife, to about a half bottle of spirits a night. He feels ambivalent about changing his habit as it 'helps him to cope'.

Intervention

❑ Refer to GP for travel immunisation prescriptions, highlighting alcohol intake.
❑ Provide verbal and written information regarding sensible drinking limits and highlight potentially dangerous situations.
❑ Give information about services available at the surgery regarding alcohol reduction/cessation programmes and details of local support groups, to include those dealing with relationship problems.

Richard attends for his travel immunisations and 6 months after his trip returns to the surgery asking for help with his drinking habit.

Second assessment

❑ Establish motivation and commitment.
❑ Set working boundaries.
❑ Establish his drinking pattern and level of dependence using in-depth assessment questionnaire, drinking diaries.
❑ Establish other substance use pattern.
❑ Establish impediments to change, identify triggers to drinking and establish alternatives to drinking.

Plan care

❑ Discuss with GP and refer for physical/clinical examination.

Intervention

☐ Discuss available/alternative treatment regimes and coping strategies.
☐ Dietary/dental advice or referral.
☐ Blood and urine sampling.
☐ Support and liaison.

In addition to his high alcohol intake Richard admits to a daily use of cocaine. After careful consideration, Richard decides to undergo detoxification. As he lives alone, has a drug and alcohol misuse problem and has no family support, he is referred to the specialist services for in-patient care during the detoxification stage of his treatment. The GP agrees to provide support via the counselling service available within the practice and a 'shared care' agreement is arranged with the specialist services. Richard is given clear explanations of the agreement and is given time to discuss his expectations and fears with the practice nurse.

Evaluation

In order to maintain a good relationship with Richard during the treatment phase he is offered the opportunity for regular follow up for clinical testing, discussion of his views and evaluation of continuity of care.

Conclusions

Many practice nurses may feel they are lacking the skills and knowledge required to deal with substance misuse problems, while others may doubt that their intervention will result in behaviour change. Such uncertainty may culminate in stereotyped attitudes towards substances misusers. However, if service delivery is to be effective, these attitudes together with the availability of resources, degree of managerial and colleague support and concerns about educational opportunities need to be addressed. The development of new nursing roles is, in part, legitimised by policies which demand increased and flexible access to health care, improved quality, closer inter- and intraprofessional working and cost effective delivery. By adapting and utilising generic skills, together with sufficient input from continuing educational programmes (Rassool 1993), practice nurses are in a pivotal position to ensure that patients receive a structured and proactive approach to health care relating to substance misuse problems.

Pessimists worried about uncovering problems which could overwhelm already stretched services offered by practice nurses would do well to consider the situation again. The underlying framework for practice nursing is the assessment, planning, organisation and evaluation of patient care (Luft 1994). Patients also have a right to be cared for by skilled and motivated professionals. If practice nurses believe unrealistic expectations are being made of them then they owe it to their patients to voice these opinions in order to influence the development of future policy. Whatever response each individual practice nurse chooses to make, she will be required to justify, measure and evaluate her action in an effort to provide an equitable and high quality service to all patients registered at her surgery.

References

Abed, R.T. & Neira-Munoz, E. (1990). A Survey of general practitioners' opinion and attitude to drug addicts and addiction. *British Journal of Addiction*, **85**, 131–6.

Anderson, P. (1987) Early interventions in general practice. In: *Helping the Problem Drinker: New Initiatives in Community Care* (eds T. Stockwell & S. Clements). Croom Helm, London.

Anderson, P. (1992) Primary care physicians and alcohol. *Journal of the Royal Society of Medicine*, **85**, 478–82.

Association of Nurses in Substance Abuse (1997) *Substance Use: Guidance on Good Clinical Practice for Nurses, Midwives and Health Visitors. Working within the Primary Health Care Teams.* ANSA, London.

Babor, T.F., Ritson, B. & Hodgson, R. (1986) Alcohol related problems in primary health care setting: a review of early intervention strategies. *British Journal of Addiction*, **81**, 23–46.

Carins, N. (1997) Culture shock. *Druglink*, **12**, 1.

Carroll, J. (1995) The negative attitudes of some general nurses towards drug misusers. *Nursing Standard*, **9**, 34.

Cooper, D. (1994) *Alcohol Home Detoxification and Assessment.* Radcliffe Medical Press, Oxford.

Department of Health (1987) *Promoting Better Health.* HMSO, London.

Department of Health (1990) *General Practice in the NHS: A New Contract.* HMSO, London.

Department of Health (1992) *Health of the Nation. A Strategy for Health for England.* HMSO, London.

English National Board. (1990) *Report of the Review Group for the Education and Training for Practice Nursing: The Challenge of Primary Health Care in the 1990s.* ENB, London.

Hyde, V. (1995). Community nursing; a unified discipline? In: *Community Nursing Dimensions and Dilemmas* (eds P. Cain, V. Hyde & E. Howkins), pp. 1–26. Arnold, London.

Kitchens, J.M. (1994) Does this patient have an alcohol problem? *Journal of the American Medical Association*, **272**, 1782–7.

Luft, S. (1994) The dynamics of practice nursing. In: *Nursing in General Practice* (eds S. Luft & M. Smith), pp. 158–86. Chapman & Hall, London.

Mayfield, D., McLeod, G. & Hall, P. (1974) The CAGE questionnaire: validation of a new alcoholism screening instrument. *American Journal of Psychiatry*, **131**, 1121–3.

Office of Population Censuses and Surveys (1995) *Morbidity Statistics from General Practice: Fourth National Study 1991–1992. Series MB5; No. 3.* HMSO, London.

Parker, J. & Gay, M. (1987). Problem drug users known to Bristol general practitioners. *Journal of the Royal College of General Practitioners*, **37**, 260–63.

Paton, A. (1994) *ABC of Alcohol,* 3rd edn. British Medical Journal Publishing Group, London.

Prochaska, J. & DiClemente, C. (1986) Towards a comprehensive model of change. In: *Training Addictive Behaviour: Process of Change* (eds W.R. Miller & N. Heather), Plenum, New York.

Rassool, G.H. (1993) Nursing and substance misuse: responding to the challenge. *Journal of Advanced Nursing,* **18,** 1401-7.

Royal College of Nursing (1991) *Practice Nursing. Leaflet 000195.* RCN, London.

Russell, M.A.H., Stapleton, J.A., Jackson, P.H., *et al.* (1978) District programme to reduce smoking: effect of clinic supported brief interventions by general practitioners. *British Medical Journal,* **295,** 1240-44.

Tettersell, M. & Luft, S. (1994). Lifestyle influences on client health. In: *Nursing in General Practice* (eds S. Luft, & M. Smith), pp. 37-57. Chapman & Hall, London.

Tackling Drugs Together (1995) *Task Force Review.* HMSO, London.

United Kingdom Central Council (1992) *The Scope of Professional Practice.* UKCC, London.

Wanigaratne, S., Wallace, W., Pullin, J., *et al.* (1990) *Relapse Prevention for Addictive Behaviours.* Blackwell Scientific Publications, Oxford.

Wells, B. (1990). Psychosocial interventions. In: *Substance Abuse and Dependence* (eds A.H. Ghodse & D. Maxwell). Macmillan Press, London.

Wenrich, M.D., Paauw, D.S., Carline, J.D., *et al.* (1995) Do primary care physicians screen patients about alcohol intake using the CAGE questions? Cited by Greener, K. (1996) Screening for alcohol abuse. *Practice Nursing,* **17,** 35-7.

Chapter 14

School Nursing and Substance Misuse

Pat Jackson & Judy McRae

Introduction

The school nurse is ideally placed to offer pupils, parents and school staff support and advice relating to substance use and misuse. They have an important role in providing one to one confidential intervention and support to individual pupils as well as small group or whole class health education activities. Schools have a statutory obligation to provide drug and alcohol education within the framework of the National Curriculum, but this is dependent on the individual schools. However, the school nurse can encourage and support schools to develop their drug education policies and related procedures to ensure that a comprehensive and holistic approach is provided to tackle substance use and misuse within and outside the school settings.

This chapter presents a brief overview of the nature and extent of substance misuse in young people. It describes the range of school nurse interventions that are applicable in the school environment. Reference is also made to the framework in which the school nurse must operate. Prior to any intervention of a sensitive nature the school nurse needs to consider their own moral code, their professional code and accountability and the school's code and policies. Case vignettes are used to illustrate specific problems that the school nurse may encounter.

Nature and extent of substance use and misuse

Research has demonstrated that on average nearly 50% of 14–15 year old pupils in school have been offered or have tried some form of illicit substance (Balding 1994; Denman Wright & Pearl 1995; Bagnall & Dilloway 1996). Denman Wright and Pearl (1995) reported on a longitudinal study carried out to monitor young people's knowledge and experience of illicit drugs between 1969 and 1994 at 5 yearly intervals. The study looked at young people's self reported levels of knowledge and experience of illicit drugs. The findings showed that the proportion of 14 to 15 year olds that knew someone taking drugs increased from 15% to 65% and that the proportion who had been offered drugs had increased from 5% to 45%. The most alarming factor was that both of these proportions had more than doubled in the period 1989 to 1994.

An American study involving 20 629 high school students looked at the 'gateway' drug effect, to determine whether there was any relationship between smoking, alcohol consumption and use of illicit substances. The results demonstrated that 20 a day cigarette smokers were three times more likely to drink alcohol and 10 to 30 times more likely to use illicit substances than non smokers (Torabi *et al.* 1993). Balding's (1994) study also makes reference to the 'gateway' effect and suggested that we should prioritise our interventions on alcohol and tobacco use in young people, as this is likely to reduce the attraction of illicit drugs. No single theory offers an explanation as to why young people take drugs. However, there is evidence that suggests that peer group pressure is a strong influencing factor (Rassool 1993; Balding 1994).

Adolescence is essentially a period in the life-span in which the individual, previously dependent on parents and carers for the development of his/her values and identity, seeks independence and attempts to establish a new and personal identity (Holt 1993). For Holt an important part of this development is risk taking behaviour such as participation in dangerous sports and experimentation with drugs and alcohol. DeBell & Wales (1996) describe a hierarchy of danger where adolescent perceptions of risk are concerned. The risk associated with behaviour is related to either short or long trem dangers. Smoking therefore poses a lower health risk in the short term than taking, say, Ecstasy, which in turn poses a lower health risk than unprotected sexual intercourse. This is an important factor to consider when developing any health promotion strategies aimed at young people.

School health service

Today, the school health service is generally accepted to be school nurse led. The aim of the service is to promote health among children and young people by working in partnership with pupils, parents, education and other agencies. The link with education is a crucial one as it is desirable to bring health and education together if children are to make optimum academic progress (Narracott *et al.* 1996).The majority of schools in the UK will have access to a school nurse. However, given that there is no nationally agreed strategy for the school nursing service, the amount and type of contact for each school will vary. Still the role of the school nurse in relation to drug misuse interventions can and should be defined.

The National Curriculum

Since the introduction of the National Curriculum in 1989 schools have had a statutory duty to provide drugs education within core subject areas, namely the science orders. In 1995 the revised National Curriculum was introduced for key stages 1, 2 and 3 and in 1996 for key stage 4; this still retains the duty on schools to provide drugs education at all four key stages within the science curriculum. The statutory duty on schools requires the following sequence to be taught:

- ❑ Key stage 1 (infant school) 'the role of drugs and medicines';
- ❑ Key stage 2 (junior school) 'that tobacco, alcohol and other drugs can have harmful effects';
- ❑ Key stage 3 (lower secondary) 'that the abuse of alcohol, solvents and other drugs affects health', 'that the body's natural defence may be enhanced by immunisation and medicines' and 'how smoking affects lung structure and gas exchange';
- ❑ Key stage 4 (upper secondary) 'the effects of solvent, alcohol, tobacco and other drugs on the body' (Department for Education 1995a).

The government's white paper Tackling Drugs Together (1995) sets out a national strategy for interventions relating to drugs misuse in which schools clearly have a vital role.

Role of the school nurse

School nurses are ideally placed to be a resource for children, parents and teachers providing research based child health related advice on a variety of topics. The role of the school nurse is unique in that the nurse can work individually with children and young people alongside and with their families, and in the classroom in partnership with teachers. The NHS Health Advisory Service put forward a proposal for a four tier model for substance use and misuse services for children and adolescents (Health Advisory Service 1996). The role of the school nurse can be identified in tier 1:

> 'Services are those which are accessible directly by the general public and which provide a first response to the needs of children and adolescents. They include education, preventative work and treatment. Service components includes the provision of information and advice in uncomplicated situations and the conduct of initial assessments of personal need and they are also important in providing advice and information to parents and schools.'

Every school age child should have access to a school nurse. The school provides an ideal opportunity for population based health interventions as the target audience is captive. The school nurse is also accessible to parents and individual school staff. The role of the school nurse in relation to substance misuse interventions is threefold:

- ❑ Pupil focused: by offering one to one support and advice and referring on to appropriate agencies as necessary;

❏ School focused: by assisting schools in the development and implementation of drug related policies and participating in school based health promotion programmes;

❏ Community focused: by acting as the 'link' health worker the school nurse provides the link between the school, home and the community; the school nurse also acts as a resource to the school in helping the school to establish links with other sources of 'expert' advice.

School nurse interventions

Pupil focused school nurse interventions in relation to drugs use and misuse can be seen to focus predominantly on adolescents. The intervention is likely to be delivered in one to one or small group settings, as well as in supporting health promotion programmes within the classroom. For the majority of primary school age children, their needs relating to raising awareness about drugs and substance misuse might be addressed within the classroom and in the context of the health promoting school (Wetton & McWhirter 1995) working with interagency collaboration.

A report published by the British Paediatric Association (1995) recommends that young people should be offered at least one general health check with the school nurse between the ages of 11 and 14 years. This should be seen as an opportunity to encourage young people to begin to take responsibility for their own health. The management of the individual's health career shifts from the parent to the young person and it is important that the young person is able to identify their own health needs. One initiative that has been developed to support this developmental process is the introduction of a pupil held health record 'health fax'. The record has been designed as a tool for health promotion messages specifically related to young people (McAleer & Jackson 1994; Jackson 1996).

The health interview provides an opportunity for one to one health promotion and discussion of issues and concerns raised by the young person as well as topical issues which have been identified in the school health profile (Department of Health 1994). Good practice can be identified if the young person and parent/carer fill in a general health questionnaire before the health interview. This is a useful way of introducing issues related to healthy life-styles and, in the interview, is a means of investigating in more depth the young person's perceptions and specific health needs (Bagnall & Dilloway 1996). Health interviews also provide a forum for young people to disclose any concerns and experiences of substance use. Health advice given to young people should be related to them as individuals and should focus on what is relevant to young people. Young people are concerned with the here and now and any long term health effects from risk taking behaviour are not likely to be heard (Royal College of General Practitioners 1996).

As well as structured health interviews young people should be offered the opportunity to seek advice and support by the provision of 'drop in' sessions by the school nurse. 'Drop ins' or 'open door' initiatives can be held in schools at break times or at the start or end of the school day. These are self referral sessions where the young person can seek out the school nurse for a variety of reasons. If the school nurse cannot offer the appropriate advice, she may need to refer the young person to another agency, with the young person's consent. When a young person independently seeks professional advice to resolve a problem, it may be an indication that they are beginning to take responsibility for their own health careers. (Department of Health 1994).

School nurses working with young people are in the privileged position of being able to work in schools and link with both pupils and teachers while remaining separate from the school's management structure. As registered nurses, school nurses have a duty to adhere to the UKCC Code of Professional Conduct which requires nurses to respect confidentiality obtained in professional practice and disclose such information only with the client's consent. However, the same document states that breaches of confidentiality in the public interest should only occur after much professional consideration and judgment. Therefore, if a school nurse suspects a young person is seeking advice on matters which are a consequence of exploitation or abuse of drugs, the school nurse may decide to disclose the information in order to protect the young person from further harm. It is good practice to counsel the young person and persuade the young person to agree to the disclosure (Brook Advisory 1996). The authors recommend that this clarification on confidentiality takes place with young people before discussions on advice.

It is this clarification on confidentiality that can often be the lynch pin to young people seeking advice from the school nurse. Young people will be reassured that any information will be treated in confidence. However, it is also important to remember that young people cannot be treated wholly as adults (Kelly 1991). Young people lack the emotional maturity to cope with independence and still need the emotional support of parents or other carers. The school nurse, therefore, should use the skills of assessment and facilitation to empower the young person to use advice/information appropriately.

Health education

The skills required for the delivery of drugs education in the classroom are transferable skills which can be used for the delivery of health education in relation to other topics. However, the knowledge base is different. It is important that teachers realise that the school nurse is not usually a qualified teacher but by virtue of his/her training has a particular expertise that will complement the skills and knowledge of teaching staff for effective classroom delivery of health education. The Department of Health

(1996) has recognised the contribution that school nurses can make in supporting school based health education programmes but also stresses that school nurses should not teach classes on their own.

School nurses should be part of a team delivering a planned and co-ordinated drugs education programme in the school setting which is led by the teaching staff (Department for Education 1996b; South Thames Regional Health Authority 1996). School nurses should not be involved in drugs education if they do not themselves feel comfortable talking about the subject. Neither should school nurses be coerced into providing 'one off' sessions to pupils. School nurses who are participating as part of a team should also be aware of the school's drug education policy and acknowledge any possible conflict with their own professional accountability.

School policies

The government White Paper, Tackling Drugs Together (1995) further requires schools to develop policies relating to drugs education and dealing with drug incidents in school. School policies in relation to drugs should not only focus on how, when, what and by whom drugs education should be delivered in the classroom but should also be developed in context with other related policies. Drugs education is about the whole ethos of the school and what is taught in the classroom should have relevance to the day to day conduct of the school. The school nurse is a key player in assisting schools to develop policies and is able to demonstrate to schools the link between such policies, the whole school ethos and ultimately academic achievement.

The Department for Education and Employment (1996) has issued guidance to schools on the management of prescribed and non prescribed legal medicines in school. The issue of administering medication in school has for most teaching staff been a source of considerable debate and anxiety – to the extent that some pupils may be denied access to school if they are taking medication for a short period of time or even denied total access to the school of their choice if they require medication for a chronic condition. If we are to teach children and young people that some drugs are necessary for health maintenance then we need to ensure that what is taught is borne out in school practice.

Smoking policies

Smoking policies in schools should also reflect what is taught in the classroom. Schools should adopt a 'smoke free zone' principle which applies to staff and visitors to the school and operates both within and out of buildings. If we are to take what was stated earlier in that research has demonstrated that attitudes and behaviour relating to smoking or alcohol have a direct influence on the use of other illicit substances, then a school's policy on smoking should be seen as a priority.

Drug policies: alcohol and illicit substances

Schools need to consider as well their role in dealing with drug related incidents in the school. Confidentiality needs to be explicitly dealt with in any policy as does the legal obligations of staff and their 'duty of care' in respect of pupils.

Case vignettes

A 15 year old girl goes to see the school nurse at the start of the afternoon lessons. The girl has taken an overdose of paracetamol at lunch time. She is also distressed about her parents being told. The following should be considered:

❑ Immediate medical treatment
❑ Confidentiality – who needs to know?
❑ Advocacy
❑ Long term support

Several children in a primary school are asthmatic. Their inhalers are kept in a locked cupboard in the head teacher's office. The school nurse is planning to raise awareness of asthma with the school staff. The following should be considered:

❑ Development of a school asthma policy
❑ Staff training on asthma and asthma medication
❑ Inhaler access for all pupils
❑ An asthma club to include parents
❑ Children's right to confidentiality

A 14 year old boy was caught playing truant from school. The school arranged a meeting with the boy's parents to inform them of their son's behaviour. The boy refused to discuss the situation with the teacher and his parents. Later the boy went to see the school nurse and disclosed that he was sniffing solvents because other boys were making him do it! He was staying away from school to avoid the other boys in his class. He felt the punishment from his parents for playing truant was preferable to the punishment for 'glue sniffing'. Consider the following:

❑ The rights of the child
❑ The welfare of the child
❑ What do the parents need to be told?
❑ What does the school need to be told?

❏ School policy on bullying
❏ Long term support for the boy

Conclusions

The school nursing service provides a primary generic service to what is essentially a healthy school age population, a population that starts school having barely left babyhood and leaves school on the brink of adulthood, a population where there is enormous potential to influence and inform. The school nurse, in recognising his/her role in relation to substance use and misuse, must also recognise their limitations. Some areas are developing a team approach to school nursing to enable skills to be used more effectively. This enables school nurses to develop specialist roles in addition to their generic role. All school nurses should have basic training in substance use with regular updating. The addition of a school nurse with specialist training in substance use would be a useful asset to schools within the team's catchment area and to school nursing colleagues.

References

Balding, J. (1994) Young people and drug-taking: facts and trends. *Education and Health*, **12**, 4.

British Paediatric Association (1995) *Report of a Joint Working Party on Health Needs of School Age Children*. The Polnay Report. BPA, London.

Brook Advisory Service (1996) *What should I do?* BAS, London.

DeBell, D. & Wales, H. (1996) Teenage smoking. *British Journal of Community Health Nursing*, **1**, 235–40.

Denman Wright, J. & Pearl, L. (1995) Knowledge and experience of young people regarding drug misuse 1969–1994. *British Medical Journal*, **310**, 20–24.

Department for Education and School Curriculum Assessment Authority (1995a) *Drug Education: Curriculum Guidance for Schools*. DFE, London.

Department for Education (1995b) *Drug Prevention in Schools*. Circular Number 4/ 95. HMSO, London.

Department for Education and Employment (1996) *Reporting children with medical needs. Circular 14/96*. HMSO, London.

Department of Health (1994) *Negotiating School Health Services*. HMSO, London.

Department of Health (1996) *Child Health in the Community NHS Executive*. HMSO, London.

Jackson, P. (1996) Health facts. A pupil held health record. *Health Education*, **96**, 8–10.

Health Advisory Service (1996) *Children and Young People Substance Misuse Services*. HMSO, London.

Holt, L. (1993) The adolescent in accident and emergency. *Nursing Standard*, **8**, 8.

Kelly, J. (1991) Caring for adolescents. *Professional Nurse*, **6**(9), 498–501.

McAleer, M. & Jackson, P. (1994) The school health fax. *Nursing Times*, **19**, 29–31.

Narracott, L., Gatehouse, D. & Baird, L. (1996) Top of the class. *Nursing Standard*, **10**, 25–6.

Rassool, G.H. (1993) Adolescents and street drugs: issues for community nurses. *Professional Care of Mother and Child*, **3**, 292–3.

Royal College of General Practitioners (1996) *Review of Teenage Health: Time for a New Direction. The Health of Adolescents in Primary Care.* RCGP, London.

South Thames Regional Health Authority (1996) *Opportunities for Health and Education to Work Together.* NHS Executive. STRHA, London.

Tackling Drugs Together (1995) *A Strategy for England 1995–1998.* HMSO, London.

Torabi, M.R., Bailey, W.J. & Majd-Jabbari, M. (1993) Cigarette smoking as a predictor of alcohol and other drug use by children and adolescents: evidence of the 'gateway' drug effect. *Journal of School Health*, **63**, 302–7.

Wetton, N. & McWhirter, J. (1995) *Health for Life: A Guide for Health Promoting Schools.* Forbes Publications, London.

Chapter 15

Substance Misuse in the Accident & Emergency Department

Fiona Jeffcock

Introduction

There are many different substances which may be misused. Those which may be presented in an Accident & Emergency (A&E) department include alcohol, drugs such as heroin and methadone (injecting), street drugs such as Ecstasy (MDMA) and cannabis, and oral prescription drugs which are misused such as hemineverin, temazepam and dihydracodeine (DF118). A&E departments are often the first place attended by patients with acute problems related to substance misuse. While there are those who have not taken a psychoactive substance intentionally, where a drink has been 'spiked', the majority have taken the substance with the intention of gaining a pleasurable effect from it. It is relatively uncommon for patients to present following single substance misuse; multiple substance misuse is the more regular occurrence.

This chapter aims to give an introduction to substance misuse as seen in the A&E department of general hospitals. It will cover the range of patients presenting following substance misuse, with the care and treatment they receive. The problems encountered by both the patients and the staff will be discussed as will the way forward in A&E departments.

Perception of health care professionals

Many health care professionals view those who misuse substances of any variety as a 'nuisance' and they are frequently labelled as such. Labelling a patient contributes to felt stigma and can reduce their feelings of self-worth and self-esteem within the community (Goffman 1963). Doctors and nurses have been overheard saying 'not another overdose', while being stretched on a busy and stressful shift. Some patients do not receive the sympathetic care they want, especially when it is a frequent attender with repeated misuse.

Patients who are likely to receive a sympathetic reception in A&E are the elderly who have attempted suicide using prescription medication.

These cases are perceived as being 'genuine' and requiring maximum nursing and medical care to prevent repeated attempts. The elderly are often alone, having been bereaved and lost long term partners, or they may be suffering from a chronic debilitating illness and can take the constant suffering no longer (Toulson 1996). Many health care professionals can 'see' relatives of their own when nursing patients and are, in the main, more sympathetic. Those receiving the least sympathy are patients who attend following the use of excess intravenous heroin, methadone or those who were using other street drugs to 'experiment'. These are usually younger people ranging from late teens to middle age (Gibbs 1990).

Dealing with an emergency

Patients who inject too much heroin or methadone may stop breathing and have a respiratory arrest, or they may become unconscious. These patients are life threatening emergencies who arrive as priorities via the ambulance service, with a courtesy call to warn of the impending arrival. This enables a department to prepare for the patient's arrival, with both medical and nursing personnel ready to receive them. Naloxone (the reversal agent) is administered by either the paramedics or the doctors at the hospital. This reverses the effect of the opiate. If the patient has had a respiratory arrest then basic life support is necessary until the naloxone takes effect. Once the patient has been roused they may become aggressive; reversing the drug also gives them withdrawal effects.

When patients become abusive and sometimes violent the police are called as protection for the staff and the other patients and to restrain the violent patient. This reduces the capacity of many doctors and nurses to be sympathetic. A patient may have had his or her life saved by a team only to then threaten them verbally or physically.

Presenting at the A&E department

The patients presenting to A&E departments are wide ranging both in age and background. Some are from the higher social classes in full time employment, while others are unemployed and homeless. The age range of those seen is generally from late teens to the late 60s; while there are those who are outside this age range, they are the exception rather than the rule. There appears to be an equal mix of males and females presenting to the department following substance misuse. Patients presenting in this way to A&E departments are seen immediately as it is life threatening; this may mean that others with urgent but not life threatening conditions are made to wait, and some may be in considerable pain.

Alcohol is often a contributing factor in many of those who attend an A&E department (Keech 1992). Alcohol intoxication may be related to more than just medical problems. Alcohol is known to be a contributing factor in social and psychological problems and it may also have legal implications. Socially the patient may become isolated due to their behaviour or drinking habits; domestic violence and potential child abuse and neglect may be involved. Following on from social isolation, the patient may become depressed and suicidal as a result. Legally, issues surrounding theft to pay for either a drug or alcohol problem may result in court appearances (Kennedy & Faugier 1989). There has been a marked increase in the number of patients attending A&E departments following misuse of a psychoactive substance. This may be due to the accessibility of alcohol and drugs on the streets. The mortality and morbidity of alcohol related problems are alarming and are on the increase (Suokas & Lonnqvist 1995). Alcohol has been shown to be a contributing factor in 61% of serious head injuries, while one in three drivers who are killed in road traffic accidents are recorded as being over the legal limit for blood alcohol levels (Keech 1992).

Many people who take an overdose present to A&E; they may be presenting of their own accord or after being encouraged by friends or family. A large proportion of these attendances occur during the evening or night. This may be due to the limited availability of voluntary organisations at these times; in addition many GPs now use deputising services and patients may not want to see a 'stranger'.

There are some patients who genuinely have taken an overdose accidentally. This most commonly occurs when someone experiences severe pain, often toothache or headache, and then takes more than the recommended dose of analgesia. When they present to A&E they usually are asking for stronger pain relief and are astonished that they have taken what constitutes an overdose and may need active treatment. The majority of those taking an overdose are intentional, as either a cry for help or a serious suicide attempt. Those who are desperate for help usually attend the department within an hour of taking the tablets or substance, after contacting a friend and telling them what has happened. The more serious attempts are sometimes only found by chance as a friend calls round and may find them unconscious and unrousable; these patients usually arrive by ambulance, whereas the others will often self present.

Types of patients

Those who take psychoactive substances are liable to fall into one of three categories: experimental, recreational or dependent. A&E departments see patients who are in all the above categories. Due to the wide variety of patients presenting to A&E, it is only possible to describe briefly in the following sections substance misusers attending the service.

Detoxification

Patients with long standing alcohol problems may present to A&E with a wish to be admitted. Depending on the hospital, those patients admitted are either placed on the general wards under the care of the physicians or on the psychiatric unit with psychiatric input. Patients admitted to the psychiatric wards often feel that there is a stigma associated with the admission and prefer the general wards for their treatment. Being admitted to a general medical ward normalises the problem and makes it more acceptable in the patient's mind.

Many patients arrive requesting detoxification while still under the influence of alcohol. These patients are seen by the medical practitioner but are told that they will not be admitted while under the influence of alcohol. Those who are serious about detoxifying are advised to see their GP the following day or return to the department in a state of sobriety. Normally the psychiatrists will not assess patients who are under the influence of alcohol, as their mental state cannot be properly ascertained (Walsh 1996).

Withdrawal

Patients may present at any time with a critical condition which is further complicated by alcohol withdrawal while they are treated in hospital. If the withdrawal is not managed well in hospital, the patient may self discharge in order to satisfy their need for alcohol. This creates a downward spiral as the diseased organ is not given a chance to repair and 'heal' and is subsequently damaged further by more alcohol. To assist with this the patient is often prescribed chlormethiazole (hemineverin) and/or diazepam orally or intravenously to counteract the withdrawal symptoms and unpleasant side effects which may be experienced.

Non compliance

A&E staff face an ethical dilemma when a patient either refuses treatment or leaves the department while considered at risk to themselves. Many hospitals have local policies to deal with this. This may include informing hospital security, the hospital manager, the patient's relatives and the police. The police will often help to find a patient although the patient may still refuse to return to the department. In certain circumstances, a patient may be put under a section of the mental health act which allows treatment to be enforced; however, this occurs only rarely.

Intoxicated with head injuries

Patients who are bought to A&E while intoxicated are often suffering from an injury. Those who cause most concern to the staff are patients with a head injury who are also drunk. Their actions may be inappropriate, their speech slurred and their recorded observations may alter, but this may be due to either the alcohol or the head injury (Flemming 1991). Misjudging this situation could cost someone their life. It is important for nurses and medical staff at all times not to treat these patients as drunks but rather as potentially life threatening head injuries. Their neurological observations should be recorded regularly and medical staff alerted if a deterioration is noted. It is also important to check their blood sugar reading (BMstix) at regular intervals as this can drop with intoxication.

Nursing care

All patients who attend A&E departments have a right to a certain standard of nursing care regardless of their complaint. However, some patients do not receive this and they are the ones who have misused either drugs or alcohol or both. Patients need to be considered as individuals and their needs assessed accordingly on their arrival at A&E departments. Patients may not always require active medical treatment but rather need quality time talking to another individual who happens to be a professional. Those who take an overdose as a cry for help always have an underlying problem.

All patients who arrive in A&E are assessed by either the triage nurse or another designated to meeting patients arriving by ambulance. A brief history is taken and a triage category is given. Under new British Association of Emergency Medicine (BAEM) (1997) guidelines this will be one of five categories, 1–5. Category 1 is the most urgent and 5 is the least. The triage category given is a statement of the urgency required for the patient as assessed by an experienced nurse. If an overdose has been taken, the triage category is usually 2 or 3 depending on what exactly has been taken. There are obviously exceptions, those requiring immediate resuscitation would be in category 1.

Once a patient is taken to a cubicle, a named nurse is responsible for a more detailed nursing assessment. This includes further history on what was taken, the quantity and when, also whether any alcohol was ingested. Although the patient has already given the history once to the ambulance crew or the triage nurse, it is usual to gain it a second time. This is to ensure that the stories match and the most accurate information is obtained regarding the quantity and time of the overdose. A baseline set of observations is always recorded so any deviation may be seen and recognised at a later time, which could indicate that the patient's condition is deteriorating. A BMstix and an ECG may also be recorded depending on the overdose.

Once a full history has been obtained the named nurse may recategorise the patient's priority. The National Poisons Unit is then contacted for advice on the recommended treatment and management of the patient. This advice is carefully documented on the patient's records for the doctor to use when planning the patient's management. The doctor will then see the patient and the appropriate treatment will be given. If the patient does not require admission on medical grounds, then their mental state is assessed by the A&E doctor. If the patient is thought to be actively suicidal, or it is during normal weekday working hours, the psychiatrist or the liaison community psychiatric nurse will be asked to come and assess the patient. Out of hours, the psychiatrist will always see the patient if they are actively suicidal. Those who are considered not to be at risk are discharged home with relatives or a friend and followed up in the community by the psychiatric liaison team. Follow up after an overdose is important as it concentrates on the psychological aspects rather than the physical (Lindars 1991). It has been shown that approximately 20% of those who attempt suicide will try again and 10% of them will be successful (O'Shea *et al.* 1986). The following two case vignettes illustrate the type of patients presenting at A&E departments, followed by nursing interventions.

Case vignette 1

Mr J, aged 36, presented to A&E at 3 am following a seizure at home in bed. He had a history of drinking a bottle of whiskey each day. Mr J appeared to have been having marital problems and had recently been issued with an ultimatum by his wife: 'give up the drink or I will leave you'. Following this, Mr J stopped drinking suddenly, within 48 hours he had an epileptic seizure and was bought to the department by the ambulance service. His wife followed shortly after in the car.

On arrival at A&E he was alert but disorientated and appeared very anxious about what had happened as he had no recall of the event. His vital signs were recorded; at this time his pulse was noted to be raised as was his blood pressure. His skin was cold and clammy and he was sweating profusely. His vital signs were recorded half hourly following his initial assessment. Mr J did not admit to the nursing staff on initial assessment that he had a drinking problem. The history of his drinking was gained from the ambulance personnel and his wife once she arrived. After examination by the doctor, blood samples were taken and intravenous access was gained. As Mr J was tachycardic an ECG was recorded at the doctor's request and he was wired to a cardiac monitor for continual monitoring of his heart rate and rhythm. Mr J was prescribed oral hemineverin tablets to help reduce his level of anxiety and his withdrawal symptoms. These were administered and appeared to have an effect after a short period of time. Once the blood results were available it became apparent that Mr J had poor renal function. He was commenced on a crystalloid intravenous infusion and referred to the on-call medical team. Following further assessment by the medical team he was admitted to a general medical ward for detoxification and careful observation of his renal function.

Mr J was fortunate in having the support of his family during what was a very difficult period. He had relied on alcohol for a number of years and required emotional support in conjunction with the physical support he received while on the ward. He was subsequently discharged from the hospital and was able to return home with support from his family, general practitioner and staff in the out-patients department.

Case vignette 2

Mr S was brought to the A&E department by the ambulance service following a priority call. His history was obtained from an accompanying friend who informed the staff that the casualty had taken an overdose. On arrival in A&E Mr S was unconscious. He was tolerating a guedel airway to maintain a patent airway; 100% oxygen was administered using a mask and reservoir bag. The paramedics had inserted a cannula into his arm for intravenous access prior to their arrival in the department. His Glasgow coma score was 3, there was no response to painful stimuli and there was no limb movement or verbal response. Mr S was hypotensive and bradycardic with a respiratory rate of 12 breaths per minute.

The friend informed the staff that Mr S had admitted on the phone to taking unknown quantities of paracetamol 500 mg, dothiepin 75 mg and diazepam 5mg tablets. The National Poisons Unit was contacted for advice and it recommended that a gastric lavage be performed. As Mr S was unconscious and without a gag reflex, an anaesthetist was called to intubate him to prevent aspiration of gastric contents while the washout was being performed. Following this procedure Mr S was referred to the duty medical team for admission. Initially, routine blood samples were taken for urea and electrolytes, a full blood count, and clotting screen; 4 hours following ingestion of the tablets, paracetamol and salicylate levels were taken. Paracetamol and salicylate levels are routinely taken on all overdose patients at 4 hours post ingestion as the levels are most accurate at this time. On the basis of this information a set standard is followed as to whether the antidote acetylcysteine (parvolex) is required for paracetamol overdoses. Mr S was known to be a heavy drinker and therefore more at risk from the effects of the paracetamol than those who have normal liver function.

Mr S was admitted to a general medical ward and kept under close observation until his mental state was assessed. Following assessment by the psychiatrist 2 days later Mr S was transferred to the psychiatric ward for further assessment and treatment.

Conclusions

Nurses are often accused of not treating patients with drug and alcohol problems in a caring and sympathetic manner, particularly when deliberate self-harm is also involved (Van den Bent-Kelly 1992). These patients are all humans and deserve every chance at leading a full and enjoyable life. Everyone experiences moments of despair, for some these become overwhelming and result in self-destructive behaviour.

Nurses are in an ideal situation to listen and spend time with those who self harm or have drug and alcohol problems. It may then lead on to those patients being able to discuss their problems and seek the necessary and appropriate help and therefore assisting with preventative measures (Kennedy & Faugier 1989; Rassool & Gafoor 1997). There needs to be an awareness of non-verbal communication to avoid a patient feeling worthless and a problem to staff and consequently labelled as 'being dif-ficult' (Bentley 1988). Work undertaken by Wright (1986) shows that staff 'need to explore their own feelings about life and death and attitudes to deliberate self-harm, then they can work with the patient objectively and effectively'. We only have one chance; life is not a rehearsal, it is for real. Everyone deserves to be treated with compassion and consideration regardless of the problem.

References:

Bentley, J. (1988) Body language: non-verbal communication and the nurse. *Nursing Standard*, **2**, 30–32.

Flemming, J. (1991) Alcohol-induced head injury. *Nursing Times*, **87**, 29–31.

Gibbs, A. (1990) Aspects of communication with people who have attempted suicide. *Journal of Advanced Nursing*, **15**, 1245–9.

Goffman, E. (1963) *Stigma: Notes on the Management of Spoiled Identity*. Penguin Books, London.

Keech, D.(1992) Drinking safely. *Nursing*, **88**, 5.

Kennedy, J. & Faugier, J. (1989) *Drugs and Alcohol Dependency Nursing*. Heinemann Nursing, London.

Lindars, J. (1991) Holistic care in parasuicide. *Nursing Times*, **87**, 15.

O'Shea, B., Falvey, J. & McCollam, C. (1986) Aspects of deliberate self-harm. *British Journal of Hospital Medicine*, **35**, 335–7.

Rassool, G.H. & Gafoor, M. (1997) *Addiction Nursing: Perspectives on Professional and Clinical Practice*. Stanley Thornes, Cheltenham.

Suokas, J. & Lonnqvist, J. (1995) Suicide attempts in which alcohol is involved: a special group in general hospital emergency rooms. *Acta Psychiatrica Scandinavia*, **91**, 36–40.

Toulson, S. (1996) The right to die: the dilemma for A&E nurses. *Professional Nurse*, **11**, 7.

Van den Bent-Kelly, D. (1992) Too busy for trivia. *Nursing*, **5**, 5.

Walsh, M. (1996) *Accident and Emergency Nursing, a New Approach*, 3rd edn. Butterworth-Heinemann , Oxford.

Wright, B. (1986) *Caring in Crisis: A Handbook of Intervention Skills for Nurses*. Churchill Livingstone, Edinburgh.

Chapter 16

HIV, Hepatitis and Substance Misuse

Helen Pritchitt and Andrew Mason

Introduction

Substance misusers with HIV or hepatitis have complex physical, mental and social problems and may be in contact with specialist drug, mental health, primary care and acute hospital services. Drug users are usually infected with HIV by sharing injecting equipment and can also be infected through unsafe sex while under the influence of drugs or from prostitution to fund a drug habit (Jaquet 1992). Substance misusers may already have a compromised immune system due to drug use, malnutrition or sleep deprivation and are more susceptible to endocarditis, hepatitis, tuberculosis and bacterial pneumonia leading to increased mortality even in non HIV infected individuals. Symptoms experienced by injecting drug users with HIV can differ from those experienced by other groups. For example, injecting drug users have a higher incidence of pulmonary tuberculosis, pneumocystis pneumonia and cryptococcal disease than gay men, and are less likely to have cytomeglovirus, Kaposi's sarcoma or *Herpes simplex* (Friedland & Selwyn 1990). Women injecting drug users with HIV have a higher incidence of sexually transmitted diseases (STDs) and cervical abnormalities (Brimlow 1994). Septicaemia, endocarditis and pneumonia may be five times higher in HIV positive injecting drug users and mortality rates up to six times higher (Selwyn *et al.*, 1988).

The aims of the chapter are to examine the problems associated with HIV, hepatitis and tuberculosis in relation to substance misuse. A brief overview of the nature and extent, disease process, treatment, infection control, testing, counselling and health education issues are presented. The role of the health care professional and the assessment and management of drug users in non specialist units are addressed. A case vignette is included to illustrate the health needs of substance misusers with HIV.

Nature and extent of HIV infection

According to the World Health Organization (WHO), it is estimated that more than 3 million people worldwide have acquired immunodeficiency syndrome (AIDS) (WHO 1994). This figure, however, does not take into account:

❑ Those who have not been reported
❑ Those who have AIDS, but have not been diagnosed
❑ People who are HIV positive and are asymptomatic
❑ Those untested for the HIV virus

The WHO (1993) estimates that 10 million people are HIV positive and that by the year 2000 up to 40 million people will be infected. The majority of HIV infection is seen in sub-Saharan Africa and developing countries where it is spread by heterosexual contact. In developed countries the majority of people with HIV infection have been homosexual men. However, there has been a rise in the number of people who have acquired the virus through heterosexual contact (Pratt 1995). In the UK 6% (881) of people who have been diagnosed as having AIDS were injecting drug users and 11% (1235) of HIV positive people are from this group. There are regional variations; for example, infections attributed to injecting drug use account for 36% of AIDS cases in Scotland but only 4% of those in England (PHLS Communicable Disease Surveillance Centre 1996). Numbers of injecting drug users in the UK with AIDS are low compared with some European countries, e.g. France, Spain and Italy (Gossop 1993).

HIV disease

HIV is a retrovirus that attacks CD4 host cell receptors. These receptors are found on macrophages, microglial cells and, most importantly, certain lymphocytes (T4 – helper cells). The HIV replicates within the cell and then destroys it. Over a period of time the immune system becomes so damaged that the infected person becomes susceptible to opportunistic infections and unusual tumours. At this stage the person has a diagnosis of AIDS.

Transmission

HIV is transmitted in five ways:

❑ Unprotected vaginal or anal intercourse
❑ Sharing contaminated needles and syringes
❑ Transfusion of contaminated blood and blood products
❑ Organ transplantation or artificial insemination
❑ From mother to baby *in utero*, at birth or via breast feeding

Disease progression

Although HIV disease progresses at different rates in individual patients it is possible to categorise the stages of disease progression:

(1)   Seroconversion illness – some people may have an acute flu like illness 2–6 weeks after being infected with HIV. A few may experience more severe symptoms such as encephalitis or meningitis. Seroconversion illness is related to the production of detectable antibodies to HIV. However, a number of people will not experience any symptoms at seroconversion.

(2)   Asymptomatic infection – during this period, which usually lasts 10–15 years (Pratt 1995) people are free of symptoms and are often unaware that they are HIV positive. The virus, however, continues to replicate and damage the immune system.

(3)   Symptomatic infection – due to immune dysfunction people may present with a variety of signs and symptoms including night sweats, fever, weight loss, diarrhoea, fatigue and lymphadenopathy. Laboratory abnormalities include:
  ❏ CD4 count less than the normal level of 200
  ❏ high viral load
  ❏ thrombocytopenia
  ❏ anaemia
  ❏ lymphopaenia

(4)   Late stage disease (AIDS) – at this stage patients present with a variety of infections, not usually seen in people with a competent immune system, known as opportunistic infections. They may also present with unusual tumours (see Table 16.1).

Table 16.1 Opportunistic infections and unusual tumours which may occur in patients with late stage AIDS.

Bacterial	Viral	Fungal	Protozoal	Tumour
Mycobacterial tuberculosis	Papovaviruses	*Candida*	*Pneumocystis carrini*	Kaposi's sarcoma
Mycobacterium avium complex	Cytomeglovirus	*Cryptococcus*	Toxoplasmosis	Non Hodgkin's lymphoma
Salmonella	Herpes (*Herpes simplex and Herpes zoster*)	*Aspergillus*	*Cryptosporidium* *Isospora*	
Shigella				Cervical cancer

There is no cure for HIV nor is there a vaccine against it. At the present time, it is accepted that people with HIV will become symptomatic and die of an AIDS related condition. There have, however, been advances in care and management and the prognosis of someone with HIV has improved considerably. This improvement has been brought about first by the use of prophylaxis against pneumocystis carinni pneumonia and other opportunistic infections. Second, combination anti retroviral therapy including protease inhibitors has been shown to reduce viral load and improve life expectancy (King 1996). However, despite these advances, HIV remains an incurable, often chronic terminal condition with periods of relative well being interrupted with periods of ill health and possible hospitalisation.

Testing

HIV testing can take place in a number of settings including genitourinary (GUM) clinics, GP surgeries, drug units, antenatal clinics and acute hospitals. People are tested for a number of reasons. Some come forward for testing if they feel they may have been at risk of contracting HIV and women are offered testing at antenatal clinics. Patients may present with symptoms that relate to immunodeficiency and HIV testing may be indicated in order to plan appropriate care, treatment and management. Guidelines on pre- and post-test counselling are available (Centres for Disease Control 1993) and informed consent must be obtained before a person is tested. It is important that anyone conducting the counselling has appropriate skills and training and that the advantages and disadvantages of having an HIV test are discussed with each individual (Pratt 1995).

Advantages of HIV test

☐ A negative test may give reassurance and encourage individuals to modify their risky behaviour.
☐ If the test is positive the condition can be monitored and anti HIV drugs and prophylaxis made available.
☐ A positive or negative test may allow women to make choices regarding having children.

Disadvantages of HIV test

☐ A negative result may give a false sense of security and high risk behaviour may not be modified.
☐ Breaches of confidentiality may have implications for relationships, family, friends, and for housing and employment.
☐ Some people may find it difficult to cope with the implications of a positive result.

The Advisory Council on the Misuse of Drugs (1993) recommends that people at risk of HIV infection be encouraged to consider having a test. Addiction nurses are in a good position to initiate discussion and even if the patient decides not to have the test there will have been the opportunity to discuss safer sex and drug using behaviour.

Drugs, pregnancy and HIV

Drug misuse can be particularly dangerous for those patients who may be pregnant. Physical withdrawal from a drug, or chaotic drug use, can be harmful to both fetus and mother, and a more gradual reduction regime is indicated (see Chapter 11). If a woman is HIV positive there is a risk that she will pass on the infection to the baby. The average rate of vertical transmission is 30–40% worldwide (Cotton 1994). The transmission rate is lower in developed countries due to better health care. Women who are HIV positive who wish to became pregnant should be advised of the risks of exposing their partner to infection and of infecting the baby. If a woman is already pregnant and is known to be HIV positive, anti-retrovirals can be given to the mother antenatally, during labour, and to the baby after it is born. This has been shown to reduce vertical trans-mission considerably. Because of the benefits of antiretroviral treatment, pregnant women, especially injecting drug users, should be offered HIV testing.

Confidentiality

Fear and prejudice regarding HIV infection remains an issue in most societies. There have been incidences of violence towards people with HIV infection and their property, as well as stigmatisation by friends, family, neighbours and colleagues. It is therefore important that a per-son's diagnosis remains confidential and it is only disclosed with their consent.

Infection control

It is known that at least four health care workers have been infected with HIV since the beginning of the epidemic and a further six may have been exposed when working abroad (PHLS 1993). The risk of becoming infected after percutaneous exposure to HIV is approximately 0.33%, compared with 30% from exposure to hepatitis B virus from a patient who is 'e' antigen positive (Heptonstall *et al.* 1993). Although the risk of acquiring HIV in a health care setting is small, it is still very real. It is therefore important that appropriate infection control precautions are adhered to. As not all patients with HIV and other blood borne viruses are aware that they are infected, a system of universal infection control should be used (see Table 16.2). In the event of occupational exposure, advice must be sought immediately.

People with HIV do not need to be cared for routinely in a single room.

Table 16.2 Universal infection control precautions.

❏ Wear gloves and aprons when dealing with blood and body fluids
❏ Wash hands before and after patient contact
❏ Clear up spillages with sodium hypoclorite or equivalent
❏ Cover cuts and grazes with waterproof dressing
❏ Dispose of needles and sharps carefully
❏ Use masks and protective goggles if there is the risk of splashing to the face

However, in certain cases a single room may be required if patients have a condition that is infectious to others, e.g. tuberculosis, or are susceptible to infection themselves.

Tuberculosis

There has been a big increase in the prevalence of pulmonary tuberculosis (TB) in New York which has been linked to HIV infection. It was found that 57% of patients with HIV and TB were injecting drug users (Friedland & Selwyn 1990). Although the rise in TB cases in the UK has been attributed to immigrants from the Indian subcontinent, there is a definite link between HIV infection and TB. There is also an increase amongst homeless people and it is known that injecting drug users are more susceptible to the disease. In the past few years there has been an emergence of multi resistant tuberculosis (MRTB) with an associated high mortality rate (Pratt 1994). It is therefore important that patients with signs and symptoms of TB are referred to a specialist team for rapid diagnosis and treatment. Basic infection control methods such as covering the mouth when coughing or sneezing should be encouraged. In a hospital setting the person must be cared for in a single room, on respiratory isolation.

The signs and symptoms of TB are:

❏ cough   ❏ night sweats
❏ weight loss   ❏ haemoptysis
❏ lethargy   ❏ fever

Hepatitis

Hepatitis means inflammation of the liver and can be caused by a number of factors including alcohol, drugs, immune disorders and infection. The main cause of hepatitis is viral infection. At present there are six main types of viral hepatitis: A, B, C, D, E and G. Hepatitis A and E are spread by the faecal oral route while the others are spread by blood and body fluids.

Hepatitis B and C are of most concern to drug users with up to 85% (Robertson 1987) being infected with HBV and 68.9% (Waller & Holmes 1995) with HCV.

Hepatitis C

Hepatitis C was first isolated in 1988. Before that this form of viral hepatitis was simply known as non A, non B hepatitis. Prevalence rates vary from country to country but on average prevalence rates are 1–3% in developed countries and 2–6 % in developing countries. Overall approximately 240 million people are thought to be infected worldwide (Dolan 1997). In the UK, prevalence is between 0.5 and 1.0% and it is suggested that HCV was rare in the UK prior to the emergence of injecting drug use in the 1960s and 1970s (Mutimer 1995).

Transmission

Unlike HIV the route of transmission of HCV is somewhat controversial. It is generally agreed that parental exposure to infected blood or blood products will lead to infection, as will the repeated use by intravenous drug users of contaminated injecting equipment (Alter 1993). Healthcare workers have been infected by sharps injuries from infected patients (Van Damme 1996). There is documented evidence that HCV can be passed on by sexual contact and there is evidence of mother to baby transmission, although some believe these do not play an important role in the spread of infection (Iwarson 1994). It has been detected in saliva and the prevalence amongst dentists is higher than expected, indicating that there may be transmission by saliva (Tibbs 1995). Interfamilial spread has been reported and people with tattoos are also at risk (Mutimer 1995). However, many people with HCV have no identifiable risk factors.

Disease progression

Once infected with HCV, only 25% of people will have symptoms of acute hepatitis, i.e. fever, abdominal pain, jaundice and malaise. Some people will mount an effective immune response and will successfully clear the virus; however, the majority of those infected will develop chronic hepatitis, with varying degrees of liver damage. It is thought that of this group 10–20% may go on to develop progressive liver disease with a 15% chance of developing liver cancer.

Treatment

At present there is no vaccination against HCV. People who are HCV positive have their liver function checked on a regular basis. They should also be advised to stop or reduce their alcohol intake. If there are signs of deteriorating liver function, a liver biopsy may be performed to assess liver changes. At this stage treatment with interferon alpha (IFN) may be considered. IFN is the only licensed treatment for HCV and is given by subcutaneous injection three times a week for 6 to 9 months. Twenty-five per cent of patients treated by IFN will become HCV negative and will regain normal liver function. Others will make an initial response but will relapse 6 months after treatment.

IFN is an expensive treatment (Shiell *et al.* 1994) and has a number of unpleasant side effects including mood changes, flu like symptoms, fatigue and lethargy. The patient has to be well motivated as the treatment is usually self administered and they need regular review in the out-patients department. There may be some concern about prescribing IFN to injecting drug users as it is felt that they may not tolerate the treatment and attend follow up appointments. It should be noted that the majority of people with HCV will suffer from only mild liver damage and it is felt that most patients will die of something other than HCV related liver disease.

Testing

Unlike HIV testing there are no clear guidelines on testing and counselling in HCV infection. Many people have been tested without their knowledge, let alone consent. As for HIV, there are serious implications in having an HCV test and there is a need for co-ordinated pre and post test counselling. Health professionals should be aware of the implications of HCV infection, its routes of transmission, preventative measures and treatment options so that these can be discussed with patients before testing takes place.

Infection control

The risk of contamination by HCV from a needlestick injury is between 0 and 10% (Germanaud *et al.* 1994) and there is documented evidence of occupationally acquired infection. Universal infection control precautions should be used to prevent transmission to healthcare workers (see Table 16.2).

Care of drug users in an acute general ward

The majority of drug users with HIV infection will require acute medical care at some point in their illness, whether it is for investigations, treatment or symptom control. All patients are entitled to the same standard of care, whatever their condition or social circumstances. There is evidence, however, that ward staff may have a negative attitude toward drug users, considering them to be manipulative and unco-operative (Carroll 1995), and there is still widespread prejudice amongst health care workers, regarding caring for people with HIV infection (Forester & Murphy 1992). To promote a positive approach towards drug users, staff need to have the skills and knowledge to feel confident in dealing with this patient group.

To provide patient centred care a careful assessment must be made. It is helpful to devise a care plan with the patient and to negotiate contracts during the admission phase so as to establish the boundaries or limitations of behaviour within the hospital setting. The patient must understand that the use of non prescription drugs will not be tolerated, although in practice this may be hard to enforce. Patients will be informed that medication will be administered to keep them comfortable and free from withdrawal symptoms. Drug dependency units or hospital liaison teams may be able to help with prescribing medication and give support and advice to staff and patients. A direct and honest approach can enhance the development of a therapeutic relationship.

Initial assessment should establish what drugs are used, their frequency of use, by what route and when the drug was last used. By doing this, appropriate interventions can be taken to prevent acute withdrawal.

Health education

As well as the advice given in the previous section, drug users with HIV and HCV will need specific advice related to their condition.

HCV

People should be encouraged to reduce their alcohol intake and, if possible, stop drinking completely. They should be advised of the risks of transmitting the virus to others and, as well adopting safer injecting and sexual behaviour, should be told not to share razors or toothbrushes. If a person is receiving interferon therapy, they will need to be taught how to receive treatment and will need support and advice in dealing with possible side effects.

HIV

People will need to attend out-patient departments on a regular basis to have their condition monitored. Many people with HIV are on complex treatment regimes which need to be taken correctly to ensure they are effective. People with chaotic lifestyles may need a lot of education and support to enable them to benefit from their treatment. There has been concern that recreational drugs may interact with anti HIV therapy (King 1997) and methadone doses may need to be adjusted. Patients should be encouraged to discuss their drug use with their doctors to ensure the safe prescribing of medication.

Weight loss and poor diet have been related to increased morbidity and mortality in individuals with HIV infection and referral to a dietician may be useful.

Palliative/terminal care

There is no cure for HIV infection and most patients will require palliative care or symptom control at the end of their illness. People may die at home, in hospital, in a generic hospice or in a specialist facility. The Griffin Project, in London, provides palliative and terminal care specifically for drug users who are HIV positive. In palliative care units, care for people with HIV is generally poor with under prescribing of morphine being an issue (Lebovits *et al.* 1994). Drug users have a higher tolerance to opiates and may require higher doses to gain an analgesic effect (Staats 1992). Unconscious patients may continue to require medication to prevent fitting and withdrawal.

Case vignette

Kate is 28 years old, unemployed and lives with her partner David and their 3 year old daughter. She has been injecting heroin since the age of 15, as well as misusing benzodiazepines and alcohol. David is also unemployed and drinks heavily. The family is well known to social services and the child is on the at risk register. Kate is HIV and HCV positive and although she has been admitted to hospital with chest infections and abscesses she has not had any HIV related illnesses. Her partner and daughter are both HIV negative. She has tried detoxification and rehabilitation and, although she had never been completely drug free, had had a relatively stable life-style since the birth of her daughter.

Six months previously Kate's sister died of an HIV related illness. This had a profound effect on Kate and she is now using up to a gramme of heroin a day, as well as alcohol and temazepam. She no longer attends the out-patient department and has stopped taking her antiretroviral treatment and PCP prophylaxis. Kate presented to the casualty department acutely unwell with shortness of breath. She appeared very thin and was anxious and agitated. A presumptive diagnosis of *Pneumocystis carinni* pneumonia was made and she was admitted to the acute HIV unit.

Health interventions

Kate was started on antibiotics and steroids to treat the pneumonia. Her respiratory rate was 40 rpm and she needed constant oxygen therapy to maintain her oxygen saturation above 95%. She was agitated and was reluctant to keep on her oxygen mask. She made constant requests for drugs. The hospital drug team were contacted and advised appropriate doses of methadone and temazepam. After 48 hours, her condition was more stable. She was seen by the dietician and a nasogastric feeding regime was begun in order to improve nutritional status. The unit coun-sellor saw Kate on a regular basis and discussed issues around the death of her sister.

She was restarted on antiretroviral drugs and the importance of PCP prophylaxis was explained to her by her key nurse. Kate was seen regularly by the drug team and joined a methadone programme on discharge. In order to facilitate safe discharge a multidisciplinary meeting was held, involving the community drug team, HIV community nurse specialist, district and hospital nurses, social services and medical staff. It was felt that Kate might benefit from respite care in a specialist unit for drug users with HIV.

Conclusions

When a person has a physical illness as well as a substance misuse problem the care and management is even more complex. Staats (1992) describes a dual or triple diagnosis of chemical dependence and HIV infection (with or without a psychiatric disorder) in people who misuse drugs which can also be related to drug users who have hepatitis. It is vital that all the health, social and other community based services work together to achieve a co-ordinated package of care for those with HIV and/or with hepatitis. Nursing patients with substance use problems and HIV in a hospital or community setting can be made easier if referral to other specialist teams takes place at an early stage in discharge planning. Some patients may not acknowledge that they have a problem with drugs and may be unwilling or unable to give up drugs at the present time, but engaging patients in some forms of treatment may reduce the risks associated with continued drug use and the problems associated with HIV .

References

Advisory Council on the Misuse of Drugs (1993) *AIDS and Drug Misuse Update.* Department of Health. HMSO, London.

Alter, M.J. (1993) The detection, transmission and outcome of hepatitis C virus infection. *Infectious Agents and Disease,* **2,** 155–66.

Brimlow, D.L. (1994) Issues affecting women and iv drug users. In: *AIDS and HIV Infection* (eds D.E.Grimes & R.M. Grimes), pp. 174–84. Mosby, St Louis.

Carroll, J. (1995) The negative attitudes of some general nurses towards drug misusers. *Nursing Standard,* **9,** 36–8.

Centres for Disease Control (1993) Technical guidance on HIV counselling. *Morbidity and Mortality Weekly Report,* 15 January, 42.

Cotton, D.J. (1994) AIDS in women. In: *Textbook of AIDS Medicine* (eds S. Broder, T. Merigan & D. Bolognesi), pp. 161–8I. Williams and Wilkins, Baltimore.

Dolan, M. (1997) *The Hepatitis C Handbook,* pp. 39–40. Catalyst Press, London.

Forester, D.A. & Murphy, P.A. (1992) Nurses' attitudes towards patients with AIDS and AIDS related risk factors. *Journal of Advanced Nursing,* **17,** 1112 –17.

Friedland, G. & Selwyn, P. (1990) Intravenous drug use and HIV infection. *AIDS Clinical Care,* **2,** 31–2.

Germanaud, J., Causse, X. & Dhumeaux, D. (1994) Transmission of hepatitis C by accidental needle stick injuries. Evaluation of the risk. *Presse Medicale,* **23,** 1078–82.

Gossop, M. (1993) *Living With Drugs,* 4th edn. Arena , Aldershot.

Heptonstall, J., Porter, K. & Gill, O.N. (1993) *Occupational transmission of HIV: summary of published reports.* PHLS internal report, September.

Iwarson, S. (1994) The natural course of chronic hepatitis C. *FEMS Microbiology Reviews,* **14,** 201–4.

Jaquet, C. (1992) Help on the streets. *Nursing Times,* **88,** 24–6.

King, E. (1996) Using protease inhibitors. *AIDS Treatment Update,* **47,** 1–3.

Lebovits, A.H., Smith, G., Maigan, M. & Lefkowitz, M. (1994) Pain in hospitalised patients with AIDS: analgesic and psychotropic medications. *Clinical Journal of Pain,* **10,** 156–61.

Mutimer, D. (1995) Epidemiology of the hepatitis C virus. *Hospital Update* (Reed Heathcare Communications), February, 3–4.

PHLS (1993) Health care workers and HIV: surveillance of occupationally acquired infection in the United Kingdom. *Communicable Diseases Report 3.*

PHLS Communicable Disease Surveillance Centre (1996) *AIDS/HIV Quarterly Surveillance Tables,* 4.

Pratt, R. (1994) Safe practice. *Nursing Times,* **90,** 64–8.

Pratt, R. (1995). *HIV & AIDS – A Strategy for Nursing Care,* 4th edn. Edward Arnold, London.

Robertson, R. (1987) *Heroin, AIDS and Society.* Hodder and Stoughton, London.

Selwyn, P.A., Feingold, A.R., Hartel, D., *et al.* (1988). Increased risk of bacterial pneumonia in HIV infected drug users without AIDS. *AIDS,* **4,** 226–72.

Shiell, A., Briggs, A . & Farrel, G.C. (1994) The cost effectiveness of alpha interferon in treatment of chronic active hepatitis C. *Medical Journal of Australia,* **160,** 268–72.

Staats, J.A.(1992) Chemical dependency. In: *HIV/AIDS A Guide to Nursing Care* (eds J. Haak Flaskerud & P.J. Ungvarski), pp. 350–74. W.B. Saunders , Philadelphia.

Tibbs, C.J. (1995) Methods of transmission of hepatitis C. *Journal of Viral Hepatitis,* **2,** 113–19.

Van Damme, P. (1996) Hepatitis A, B and C occupational hazards. *Occupational Health*, **48**, 282–3.

Waller, T. & Holmes, R. (1995) Hepatitis C: time to wake up. *Druglink*, **18**, 7–9.

World Health Organization Global Programme on AIDS (1994) GPA publishes new HIV/AIDS data. *Global AIDS News – The Newsletter of the WHO/GPA*, **1**, 11–12.

World Health Organization (1993) Press release. WHO/69 (7 September). WHO, Geneva.

Part 4
Addiction Nursing: Specialist Responses

Chapter 17

Alcohol: Community Detoxification and Clinical Care

Mike Gafoor and G. Hussein Rassool

Introduction

Since the late 1970s, alcohol consumption in the UK has roughly doubled and current figures show that 27% of men and 13% of women are drinking above the recommended safe levels of 21 units and 14 units respectively per week (Alcohol Concern 1996). The medical and social costs incurred by society through alcohol misuse are alarmingly high. In the UK, the use of alcohol is associated with approximately between 8700 and 33 000 premature deaths each year (Godfrey & Maynard 1992), and it is a major factor in social problems such as homelessness, unemployment, domestic violence, marital breakdown and child abuse.

Teenage drinking is also on the increase. It is estimated that of the 3 million young people aged between 11 and 15 years, 17% are regular weekly drinkers. There has been concern expressed in the media and by the public about 'alcopops' and the cynical targeting of young people by the alcohol industry. It seems that the sweetened taste of alcopops blurs the distinction between alcoholic and non alcoholic beverages, making it more appealing to large numbers of young people. However, as yet there is little evidence to demonstrate a positive link between alcopops and an increase in teenage drinking. Indeed given the integral role which alcohol plays in our society, it could be argued that alcopops with a relatively low alcohol content might be a safer way to teach young people to drink alcohol in a sensible and controlled way.

This chapter aims to address and examine issues related to home and community detoxification for problem drinkers and the appropriate clinical interventions. It will describe the assessment, clinical care and guidelines to detoxify safely and effectively a patient who is dependent on alcohol. A case vignette will illustrate the use of Peplau's model of care with specific nursing interventions.

What is detoxification?

Stockwell (1987) defined detoxification as 'a treatment designed to control both medical and psychological complications which may occur temporarily after a period of heavy and sustained alcohol use'. It may be carried out in hospital, or in a community setting such as the patient's home or at a day centre. Community detoxification enables patients to undergo a supervised withdrawal from a drug which they are physically dependent upon, while experiencing minimum withdrawal symptoms and medical complications. Detoxification also allows the individual an opportunity to reflect upon the negative consequences associated with their substance misuse and to take up additional offers of interventions. In this context, detoxification can be regarded as a prelude to further social and psychological help aimed at influencing and motivating the problem drinkers to change their behaviours.

Rationale for community alcohol detoxification

Community detoxification is based on the principle that the patient remains in their own natural environment. This facilitates a more accurate assessment of factors which precede drinking behaviour as well as enabling the patient to test out new coping strategies in their natural environment. This approach is rooted in social learning theory which views drinking as a learned behaviour in response to environmental and social cues.

It has also been suggested that keeping the patient in their own natural environment allows for a more holistic approach in helping him. In this way, resources, such as GP, family and self-help groups, are mobilised and used more effectively. Some critics of community detoxification programmes argue that patients remain in an environment which might be perpetuating alcohol misuse, and families do not have any respite. It is also suggested that some patients may not view their problems as severe if treated at home and may also hold doubts over the effectiveness of home treatment. However, research studies have shown that community detoxification is not only as safe and effective as in-patient treatment, but is also more cost effective (Stockwell *et al.* 1990, 1991) This finding, along with the high cost of in-patient care, prompted a rapid expansion in community detoxification programmes, with addiction nurses taking the lead role in the development of such therapeutic programmes.

The potential benefits of community detoxification to a problem drinker may be summarised as follows:

❑ Treatment takes place in a familiar environment with the support of the family network and friends.
❑ The patient is able to resist environmental cues to drinking and to develop new coping strategies.
❑ The stigma of admission to a specialist unit or psychiatric hospital is disengaged.
❑ A more accessible and flexible service is provided, which encourages

the problem drinker to seek help at an early stage of their drinking career.

❏ The patient can remain at work during treatment interventions.
❏ More problem drinkers can be recruited for detoxification rather than being on a waiting list for in-patient treatment.

The alcohol withdrawal syndrome

The alcohol withdrawal syndrome usually occurs in patients physically dependent on alcohol within 6–24 hours after their last drink and peaks within 24–48 hours. It is characterised by tremors, sweating, nausea, vomiting, restlessness and anxiety, tachycardia and systolic hypertension. Some patients may experience more serious symptoms such as epileptic seizures and delirium tremens (DTs). With DTs, the patient may become confused, disorientated and experience auditory and visual hallucinations. This is a potentially serious medical condition and, if untreated, may result in death from hypothermia and cardiovascular collapse (Jaffe 1992). The symptoms of alcohol withdrawal are self-limiting and usually disappear after 5–7 days.

Assessment for community detoxification

It is important to carry out a full and comprehensive assessment before selecting a patient who wishes to undergo alcohol detoxification in his home environment. In general terms, community detoxification may be considered for individuals who experience mild to moderate withdrawal symptoms and who live in a stable home environment and can rely on support from relatives, neighbours or friends. Detoxification in the community should not be considered for severely dependent drinkers, especially those with a history of medical and psychiatric complications, for example fits, DTs or poor physical state. It is also unsuitable for patients who live alone or in unstable accommodation with little access to social support. A summary of the exclusion criteria is provided below:

❏ A history of mental health problems, including overdose, self-harm and polydrug users.
❏ A history of fully developed DTs (e.g. fits, hallucinations).
❏ A history of serious physical ill health including fits/epilepsy.
❏ A lack of or little social support, i.e. living alone or homelessness/no fixed abode.
❏ Difficulties in management as an out-patient or failure of a previous home detoxification programme.
❏ Refusal to adhere to the health and safety of home detoxification.
❏ Living with a partner or significant other who is misusing drugs or

alcohol and is perceived as being dependent on the psychoactive sub-stance(s).

A full alcohol history and the use of screening instruments such as the severity of alcohol dependence questionnaire (SADQ) will assist in deter-mining the degree of alcohol dependence and the nature and severity of withdrawal symptoms. The assessment should cover the following areas:

❑ The nature and extent of withdrawal symptoms.
❑ Any history of medical and psychiatric complications, e.g. fits, DTs, attempted suicide or overdoses.
❑ Whether the home environment is stable.
❑ The degree of support available.
❑ Whether the patient agrees to undergo detoxification at home.
❑ Failure of previous home detoxification programmes.

Lay and professional roles

The roles of both addiction nurses and the family are the key elements in the home detoxification process for an effective outcome of the intervention strategies. Before embarking on the detoxification programme, it is important to clarify the role of the patient, family or carer and professionals involved such as GP and addiction nurse. Effective communication and liaison are key elements in ensuring an effective outcome. During a com-munity detoxification in a home environment it is the patient who experiences the withdrawal and the family (carer) who provides the sup-port and care in the absence of the clinician (Derage 1994). Prior to a home detoxification, both the patient and the carer are consulted, and the process of detoxification from alcohol and subsequent follow up and after care are discussed.

This strategy enables the strengthening of the family support system and the provision of adequate information about the treatment for the patient and the family. The implementation of home detoxification is unworkable if the social network and support system are not intact. Furthermore, Orford and Wauman (1992) stated that it is the use of the strengthened social support system which may be valuable in further treatment and rehabilitation.

General practitioners are well placed to provide detoxification in the community while maintaining medical responsibility and the addiction nurse has both consultative and clinical responsibility for implementation of intervention strategies. It is important to keep the patient's GP fully informed and to determine the degree of their involvement during the procedure and to advise about the prescribing of any medication.

As most addiction nurses work during week days, it is perhaps best to commence the detoxification on a Monday morning to ensure maximum staff supervision during the acute stages of withdrawal. The patient should be told to stop drinking alcohol from midnight and breathalysed to ensure that they are alcohol free before any medication is administered. In addition, patients should be warned against the risks of driving on medication and encouraged to take fluids, a light diet and plenty of rest. The following guidelines for the addiction nurse are useful to ensure that a safe and effective community alcohol detoxification is achieved:

❑ Explain the procedures simply and clearly to the patient, family member or friend, stressing the need to avoid taking alcoholic beverages with any medication prescribed.
❑ Ask the patient to be alcohol free for at least 6 hours before the start of treatment and seek written consent for detoxification.
❑ Liaise with the GP and advise on the medication regime.
❑ Visit twice daily during the initial 72 hours to monitor vital signs, medication and withdrawal symptoms.
❑ Provide reassurance and psychological support.
❑ Reduce visits to once daily and liaise with the GP.
❑ Provide on going counselling, support and encouragement.

Clinical care and management

The objectives of drug treatment in alcohol withdrawal are:

❑ The relief of subjective symptoms
❑ The prevention or treatment of more serious complications such as seizures or arrhythmias and
❑ Preparation for long term rehabilitation

Medication regime

Chlordiazepoxide or diazepam is usually the drug of choice in community alcohol detoxification because they are much safer in overdoses and have an anti-convulsant effect. The latter function helps to safeguard against seizures. However, there is always a risk of dependence and care should be taken to ensure the patient is not prescribed these drugs for longer than the period of detoxification. A recommended prescribing regime for chlordiazepoxide is as follows:

Day 1: 40 mg qds
    2: 30 mg qds
    3: 30 mg qds
    4: 20 mg qds
    5: 20 mg bd
    6: 10 mg bd
    7: 10 mg od

The importance of follow-up care

The treatment and follow-up programme aim to offer a wide variety of alternative ways of dealing with psychological dependence, so enabling a drug-free behaviour and life-style. Ito and Donovan (1986) stated that a well planned programme for continued assistance will increase the patient's chances of a successful long-term outcome. Relapse prevention is an integral part of any after care programme for the problem drinker. It enables the client to identify high risk situations or triggers which can lead to problem drinking and to manage these by developing alternative coping skills and strategies. Such triggers might be as a result of internal or external factors or a combination of both, and can include boredom, low mood, interpersonal conflicts, social pressure, etc. Relapse prevention is based on social learning theory and facilitates the development of new patterns of thinking and lifestyle changes to assist the client in either abstaining or controlling his or her drinking. It can be incorporated into both group and individual focused after care programmes.

Nursing model for community detoxification

Peplau's (1988) interpersonal model of care appeals to the practice of addiction nursing because it is directed towards a structured, needs directed and therapeutic interaction between the nurse and the patient. Its value lies in the role the nurse may undertake within the various phases of the nurse–patient relationship. These roles include: stranger, teacher, counsellor, leader resource person, clinician and surrogate (Marriner-Tomey 1994). This model allows the problem drinker to be the central focus of attention and to take an active part in the detoxification process, treatment and rehabilitation and thus enables the patient to remain in control of the situation rather than adopt a passive role (Torres 1986). The rationale for the choice of this model is based on its optimistic framework with the view of a positive evaluation of human nature and a belief in the client's potential for personal growth. In this context both the patient and the nurse are capable of personal growth and development. An added feature of Peplau's model of nursing is that its stages can be directly linked to the systematic approach to nursing care in relation to assessment, planning, implementation and evaluation. Peplau identified four phases in the model and acknowledged that these phases overlap and interact as the process evolves. These four phases are: orientation, identification, exploitation and resolution.

Case vignette

Jane is 36, married with two young children and works part-time as a cashier in the local supermarket. Her alcohol consumption increased 6 years ago when she began drinking a bottle of wine in the evenings after putting the children to bed. Over the past year Jane began to experience alcohol withdrawal symptoms and commenced on early morning drinking to stave off the shakes, nausea and vomiting. She was now drinking half a bottle of vodka daily and presented with her partner to her general practitioner complaining of low mood, anxiety, poor memory and concentration. Her drinking had led to frequent arguments within the family and Jane's supervisor was unhappy with her work performance and absenteeism.

On assessment, Jane scored a high rating on the severity of alcohol dependence questionnaire (SADQ) and blood tests revealed a gamma glutamyl transferase (gamma GT) of 210 (therapeutic range <50) and a raised mean corpuscular volume (MCV) of 105 (therapeutic range = 85). Jane was willing to undergo a home detoxification and her partner agreed to take time off to support her during the detoxification process and after care. Jane was referred to the local community substance misuse team.

Nursing approaches and interventions using Peplau's model

In the orientation stage, the addiction nurse and Jane meet as strangers and it is the time to establish rapport, trust and mutual respect. A brief or initial assessment is made at this stage and roles are clarified. It is during the identification phase, with improved interpersonal interactions, that enables Jane to acknowledge the health related problems, i.e. alcohol problems, and begin to identify needs and problems.

The third phase, the exploitation phase, is the implementation of other therapeutic intervention strategies. In the context of alcohol detoxification, there would be a need for nursing care and counselling with medical and pharmacological treatment. During the final phase, the resolution phase, the addiction nurse and Jane work towards the termination of the nurse–patient relationship. However, in addiction nursing, this relationship is not severed totally. The addiction nurse (community) will remain in contact with Jane and implement a rehabilitation and after care programme such as relapse prevention. It is important for the addiction nurse, through the process of clinical supervision, to reflect and evaluate the dynamics of the inter-personal and therapeutic process with this particular patient (Rassool 1997).

A summary of the key problems/needs, expected outcome and nurse (or patient) intervention is provided in Table 17.1.

Conclusions

It is suggested that community based alcohol treatment programmes are more acceptable to patients because they are more accessible and less stigmatised than hospital based services (Orford & Wauman 1992). Community alcohol detoxification can be carried out safely and effectively with

Table 17.1 Key areas of the care plan.

Needs problems	Expected outcome	Nursing intervention
Poor physical health	Improvement in daily intake of nutrition	Assessment of daily intake of nutrients
Fear of withdrawal symptoms	Prevention of withdrawal symptoms	Health information/counselling
Low self-esteem	Improvement in self-worth by adoption of more positive attitude	Counselling
Lack of assertive skills	Development of assertive skills	Counselling and other behavioural techniques
Anxiety	Control of anxiety	Implementing anxiety/stress management
Boredom		Encourage participation in alternative leisure activities
Detoxification	Patient will not experience any physical distress and discomfort while undergoing detoxification	Explain the role of medication in facilitating detoxification and overcoming withdrawal. Ensure adequate medication cover
Dealing with grief reaction	Resolution of grieving process	Counselling
Relapse	Prevention of relapse or chaotic drinking pattern	Relapse prevention

careful assessment and proper planning. By allowing for the patient to remain in his or her own environment, there are special clinical benefits in helping the patient to develop new coping strategies and mobilising support from friends, family and GP. However, not everyone can be detoxified safely in the community, and careful assessment and planning are required before a patient is considered for home detoxification. In-patient treatment should be considered for those patients who are severely dependent on alcohol and who have a history of medical and psychiatric complications or for those without any form of social support or stable accommodation.

References

Alcohol Concern (1996) *Alcohol Consumption: Facts and Figures.* Alcohol Concern, London.

Derage, S. (1994) *Detoxification from alcohol at home: a preliminary and retrospective evaluation of carer's needs*. Unpublished Project submitted for the Diploma in Addictive Behaviour, Centre for Addiction Studies, Department of Psychiatry of Addictive Behaviour, St George's Hospital Medical School, London.

Godfrey, C. & Maynard, A. (1992) *A Health Strategy for Alcohol*. Centre for Health Economics, University of York, York.

Ito, J.R. & Donovan, D.M. (1986) Aftercare in alcoholism treatment: a review. In: *Treating Addictive Behaviours: Processes of Change* (eds W.R. Miller & N. Heather). Plenum Press, New York.

Jaffe, J.H. (1992) Drug addiction and drug abuse. In: *Goodman and Gilman's The Pharmacological Basis of Therapeutics* (eds A.G. Gillman, T.W. Rall, A.S. Nies & P. Taylor), pp. 522–73, 8th edn. Pergamon Press, New York.

Marriner-Tomey A. (1994) *Nursing Theorists and their Work*, 3rd edn. Mosby Year Book, St Louis.

Orford, J. & Wauman, T. (1992) *Alcohol Detoxification Services, A Review*. Exeter Community Team. University of Exeter, Exeter Health Authority. Prepared for the Department of Health and Social Security.

Peplau, H.E. (1988) *Interpersonal Relationships in Nursing: A Conceptual Frame of Reference for Psychodynamic Nursing*. Macmillan, London.

Rassool, G.H. (1997) Clinical supervision. In: *Addiction Nursing: Perspectives on Professional and Clinical Practice* (eds G.H. Rassool & M. Gafoor), pp. 227–36. Stanley Thornes, Cheltenham.

Stockwell, T. (1987) The Exeter Home Detoxification Project. In: *Helping the Problem Drinker: A New Initiative in Community Care* (eds T. Stockwell & S. Clements). Croom Helm, London.

Stockwell, T., Bolt, L., Milner, I., *et al.* (1990) Home detoxification for problem drinkers: acceptability, clients, relatives, general practitioners and outcome after 60 days. *British Journal of Addiction*, **85**, 61–70.

Stockwell, T., Bolt, L., Russell, G., *et al.* (1991) Home detoxification from alcohol: its safety and efficacy in comparison to inpatient care. *Alcohol & Alcoholism*, **26**, 645–50.

Torres, G. (1986) *Theoretical Foundations of Nursing*. Appleton Century Crofts, New York.

Chapter 18
Benzodiazepines: Clinical Care and Nursing Interventions

Mike Gafoor

Introduction

Benzodiazepines, also commonly known as minor tranquillisers, are the most widely prescribed psychotropic drugs in the UK. They were first introduced into clinical practice in the early 1960s as a safer alternative to barbiturates; they were considered less dangerous in overdose and less likely to be abused. Benzodiazepines are therapeutically useful in the treatment of anxiety and insomnia, and are also effective as antiepileptic and muscle relaxant drugs. However, the indications for their use have widened to include a variety of physical conditions and non specific symptoms: for example, backache, headache, tiredness, tension, anxiety and depression. Between 1974 and 1985, annual prescriptions dispensed for benzodiazepines ranged from 25 million to 31million (Taylor 1987). This period, often referred to as 'the tranquillising era', was also noted for the use of tranquillisers for treating people presenting with personal and interpersonal problems such as feelings of unhappiness and relationship and financial difficulties. Doctors were criticised by the public and the media for prescribing these drugs too easily and for not informing patients of the danger of dependence (Tyrer 1984). The medical profession, in their defence, argued they were merely complying with patients' expectations for 'a pill for every ill'.

As concerns grew over the problems associated with the long term use of these drugs, the Government passed new legalisation in 1985 restricting the range of benzodiazepines which could be prescribed under the National Health Service from the existing 18 to 7 types. This was followed by guidelines on the safe use of these drugs by the Committee on the Safety of Medicines (1988) and, by 1990, the number of prescriptions had fallen to 18 million (King 1992). The most frequently prescribed benzodiazepines in the UK are diazepam, temazepam, lorazepam, nitrazepam and oxazepam (see Table 18.1).

The decline in the popularity of the use of benzodiazepines has been almost as spectacular as their acceptance into clinical practice.This chapter will describe the main problems associated with the long term use of

Table 18.1 Types of benzodiazepines.

Anxiolytics (minor tranquillisers)	Anxiolytic and occasional hypnotic	Hypnotics (sleeping pills)
Chlordiazepoxide Oxazepam Lorazepam	Diazepam	Nitrazepam Temazepam Triazolam Flurazepam

benzodiazepines and outline the main therapeutic interventions required to get patients off these drugs. A case vignette and the appropriate interventions are presented.

Nature and extent

The peak period for benzodiazepines prescribing was in the late 1970s, with more than 30 million prescriptions written per year, and while there has been a downward trend in their use in recent years, more than 20 million prescriptions were still written for these drugs in 1990. It has been estimated that there are about 1.2 million long term benzodiazepine users in the UK (Ashton & Golding 1989) and of these approximately 400 000 will have difficulties with withdrawal symptoms.

It would appear that long term benzodiazepine users fall into four broad groups:

❑ The first group consists of people with physical problems, for example neurological and musculoskeletal disorders. These patients do not tend to misuse their medication and have fewer symptoms if their medication is withdrawn.
❑ The second and younger group of users is those with psychiatric symptoms such as anxiety and emotional distress. It has been found that personality characteristics and psychiatric symptoms are strongly correlated with the development of withdrawal symptoms (Tyrer 1990) and this category of patients tends to experience more difficulties coming off benzodiazepines.
❑ The third and largest group of benzodiazepine users consists of people with chronic sleeping difficulties and elderly people make up the largest proportion of this category. Approximately 15% of the elderly population take a hypnotic drug each night and the older the patient, the more likely they will be prescribed a sleeping tablet (Morgan *et al.* 1988).
❑ Finally the use of benzodiazepines is common among illicit drug users and between 37% and 50% of them reported regular use (Darke *et al.* 1994). These patients differ from those of the other groups in that they are often younger, more socially disorganised and take considerably higher doses of benzodiazepines.

Women are twice as likely than men to be prescribed benzodiazepines. Taylor (1987) estimated that the 13 million British women aged over 40 years old receive about 60% of all benzodiazepines prescribed for the UK population and of these the five million women aged over 65 years consume about 40% of all prescribed benzodiazepines.

Nature of problems

The most serious problem associated with the long term use of benzodiazepines is dependence and up to a third of long term users will develop a physical withdrawal syndrome if the drug is discontinued (Lader & Morton 1991). This usually occurs within 2 to 3 days after the last dose but may take up to 10 days to appear if the drug taken is a long acting one, for example diazepam or Librium (chlordiazepoxide). The symptoms may last between 1 and 6 weeks but some can persist for several months later (Petursson 1994). The withdrawal syndrome is typically characterised by tremor, sweating, palpitations, sleep disturbances, panic attacks, irritability, tension, increased anxiety and various perceptual changes, such as tingling sensations, photophobia and hypersensitivity to touch and pain. Some patients, particularly those taking large doses of benzodiazepines, may suffer from more serious problems such as seizures, hallucinations and confusional states.

Another problem associated with long term use of benzodiazepines is their adverse effects on cognitive function, and the patient's ability to think clearly and learn new information is impaired. They often complain of a poor memory for everyday events and find it difficult to sustain attention for any length of time. This may result in a loss of self-confidence and self-esteem, and many patients do suffer with feelings of depression. Emotional reactions such as increased aggressiveness and hostility feelings are present in a small number of cases and uncharacteristic behaviour, for example shoplifting and sexual promiscuity, has been reported by some patients.

The elderly are particularly at risk of the adverse effects of benzodiazepines due to decreased metabolic clearance and they may suffer from drowsiness and confusion resulting in accidents and falls. This is an obvious concern given that the elderly represents a high usage group.

The use of benzodiazepines is common among illicit drug users and research has shown a positive link between benzodiazepines use and HIV risk taking behaviour among injecting drug users (Darke *et al.* 1992). These patients are more likely to inject and share equipment more frequently and have higher levels of physical, social and psychological problems (Darke *et al.* 1994). The injecting of temazepam capsules resulting in serious health risks has recently led to a change in the law banning their use and making it illegal to possess the tablets without a prescription. Finally, although comparatively safe in overdoses, benzodiazepines can be fatal when taken in large doses with other sedative type drugs such as barbiturates and alcohol.

Summary of problems

- Side effects include headaches, blurred vision, poor concentration and memory, irritability and lethargy.
- Withdrawal symptoms include anxiety, panic attacks, insomnia, perceptual disturbances, fits, aches and pains.
- Poor memory and concentration, difficulty in thinking.
- Confusion and risks of falls and accidents in elderly patients.
- HIV risk taking behaviour in polydrug users.

Clinical care and nursing interventions

Preparing a client for withdrawal

Nurses and other health care workers have an important role in developing health promotion strategies to help their patients avoid or reduce benzodiazepine use. Patients who are taking these medications regularly on a long term basis should be informed of the risks of dependence and other adverse effects and should be provided with advice and help in withdrawal. The Government's *Health of the Nation* (Department of Health 1992) document highlights the need to 'improve the education of primary care teams about non-prescribing interventions in the management of anxiety disorders and in graded withdrawal of benzodiazepines in chronic users'.

Before embarking on a withdrawal programme, the addiction nurse should carry out a careful assessment to establish the type and dosage as well as the reasons for taking benzodiazepines and duration of use. In addition, information regarding the patient's lifestyle, personality and the degree of support available would help the nurse to develop a withdrawal programme which matches the client's individual needs. Most patients are apprehensive of the withdrawal process and their ability to cope without their medication. The nurse can help to reassure patients by emphasising the benefits of coming off benzodiazepines and by providing clear and accurate information on the nature and type of withdrawal symptoms they are likely to experience. This is important since many patients may fear that their symptoms might indicate the onset of a physical or psychiatric illness. Although nurses should encourage patients to come off benzodiazepines, they should not force patients to do so as this could prevent a successful outcome. Patients on high doses or with a history of seizures or psychotic reactions during previous attempts to withdraw may be more safely treated in hospital.

Withdrawal programme

The use of a long acting benzodiazepine such as diazepam is widely accepted as the most effective way of withdrawing patients because it leaves the system gradually and therefore slows down the onset of withdrawal symptoms. Short acting benzodiazepines, on the other hand, may cause more abrupt and severe withdrawal reactions. Table 18.2 shows the dosages of other benzediazepines which are equivalent to 5 mg diazepam.

Table 18.2 Dosages of benzodiazepines approximately equivalent to 5 mg diazepam.

Drug	Dose (mg)
Chlordiazepoxide	15
Lorazepam	0.5
Nitrazepam	5
Oxazepam	15
Temazepam	10

It is important for the client to feel in charge of the withdrawal procedure in order to increase their confidence and self-efficacy. This can be achieved by allowing them to control the reduction at a rate which is comfortable. The duration of a typical withdrawal period is 6 to 8 weeks, but this can be extended for a few months for patients experiencing severe symptoms. However, too prolonged a withdrawal programme can be counterproductive with some patients who might become unduly preoccupied with their symptoms.

Patients on high doses can make bigger reductions initially while those on a daily dose of 20–40 mg can reduce by 1–2 mg every 1–2 weeks. The use of liquid diazepam is sometimes indicated, especially during the latter stages of withdrawal so that smaller doses can be more easily taken. Many patients will experience anxiety symptoms and difficulties in sleeping regardless of the rate of reduction. These can be helped with non-pharmacological methods – the provision of counselling and psychological support as well as practical advice such as the use of relaxation tapes and anxiety and sleep management. The degree of support and intervention will vary with different patients and other approaches such as yoga, massage, aromatherapy and physical exercises can also help to reduce symptoms. Those patients who are experiencing more severe withdrawal symptoms, e.g. panic attacks, agoraphobia, depression, may require the involvement of a psychologist, psychiatrist or specialist addiction nurse. Self-help groups run for benzodiazepine users can also be helpful, especially for those patients who require ongoing support after completion of a withdrawal programme.

Summary of management of benzodiazepine withdrawal

❑ Advise patients of the benefits of coming off benzodiazepines and educate them on the nature and type of withdrawal symptoms they might experience.

❑ Substitute with an equivalent dose of diazepam to stabilise the patient's condition.

❑ Agree with the patient on a timetable for withdrawal (usually 6–8 weeks).

❑ Reduce by 1–2 mg every 1–2 weeks.

❑ Monitor and titrate the reduction rate according to the patient's symptoms.

❑ Provide help and support to cope with symptoms such as anxiety, stress and difficulty sleeping.

Case vignette

Susan is a 45 year old teacher who visited her GP shortly after the break up of her marriage complaining of difficulty in sleeping, loss of appetite and lack of interest. She was prescribed lorazepam 2 mg daily and temazepam 20 mg nocte and her symptoms improved sufficiently for her to return to work a few weeks later. Over the next 5 years, her use of lorazepam gradually increased to 4 mg daily and this was obtained mainly through repeat prescriptions. Susan started to experience symptoms such as blurred vision, poor memory and unsteadiness on her feet. She also found it difficult to concentrate and had experienced panic attacks in the supermarket. Her previous GP was no longer working with the practice and his successor felt that Susan's symptoms were related to her use of benzodiazepines. They both agreed on a withdrawal plan. This involved substituting her medication with diazepam and stabilising her on 60 mg daily in divided doses.

Health interventions

Susan was encouraged to attend once weekly for counselling sessions with the practice nurse. She managed to reduce the diazepam by 10 mg weekly for the first 4 weeks before experiencing symptoms such as headaches, tremors, aches and pains. She also felt emotionally sensitive and became tearful easily. At this stage, further reduction was stopped and restarted a week later with smaller decrements of 2 mg weekly. Susan was taught anxiety management techniques by the nurse and was provided with a relaxation tape to use whenever she became tense and anxious. She was advised against excessive coffee and alcohol intake and encouraged to keep herself occupied during the day. She joined a local aerobic class and her sleep pattern gradually returned to normal. Over the following weeks

Susan was able to discuss her feelings with the practice nurse and felt less guilty over the breakdown of her marriage. She regained her self confidence and successfully came off benzodiazepines a few months later.

Discussion

It is possible that Susan was put on benzodiazepines unnecessarily and her symptoms of sleep disturbance, loss of appetite and interest might have resolved with individual counselling. Her tolerance to the drugs increased over a 5 year period where she required larger amounts in order to get the same effect from her medication. This resulted in Susan developing both side-effects and withdrawal symptoms of benzodiazepines, for example blurred vision, memory problems, anxiety and panic attacks. Her withdrawal from these drugs was precipitated by a new GP and made easier to cope with by substituting lorazepam and temazepam with the long acting diazepam.

Conclusions

Benzodiazepines were hailed as wonder drugs when they were first introduced into clinical practice and over the next three decades were widely prescribed for a variety of physical and psychological conditions. However, in recent years, concerns over their use, misuse and dependence liability have intensified and long term users are encouraged to withdraw gradually. Nurses are ideally placed to educate patients on the health risks associated with benzodiazepines and to help them to reduce or come off these drugs. This can be achieved by adopting a sympathetic response and providing clear and accurate information as well as encouraging behavioural changes with the use of techniques such as motivational interviewing. Patients are more likely to undergo withdrawal from their medication if they feel confident that they can cope without it. A stepwise reduction of the use of a long acting benzodiazepine, e.g. diazepam, and the teaching of alternative coping strategies to deal with anxiety, stress and sleep difficulties appear to be the best method of treating people with benzodiazepine dependence. Complementary therapies, for example acupuncture, aromatherapy and reflexology, are used by addiction nurses for the purposes of detoxification, massage, relaxation, stress reduction, pain relief and palliative care (McDonald & Rassool 1997).

References

Ashton, H. & Golding, J.F. (1989) Tranquillisers, prevalence, predictors and possible consequences, data from a large UK survey. *British Journal of Addiction*, **84**, 541–6.

Committee on the Safety of Medicines (1988) Benzodiazepines, dependence and withdrawal symptoms. *Current Problems*, **21**, 1–2.

Darke, S., Hall, W., Ross, M.W., *et al.* (1992) Benzodiazepine use and HIV risk-taking behaviour among injecting drug users. *Drug and Alcohol Dependence*, **31**, 31–6.

Darke, S., Ross, J. & Cohen, J. (1994) The use of benzodiazepines among regular amphetamine users. *Addiction*, **89**, 1683–90.

Department of Health (1992) *The Health of the Nation: A Strategy for Health in England.* HMSO, London.

King, M. (1992) Is there still a role for benzodiazepines in general practice? *British Journal of Medical Practice*, **42**, 202–5.

Lader, M. & Morton, S. (1991) Benzodiazepine problems. *British Journal of Addiction*, **86**, 823–8.

Morgan, K., Dallosso, H., Ebrahim, S., *et al.* (1988) Prevalence, frequency and duration of hypnotic use among the elderly living at home. *British Medical Journal*, **296**, 601–2.

Petursson, H. (1994) The benzodiazepine withdrawal syndrome. *Addiction*, **89**, 1455–9.

McDonald, L. & Rassool, G.H. (1997) Complementary therapies in addiction nursing practice. In: *Addiction Nursing: Perspectives on Professional and Clinical Practice* (eds G.H. Rassool & M. Gafoor). Stanley Thornes, Cheltenham.

Taylor, D. (1987) Current usage of benzodiazepines in Britain. In: *The Benzodiazepines in Current Clinical Practice – International Congress and Symposium Series, No 114* (eds H. Freeman & Y. Rue).

Tyrer, P.J. (1984) Benzodiazepines on trial. *British Medical Journal*, **288**, 1101–2.

Tyrer, P.J. (1990) Any questions? *British Medical Journal*, **301**, 1084.

Chapter 19

Stimulants: Clinical Care and Nursing Interventions

Mike Flanagan

Introduction

Stimulants, such as cocaine and amphetamines, are psychoactive substances that excite the central nervous system. Some stimulants, such as caffeine and nicotine, are legally available, while others, the focus of this chapter, are controlled by national and international laws. A comparatively recent addition to the range of stimulants available in the UK is the synthetic 'designer drug' Ecstasy, a stimulant with hallucinogenic properties. There has also been an increase in recent years of the importation of khat, an East African plant which is chewed for its stimulating effect. This drug is not yet controlled under existing laws in the UK.

This chapter aims to discuss the misuse of stimulant drugs, focusing on amphetamine and cocaine, conveying the changing nature of stimulant misuse over the years. The desired and undesired effects of stimulants and the range of psychological, social and pharmacological treatments will be examined. A case vignette will demonstrate how stimulant use can precipitate contact with statutory services.

Background and nature of stimulant misuse

Amphetamine was first synthesised in 1887, but was not used pharmaceutically until 1930 when it was marketed as a bronchial dilator. The pleasurable effect of amphetamine soon resulted in recreational rather than therapeutic use, replacing cocaine as the primary stimulant of misuse. In the 1960s, the illicit use of pharmaceutical amphetamine preparations increased. Nowadays, because of their limited therapeutic uses, diverted pharmaceutical amphetamines have been mostly replaced on the illicit market by 'street speed'. The use of amphetamine further escalated alongside Ecstasy from the late 1980s as the rave scene flourished. The change in youth culture resulted in drug use, particularly stimulants, becoming associated with mainstream entertainment rather than being a subcultural activity. Amphetamine is less expensive than cocaine and has a longer duration of action. The majority of amphetamine is illicitly produced and sold as a white powder, 'speed'. There are three types of amphetamine: benzedrine, dexamphetamine and methamphetamine, with the latter being the most potent. Most street speed is benzedrine, but illicit supplies of methamphetamine seem to be increasing and this can be in a smokable preparation known as 'ice'.

Cocaine, extracted from the leaves of the coca bush, was a common ingredient in tonics and other medicinal preparations. Freud was reputed to have been an advocate of cocaine, recommending it as a cure for morphine addiction. The practice of smoking cocaine (known as freebasing or crack smoking) started in America in the 1970s and by the late 1980s was regarded as the number one social and public health problem facing the USA (Gallup Poll 1989; ABC Poll 1989). Kleber (1988) warned of epidemic cocaine use spreading from the USA to England. While the scale of cocaine misuse in the UK has yet to match US levels, there has been a radical change in the way cocaine has been distributed and sold. Crack made a well publicised entry to the illicit market, and this has resulted in widespread addiction and associated violence (International Narcotics Control Board 1995).

Sometimes categorised as a 'designer drug', Ecstasy, methylene dioxymethamphetamine, otherwise referred to as MDMA, is a synthetically produced derivative of amphetamine with hallucinogenic properties. Widely used in America since the 1970s, Ecstasy has been available in the UK since the mid 1980s. It has become a well publicised part of the rave and club dance scene and is now part of the 'normal' weekend experience for hundreds of thousands of young people across the country.

Khat, *Catha edulis*, indigenous to East Africa, has a stimulant effect and has been used in Ethiopia, Somalia and the Yemen Republics for generations as an aid to socialisation, much as alcohol is used in Western society for these purposes.

Problems and issues

The desired effects of the different stimulants have been described in Chapter 4. Their ability to cause severe mood disturbances and acute psychotic phenomena have been understood for many years (Connell 1958). The following manifestations can apply to amphetamine and cocaine, but are usually more protracted in the case of amphetamine due to the longer half life. With continued 'binge' use over days, the euphoria may become the opposing mood state referred to as dysphoria. Hallucinations can occur, even after a single dose, and may manifest themselves in several modalities. Typically, voices (auditory), sparkling lights in the peripheral vision, (visual), or the feeling of insects under the skin (tactile), can occur. Paranoid thoughts may also occur, but insight into the condition is usually impaired rather than lost.

There are many toxic effects of stimulants, but most striking is the development of amphetamine/cocaine psychosis with repeated use of high doses. It is characterised by mounting anxiety, paranoia, persecutory delusions, stereotyped behaviour and auditory, visual and tactile hallucinations (Schuster & Gust 1993). Insight is absent and violence may occur. This type of psychotic reaction can occur with any route of administration but seems most marked when the drug is smoked (Manschreck *et al.* 1987). The characteristic feature of amphetamine/cocaine psychosis is the absence of confusion or disorientation, but it still may be difficult to distinguish from schizophrenia (Ghodes 1995). The condition is self-limiting with symptoms subsiding with abstinence from the causative stimulant.

It is a common assumption that with such undesirable effects stimulant users would just give up. However, the original euphoric effect of the drug seems to be remembered clearly. As stimulant use becomes more compulsive, the drug's effect becomes associated in the user's mind with certain places, feelings, objects or occasions. Example of these 'cues', as they are known, may be a dealer's road or a particular item of drug-using paraphernalia. Exposure to cues can precipitate intense craving and renewed stimulant use. Once 'learnt', they can continue to precipitate a powerful craving long after the stimulant was last used. This craving often overrides any recollection of adverse effect. There is a growing understanding of the importance to address this phenomenon in the treatment of stimulant and other drug dependence.

Stimulant withdrawal

A degree of controversy surrounds the existence of a stimulant withdrawal syndrome. Stimulants are not considered to be physically addictive but can produce strong psychological dependence. Many symptoms experienced by users as they come down after a weekend up on stimulants are normal responses to lack of food and sleep. Most research supports the existence of a dependence syndrome (Topp & Mattick 1997). Gawin and Ellinwood (1988, 1990) described three distinct phases of the cocaine abstinence syndrome: crash, withdrawal and extinction. The syndrome is thought to be due to a depletion of the neurotransmitters responsible for regulating mood.

Crash occurs following a prolonged period of stimulant use and is characterised by agitated depression and cocaine craving. The user may seek relief from sedative hypnotics such as benzodiazepines, opiates or alcohol. The risk of suicide is most significant at this stage. A period of prolonged sleep (hypersomnolence) usually follows, with recovery in 1 to 40 hours, and is probably explained by rebound serotonergic activity (Tutton & Crayton 1993). On waking, mood is usually normal but dysphoria can continue.

Withdrawal is characterised by 24–48 hours of stable mood (euthymia) following recovery from the crash then progresses to a state of anhedonia, dysphoria, anxiety, irritability and stimulant craving, worsening over the next 12–96 hours. The experience of this unpleasant state is a contrast to recent experiences of euphoria and, coupled with exposure to conditioned cues, may result in a relapsing cycle.

The *extinction* phase sees the mood and other symptoms returning to normal as long as abstinence is maintained throughout the first two phases. Cocaine craving can still be triggered by cues. Extinction only occurs if conditioned cues are not rewarded.

Clinical care and therapeutic interventions

General principles

Therapeutic interventions should be flexible, responsive and multimodal. The aim is to address the complexity of biochemical, psychological and social factors which perpetuate stimulant use. A range of treatment approaches and opportunistic interventions are used and will be described in a later section, but there is no generally accepted treatment protocol. There are a variety of reasons why stimulant use can precipitate contact with health services. People are often most suggestible to change at times of crisis, so many addiction nurses and other professionals are routinely in the prime position to facilitate change with opportunistic interventions. Being informed about health and other effects, and where to go for help, enables informed choice over future substance use. These 'brief interventions' have been found to result in lasting health benefits with alcohol misusers (Anderson 1993).

Detoxification from stimulants

There is a lack of consensus over the existence of a stimulant withdrawal syndrome and no specific detoxification protocol for stimulant withdrawal (Feigenbaun & Allen 1996). In most cases, stimulant withdrawal does not require any medical intervention; it is an accepted part of the user's week. In some cases, particularly high dose crack users with severe dependence and withdrawal symptoms, intervention is required. Careful assessment is necessary in order to instigate appropriate treatment. There is no place for replacement prescribing, as methadone is used to detoxify from opiates. The client should be advised to stop using the drug abruptly.

Ghodes (1995) outlined a treatment plan advocating oral or intravenous diazepam to settle agitation. Psychotic symptoms secondary to stimulant use are self limiting and should settle in a few days. Phenothaizines should only be used in severe or protracted cases and should be used with caution if the client is dependent on alcohol or another sedative-hypnotic due to their epilepticogenic effect. Suicide is a real risk during stimulant with-drawal due to intense dysphoria. Depressive symptoms should be moni-tored. Hospital in-patient treatment must be responsive if a client is deemed to be at risk of deliberate self-harm.

Specialist interventions

Due to the compulsive nature of stimulant dependence and its potential for impairing neurological functioning, there is general agreement that absti-nence should be the main aim of treatment (Strang *et al.* 1993; Schuckit 1994). Controlled use should not be advised due to the likelihood of this leading to further compulsive use (Washton 1987). Treatment follows a number of stages from assessment to detoxification and to relapse pre-vention. The initial interview is an important opportunity to engage the individual and motivational interviewing (Miller 1983) is a widely accep-ted therapeutic technique with the aim to 'reframe' the problem in the individual's mind, generating cognitive dissonance resulting in motivation to change substance use behaviour.

It is essential to address cue precipitated craving in treatment pro-grammes meaningfully. These treatments have a theoretical basis in learning theory. For a review see Drummond *et al.* (1995). Childress *et al.* (1987) reported a significant reduction in craving reported by opiate and cocaine dependent patients after 20, one hour sessions being exposed to conditioned stimuli (cues). In a study of cue exposure treatment in opiate and cocaine dependence, Dawe and Powell (1995) concluded that cue exposure did not yield any additional benefits, but recommended further research into those specific components of cue exposure which can facili-tate behavioural change.

An alternative treatment evaluated for crack/cocaine detoxification is acupuncture (Lipton *et al.* 1994). Over a one month period, a sample of 150 treatment seeking cocaine abusers were randomly assigned to one of two treatment groups. The first received acupuncture at the correct ear location, while the second received acupuncture at ear locations not used for drug use treatment. Urine results favoured the experimental group, but self-report and retention in treatment were comparable. Being a single blind trial, one cannot discount the possibility of bias being conveyed from the acupuncturist to the control group. This approach may gain scientific approval and become a valuable addition to a comprehensive range of services.

Strang *et al.* (1993) described a comprehensive treatment repertoire which includes the following:

❏ Harm reduction strategies, clear education about the effects of cocaine, safer drug use practices and needle exchange.

❏ Use of Miller's modal of motivational interviewing to facilitate the consideration of change.
❏ Symptomatology of cocaine withdrawal is managed by understanding and support from the therapist.
❏ Relapse prevention work is based on the cognitive behavioural model (Marlatt & Gordon 1984). High risk situations are pinpointed and new coping skills are acquired and practised.
❏ The use of cue exposure techniques to break the stimulus–response relationship.
❏ Individual psychotherapy for specific cases, such as those with a history of traumatic past events, sexual abuse or early parental loss, for example, or other developmental disruptions.
❏ Adjunctive tricyclic antidepressant medication, usually desipramine.
❏ Family therapy.
❏ Twelve step programmes.
❏ Therapeutic communities and rehabilitation units.

Carroll *et al.* (1994) compared treatment outcome between pharmacological and psychotherapeutic treatment interventions by randomly assigning cocaine abusers to different treatment models. The results confirm the need for a comprehensive treatment approach as patients exhibiting different severity of dependence responded to different treatment combinations in different ways. For example, patients with lower severity of dependence responded more favourably to desipramine therapy (a tricyclic antidepressant) than the severely dependent, who responded more favourably to relapse prevention. Until better matching techniques have been developed, a comprehensive range of treatment modalities is the gold standard.

Role of drugs in relapse prevention

The binge–crash nature of escalating stimulant intake results in progressively less fulfilling and more disturbing highs, with a corresponding crash period. The stark contrast of euphoria to dysphoria is a manifestation of changes in levels of neurotransmitters. The most promising results have been with two dopamine agonist drugs, desipramine and bromocriptine and these have been found to be most effective as adjunctive treatment for cocaine dependence. Bromocriptine seems most helpful in the first 1 to 2 weeks of treatment by improving mood and decreasing craving. Desipramine could become the treatment of choice for the anhedonia that persists for weeks after the initiation of abstinence (Tutton & Crayton 1993).

The use of antidepressant medication in the treatment of stimulant misuse has yet to achieve general acceptance. In most cases, mood has returned to normal before the antidepressant has reached therapeutic levels. The discovery of specific stimulant antagonists, with an action similar to that of naltrexone with heroin addicts, would provide a more effective adjunct to treatment than the medications studied so far. Schuckit (1997) comments how advances are being made in the development of such a drug. However, despite the cost effectiveness of pharmacological agents compared with psychological treatments, they must remain an adjunct rather than a panacea for cocaine dependence.

Case vignette

This case illustrates how stimulant users can come into contact with statutory services and the subsequent responses.

Heather, who is 19 years old, is taken to A & E by a friend in the early hours of the morning. She is a regular amphetamine user and had been taking speed intranasally over the previous 2 days. She is preoccupied by concerns that an individual wishes her harm. The casualty officer contacts the duty psychiatrist for an assessment of Heather's mental state. Following assessment, the duty psychiatrist recommends that Heather is admitted to the acute psychiatric unit for observation and makes a referral to the community drug and alcohol team. After a short stay on the ward, she gradually gains insight into the cause of her persecutory beliefs and benefits from the opportunity to talk through her experiences with her keyworker from the community drug and alcohol team.

Health interventions

❑ Wherever possible, nurse in a calm, non stimulating environment.
❑ Ensure adequate dietary intake, fluid and rest.
❑ Clearly explain the reasons and procedure for all interventions.
❑ Administer medication until psychotic symptoms subside.
❑ Monitor mood and provide support during the crash and withdrawal phases.
❑ Be aware of the possibility of deliberate self-harm or suicide.
❑ Use urinalysis to confirm or identify drug use.
❑ Encourage Heather to talk about her recent experiences, concerns and drug use.
❑ Avoid getting into disputes about the reality of her beliefs, but provide reassurance and avoid reinforcing paranoid beliefs.
❑ Encourage Heather to identify what she hopes to change about her drug use.
❑ Educate about the effects of amphetamine if the client is receptive.
❑ Ensure follow up. Use the care programme approach to clarify roles and responsibilities in the overall care.

Discussion

This illustrates how stimulant users can present for help. Carefully timed interventions can help to engage the person into treatment. An assertive approach and the involvement of friends or relatives enable diagnosis and informal admission. Heather required symptomatic drug treatment (chlorpromazine) during the withdrawal period. Advances are being made to develop pharmacological treatments that help in relapse prevention. At this stage, post-detoxification interventions are essentially psychological and social. The use of motivational interviewing when Heather's focus of attention was on her drug use enabled her to take responsibility for her problems. This is an evidence based approach that could be effectively employed by many nurses and other professionals. Specialist drug teams may use this and other cognitive behavioural approaches such as Marlatt's model of relapse prevention and cue exposure therapy. These are relatively new techniques which have yet to be incorporated into everyday practice for many in the substance misuse field.

Conclusions

High dose stimulant and crack users may require admission under the Mental Health Act in cases where the risk of self-harm is significant and informal admission is refused. Front line staff need to be able to identify signs and symptoms of drug misuse to instigate appropriate treatment, highlighting a need for pre- and post-basic training on skills, attitude and knowledge related to drug misuse. Liaison is essential between departments so there can be continuity of care, and it is important for there to be a mutual understanding of responsibility for care between community mental health teams and community drug and alcohol teams. Where role boundaries are not clear, services may fail to meet the needs of the patient and the patient may fail to engage.

References

ABC Poll (1989) Reported in the *Washington Post*, 29 August.

Anderson, P. (1993) Management of alcohol problems: the role of the general practitioner. *Alcohol & Alcoholism*, **28**, 263–72.

Carroll, K.M. , Rounsaville, B.J., Gorden, L.T., *et al.* (1994) Psychotherapy and pharmacotherapy for ambulatory cocaine abusers. *Archives of General Psychiatry*, **51**, 177–87.

Childress, A.R., Ehrman, R., McLellan, A.T. & O'Brien, C.P. (1987) Conditioned craving and arousal in cocaine addiction. In: *Problems of Drug Dependence: NIDA Research Monograph Series*, 74–80. National Institute on Drug Abuse, Rockville, Maryland.

Connell, P. (1958) *Amphetamine Psychosis*. Institute of Psychiatry, Maudsley Monographs No 5. Oxford University Press, London.

Dawe, S. & Powell, J.H. (1995) Cue exposure treatment in opiate and cocaine dependence. In: *Addictive Behaviour: Cue Exposure, Theory and practice* (eds D.C. Drummond, S.T. Tiffany, S. Glautier & B. Remington), pp. 197–209. John Wiley, Chichester.

Drummond, D.C., Tiffany, S.T., Glautier, S. & Remington, B. (1995) Cue exposure in understanding and treating addictive behaviours. In: *Addictive Behaviour: Cue Exposure, Theory and Practice* (eds D.C. Drummond, S.T. Tiffany, S. Glautier & B. Remington). John Wiley, Chichester.

Feigenbaum, J.C. & Allen, K.M. (1996) Detoxification. In: *Nursing Care of the Addicted Client* (ed. B.K.M. Allen), pp. 139–75. Lippincott, Philadelphia.

Gallup Poll (1989) July and August reports in *USA Today*.

Gawin, F.H. & Ellinwood E.H. (1988) Cocaine and other stimulants: actions, abuse and treatment. *New England Medical Journal*, **318**, 1173–82.

Gawin, F. & Ellinwood, E.H. (1990) Cocaine abuse treatment: open pilot trial with desipramine and lithium carbonate. *Archives of General Psychiatry*, **41**, 903–9.

Ghodes, A.H. (1995) *Drugs and Addictive Behaviour: A Guide to Treatment*, 2nd edn. Blackwell Science, Oxford.

International Narcotics Control Board. (1995) *Report of The International Narcotics Control Board for 1994*, paragraph 300. United Nations, New York.

Kleber, H.D. (1988) Epidemic cocaine abuse: America's present, Britain's future? *British Journal of Addiction*, **83**, 1359–71.

Lipton, D.S., Brewington, V. & Smith, M. (1994) Acupuncture for crack–cocaine detoxification: experimental evaluation of efficacy. *Journal of Substance Abuse Treatment*, **1**, 205–15.

Manschreck, T.C., Allen, D.F. & Neville, M. (1987) Freebase psychosis: cases from a Bahamian epidemic of cocaine abuse. *Psychiatry*, **28**, 555–64.

Marlatt, G.A. & Gordon, W.H. (1984) Relapse prevention: introduction and overview of the modal. *British Journal of Addiction*, **79**, 261–73.

Miller, W. (1983) Motivational interviewing with problem drinkers. *Behavioural Psychotherapy*, **11**, 147–72.

Misuse of Drugs Act (1971) HMSO, London.

Schuckit, M.A. (1994) The treatment of stimulant dependence. *Addiction*, **89**, 1559–63.

Schuckit, M.A. (1997) Science, medicine, and the future. Substance use disorders. *British Medical Journal*, **314**, 1606.

Schuster, H. & Gust, S.W. (1993) Cocaine: challenges to research. In: *Drugs, Alcohol and Tobacco: Making the Science and Policy Connections* (eds G. Edwards, J. Strang & J.H. Jaffe), pp. 146–55. Oxford University Press, Oxford.

Strang, J., Farrell, M. & Unnithan, S. (1993) Treatment of cocaine abuse: exploring the condition and selecting the response. In: *Cocaine and Crack: Supply and Use* (ed. P. Bean). Macmillan Press, Basingstoke.

Topp, L. & Mattick, R.P. (1997) Validation of the amphetamine dependence syndrome and the SAMDQ. *Addiction*, **92**, 151–62.

Tutton, C.S. & Crayton, J.W. (1993) Current pharmacotherapies for cocaine abuse: a review. *Journal of Addictive Diseases*, **12**, 109–27.

Washton, A. (1987) Outpatient treatment techniques. In: *Cocaine: A Clinician's Handbook* (eds A. Washton & M. Gold), pp. 106–7. Guildford Press, New York.

Chapter 20

Opiate and Polydrug Use: Clinical Care and Nursing Interventions

Mike Gafoor

Introduction

In recent years, polydrug use or multiple drug taking has become a common feature with opiate users. Health care workers are more likely to come across the polydrug using patient than someone who is just taking heroin. The term polydrug use may be defined as a pattern of drug taking involving the use of more than one drug taken together or in rapid sequence of each other (Royal College of Psychiatrists 1987). Drugs such as benzodiazepines, amphetamines, cocaine and alcohol are frequently used in various combinations, either to complement the effects of opiates or to alleviate withdrawal symptoms.

As a group, polydrug users present many challenges to health care workers. Research has also shown them to have more complex physical, social and psychological needs than other drug users (Darke *et al.* 1993). They often fail to attend follow up appointments and, when they do attend, are frequently in a state of intoxication or withdrawal. In addition, the polydrug using patient tends to be drug seeking in behaviour and may exaggerate their drug use in order to obtain a prescription. Consequently they are susceptible to serious drug interactions with prescribed medication and drug overdoses. It is therefore important that nurses working in a primary care setting are able to understand the health needs of this patient group and to develop a model of clinical management to address such needs adequately.

This chapter will examine the extent of opiate use and describe the nature of problems experienced by polydrug opiate users. It will also outline the main treatment strategies and nursing interventions.

Nature and extent

It is difficult to be precise on the number of opiate users in the UK, as drug misuse is frequently a clandestine activity and is not routinely reported. Until May 1997, all doctors were legally obliged to notify anyone who was known or suspected to be addicted to opiates or cocaine; this requirement for doctors to send the particulars of drug addicts to the Home Office was revoked by the 1997 Regulations on the Misuse of Drugs. However, community studies suggest that for every drug misuser who presents to services, another five to ten do not. Hence if this factor is applied to the latest home office figures which showed 33 804 opiate users notified in 1995 (Home Office Statistical Bulletin 1996) the true extent of the problem lies between 169 000 and 338 000. The Home Office statistics also indicated that the number of heroin users notified showed a steady rise from 15 086 in 1991 to 24 530 in 1995, with a 25% increase in users under 21 years old.

The pattern of polydrug use varies greatly, with different cultures existing within the drug using population. In Scotland, for example, the majority of opiate users are injectors and heroin is often mixed with drugs such as diazepam, temazepam and alcohol (Hammersley *et al.* 1995). Similarly, Perera *et al.* (1987) found that 90% of mainly heroin addicts used benzodiazepines either to boost the effects of opiates or to alleviate anxiety and sleeping problems. However, Darke and Hall (1995) found that amphetamine use was more common in a sample of heroin users. As well as the pharmacological reasons, factors such as availability, price, purity as well as the social and cultural meanings attached to different types of drugs may determine what drug is taken and how. Although opiate users come from all sections of society, there are strong links which exist between heroin use, social deprivation and unemployment (Pearson 1987). The typical profile of an opiate polydrug user is someone who is young, male, not in treatment, injects and recently borrowed injecting equipment (Darke & Hall 1995).

Nature of problems

Physical

The health risks experienced by drug users depend upon factors such as dosage, quantity, duration of use and route of administration. Strictly speaking pharmaceutical heroin can be taken for long periods without any obvious ill-effects. Street heroin, however, is often mixed or 'cut' with other drugs to increase its bulk and in the past harmful substances such as brick dust and bicarbonate of soda have been used. Most of the medical problems such as hepatitis, thrombophlebitis, abscesses, endocarditis, septicaemia and HIV are caused by unsterile injecting techniques and sharing injecting equipment. Sometimes tablets are crushed and injected, resulting in blockage to the blood supply and gangrene of the limbs. Polydrug users, particularly those who inject benzodiazepines, are a high risk group for HIV and hepatitis B and C, as they tend to inject more frequently and are more likely to be involved in needle sharing and unsafe sexual practices (Klee *et al.* 1990).

Drug overdoses involving the combined use of opiates with other central nervous system (CNS) depressant drugs such as alcohol, barbiturates and benzodiazepines are a common problem among polydrug opiate users. Accidental overdose may also occur if an unusually high purity of heroin is used or the drug user returns to opiate use after a period of abstinence. Death is usually due to respiratory failure and inhalation of vomit. The drug naloxone is an opiate antagonist that is used in opiate overdose.

Sexual dysfunction is another problem commonly associated with opiate use, and decreased libido and impotence are frequently reported by users. Female users may suffer with menstrual irregularities such as amenhorrea due to the inhibiting effect of opiates on the menstrual cycle. However, pregnancy may still occur and the continued use of opiates during pregnancy can lead to premature labour and fetal distress. Babies born to opiate dependent mothers are likely to suffer from withdrawal symptoms and require treatment at birth. Opiates can also slow down the passage of food in the intestine by their effects on the gastrointestinal tract, and many users suffer from persistent constipation. They often lead a chaotic life-style and neglect diet and personal hygiene, which makes them more vulnerable to physical problems.

Psychological

The rate of psychiatric morbidity among opiate users is twice that of the general population and depression, anxiety and antisocial personality disorder are the most common psychiatric disorders (Darke *et al.* 1992). Opiate users who are also dependent on other CNS depressant drugs, for example, alcohol, barbiturates and benzodiazepines, frequently experience depressive symptoms such as low mood, poor appetite, sleep disturbance and suicidal ideas. Substance misuse and depression have been found to be associated with suicide more often than any other psychiatric disorder (Murphy 1988) and death rates have been estimated to be around 15%. Restlessness, irritability, and aggressive behaviour may result from either intoxication or withdrawal of sedative type drugs and many patients suffer with memory impairment. Anxiety and panic attacks may result with the long term use of benzodiazepines, amphetamines, cannabis and alcohol.

Social problems

As the polydrug user becomes more immersed in a substance misuse lifestyle, he or she is unable to meet family, work and social commitments. This may result in unemployment, housing and family problems. The patient may also become involved in activities such as stealing and prostitution to fund an increasing drug habit and legal difficulties may ensue. A study carried out on heroin users attending a drug treatment unit in

Liverpool showed that 90% of them were involved in shoplifting or burglary in order to finance their opiate habit (Fazey 1987). Drug users are often perceived as weak-willed individuals and may suffer from social prejudice and negative stereotyping. This can lead to them feeling socially marginalised and alienated from society. Although drug use in itself does not equate with poor child care, research from the USA has shown substance misuse to be a major factor in child abuse and neglect (Children's Defense Fund 1992).

Problems of dependence and withdrawal

The regular use of opiates may result in the development of physical and psychological dependence. Physical dependence is characterised by the development of tolerance whereby an increasing amount of the drug is required to experience its pleasurable effects and the user experiences withdrawal symptoms if the drug is reduced or stopped. Psychological dependence is considered by many drug users to be the most difficult part of coming off drugs and it has been described as 'an overriding compulsion to take a drug despite the knowledge of its harmful consequences' (Ghodse 1995). The physical withdrawal symptoms of opiates are similar to a bout of flu and vary in severity according to the dosage, duration of use and expectations of the user. With heroin, these can appear 6–12 hours after the last dose and with methadone, which has a much longer half-life, 24–48 hours after the last dose. The opiate withdrawal syndrome consists of a wide range of signs and symptoms that include:

❑ Abdominal cramps and diarrhoea
❑ Muscle aches
❑ Dilated pupils
❑ Runny nose and eyes
❑ Hot and cold flushes
❑ Anxiety and restlessness

Opiate users who are also dependent on drugs such as barbiturates or benzodiazepines would have additional withdrawal symptoms such as tremors, perceptual disturbances and, in some cases, withdrawal seizures.

Assessment

The purpose of assessment is to identify the nature and severity of the individual's drug use and to develop with the patient a care plan to meet his/her physical, psychological and social needs. Assessment is more than a data collection process as it enables the nurse to establish a therapeutic relationship with the patient by listening to his/her concerns and gaining an understanding of what help is required to meet those concerns. It should be seen as an ongoing process that provides an opportunity in helping patients to understand the effects of various psychoactive substances and how to avoid the harm associated with their misuse (for example HIV and hepatitis B and C infections, overdoses).

Polydrug users often fail to attend follow up appointments and it is important that health education is provided at the earliest contact and continues throughout treatment. The use of motivational interviewing techniques whereby the patient is asked to draw up a personal inventory of both the positive and negative aspects of substance use can help to increase his/her insight and motivation. It can also identify the important issues from the patient's perspective and contribute towards mutual goal setting between the nurse and the patient. A good knowledge base regarding the physical, social and psychological consequences of substance misuse and the resources that are available locally will help towards achieving a satisfactory assessment and care plan.

The nurse should aim to acquire the following information from the patient at the assessment interview.

❑ Drugs: types, dose (amounts, cost), frequency, how long, route of administration (history of HIV risk taking behaviour), nature of problems (physical, social and psychological), signs of intoxication or withdrawal, details of previous treatment and perception of help required.
❑ Alcohol: number of units, frequency and duration of use, withdrawal symptoms and complications.

In addition the addiction nurse should observe the patient for signs of withdrawal and intoxication and the presence of any injecting 'track' marks. Additional information (with the patient's permission) from friends and relatives along with urinalysis will aid the assessment process.

Medical management

Polydrug opiate users may require help with medication either to detoxify or to stabilise their drug use. Methadone (a synthetic opiate) is the most common drug used in the treatment of opiate addiction. It is usually prescribed in oral liquid form and dispensed on a daily basis. The rationale behind the use of methadone is to help to move patients away from injecting street drugs and to stabilise their lifestyle. Many GPs are willing to prescribe oral methadone to opiate users provided it is on a time limited basis and there is clinical support from the local drug service. Once it is established that the patient is physically dependent on opiates, he or she is then stabilised on a dose of methadone which will adequately suppress any withdrawal symptoms but does not make the patient become intoxicated. The stabilisation procedure may be carried out as either an in-patient or out-patient and is necessary since the purity of illicit opiates may vary and patients may not give an accurate history of their drug use. In the UK, the starting dose of methadone is usually between 20 and 60 mg and this is gradually reduced to zero over an agreed period of time.

Polydrug opiate users may also be dependent on other drugs such as benzodiazepines or alcohol. Alcohol detoxification in most cases (except in patients with a history of seizures or serious physical or psychiatric conditions) can be carried out as an out-patient using a benzodiazepine drug such as Valium or Librium. Benzodiazepine withdrawal is usually achieved by converting to a long acting drug like Valium and reducing the dosage every 2–3 weeks. It is better to withdraw the patient from any sedative drugs first before attempting to reduce his/her methadone.

Admission to hospital may be necessary for some polydrug users to stabilise their medication needs or for safer detoxification, particularly if there is a risk of withdrawal seizures. The drug naltrexone which blocks the effects of opiates may be used to prevent relapse in patients who are opiate free, while antabuse is commonly prescribed for alcohol dependent patients who wish to remain abstinent. Some opiate users may decline the use of opiate drugs and non opiate medication such as thioridazine, Lomotil (co-phenotrope) and propanolol may be used to provide symptomatic relief of withdrawal symptoms.

Psycho-social support

Polydrug opiate users tend to view their drug problems purely in pharmacological terms and may pressurise staff for medication. It is necessary to establish a therapeutic relationship with the patient for any prescription offered to achieve full benefits. Such a relationship should be based on trust, understanding, respect and empathy. Counselling and support are important both during and after withdrawal from medication. The addiction nurse can help the patient to identify and cope with high risk situations or cues which might lead to relapse of substance misuse. Some patients may require help to deal with problems such as anxiety and sleeplessness, while others need more practical help to deal with issues such as homelessness and unemployment. Counselling sessions can be used to explore underlying emotional conflicts and to provide an opportunity to set mutually agreed goals that will help the patient to stay off drugs and improve their self-esteem.

Polydrug users often have problems such as homelessness and unemployment, and may return to drug use through boredom or an inability to move away from a drug oriented lifestyle. Helping them to develop new interests and relationships is an important aspect of preventing them from returning to drugs. The involvement of a social worker to assist with housing and benefit issues as well as practical help in finding suitable employment are sometimes necessary. For a few patients, a period of stay in a residential rehabilitation facility might be the only way in which they are able to achieve a drug free lifestyle.

Case vignette

Jane is 25 years old and recently returned to live with her parents after a period of living in 'squats'. She has a long history of drug misuse since the age of 13 when she was taken into care for continuous truanting from school. In the past she has used solvents, crack cocaine, amphetamines, LSD and Ecstasy on a regular basis before being introduced to heroin injecting 4 years ago. She spends approximately £40 per day on her habit which she funds by shoplifting and by exchanging sex for drugs. Jane has also been taking varying amounts of temazepam tablets daily for the past year which she obtains from her GP and buys off the streets. She has had several admissions to the A&E department with drug overdoses and after being beaten up by her boyfriend, himself a heroin addict. Jane presented to her GP complaining of panic attacks, low mood and sleeplessness. She wanted some more temazepam tablets but instead was asked to see the practice counsellor who then arranged for a joint assessment with the addiction nurse specialist.

Clinical management and nursing interventions

On assessment, it became apparent that Jane's symptoms were due to benzodiazepine withdrawal and she agreed to undertake a gradual withdrawal programme from both benzodiazepines and opiates. Jane was stabilised on 30 mg diazepam and 30 mg oral methadone linctus daily, which was gradually reduced over a 3 month period. The nursing assessment revealed the nature of Jane's dependence on opiates and benzodiazepines along with her psychological problems. She was provided with health education on the risks associated with injecting drug use and unsafe sexual practices. The addiction specialist nurse advised the GP on medication needs and, after stabilisation, Jane was helped by the practice nurse to withdraw gradually from benzodiazepines and methadone. In addition, Jane received counselling and support to deal with unresolved emotional difficulties over her parents' separation and was taught anxiety management and relaxation exercises. Her self esteem and confidence improved sufficiently to enable her to get a job and to make changes in her relationship. She is currently in a new and stable relationship.

Conclusions

Polydrug use is common among opiate users and this group of patients usually have complex health and social needs. They are often difficult to engage in treatment due to a chaotic lifestyle and drug seeking behaviour. Nurses in both hospital and community settings can play an important role in the assessment, management and care of the polydrug opiate user. A good background knowledge on the range of commonly used illicit substances and their effects will help the nurse to understand the nature of the patient's problems. Therapeutic skills in assessment, counselling, stress management and health promotion are important in helping the polydrug using patient either to abstain or to stabilise his/her use of substances. In some cases, clinical support and training from specialist substance misuse agencies may be necessary.

References

Advisory Council on the Misuse of Drugs (1988) *Aids and Drugs Misuse*. Part 1. HMSO, London.

Children's Defense Fund (1992) *The State of America's Children, 1992*. Children's Defense Fund, Washington DC.

Darke, S. & Hall, W. (1995) Levels and correlates of polydrug use among heroin users and regular amphetamine users. *Drug and Alcohol Dependence*, **39**, 231–5.

Darke, S., Wodak, A., Hall, W., *et al.* (1992) Prevalence and predictors of psychopathology among opioid users. *British Journal of Addiction*, **87**, 771–6.

Darke, S., Swift, W., Hall, W. & Ross, M. (1993) Drug use, HIV risk-taking and psychosocial correlates of benzodiazepine use among methadone maintenance patients. *Drug and Alcohol Dependence*, **34**, 67–70.

Fazey, C.S.J. (1987) *The evaluation of the Liverpool drug dependency clinic*. Report to the Mersey Regional Health Authority.

Ghodse, A.H. (1995) *Drugs and Addictive Behaviour: A Guide to Treatment*, 2nd edn. Blackwell Scientific Publications, Oxford.

Hammersley, R., Cassidy, M.T. & Oliver, J. (1995) Drugs associated with drug-related deaths in Edinburgh and Glasgow, November 1990 to October 1992. *Addiction*, **90**, 959–65.

Home Office Statistical Bulletin (1996) *Statistics of Drug Addicts notified to the Home Office, United Kingdom*, 1995. HMSO, London.

Klee, H., Faugier, J., Hayes, C., *et al.* (1990) AIDS-related behaviour, polydrug use and temazepam. *British Journal of Addiction*, **85**, 1125–32.

Murphy, G.E. (1988) Suicide and substance abuse. *Archives of General Psychiatry*, **45**, 593–4.

Pearson, G. (1987) Social deprivation, unemployment and patterns of heroin use. In: *A Land Fit For Heroin* (eds N. Dorn & N. South). MacMillan, London.

Perera, K.M.H., Tulley, M. & Jenner, F.A. (1987) The use of benzodiazepines among drug addicts. *British Journal of Addiction*, **82**, 511–15.

Royal College of Psychiatrists (1987) *Drug Scenes: A Report on Drugs and Drug Dependence*. Gaskell, London.

Chapter 21
Nicotine Addiction: Health Care Interventions

Carol Mills

Introduction

Smoking is a major cause of death and disability in the UK and the Western world as a whole (Callum *et al.* 1992). Recent figures suggest that the smoking-related death rate is increasing and now stands at approximately 120 000 deaths per year with about half of these occurring before or during middle age. Half of all lifelong smokers die as a result of smoking (West 1997). Facilities for providing an effective cessation counselling service vary from district to district and are completely non existent in many district health authorities in the UK. Therefore the needs of the 70% of smokers who want to quit are not being met as most areas do not have a centralised cessation service. The only resource for potential 'quitters' is 'Quitline', the telephone smoking cessation counselling and advice service.

Many health professionals are not prepared to deal with patients wishing to quit nor do they understand the nature of nicotine addiction. There is also the difficulty of when to advocate the use of nicotine replacement therapy (NRT). A clinic or group setting ensures that adequate instruction on appropriate use of NRT can be provided. An assessment interview is the ideal situation to discuss a patient's dependency on cigarettes and the motivation to quit and also determine the method of NRT and contraindications to its use (Anthonisen *et al.* 1994). NRT as an effective component of the intervention can almost double the long term abstinence rates from 16% to 27% (Foulds 1993).

The aims of this chapter are to describe a smoking cessation service in action and the methods of interventions that can be utilised at both individual or group level. Two case studies are presented to describe the process of enabling smokers to quit.

A smoking cessation service

This section will describe some of the main methods used in a smoking cessation service and is based on the development of such a service at St

George's Healthcare NHS Trust, London. A smoking cessation service should include both motivational and treatment intervention strategies and encompass an easily accessible facility for patients. The aims of the service are to provide an accessible, effective smoking cessation counselling service for staff, patients and the local community and to deliver training and information on smoking cessation to health professionals.

All potential quitters attend an assessment interview and join either group therapy sessions or a one to one session. Group meetings are weekly over 5 weeks; one to one therapy may last longer depending on the patient's needs. At the first session, members are encouraged to quit smoking and to use transdermal nicotine patches, full strength for 6 weeks then reduce the strength to a lower dose if desired. Follow-up contact is made at 8 and 12 weeks and again at 6 and 12 months to establish if the patient is still abstinent. In the context of this chapter, NRT refers to transdermal nicotine patches and nicotine gum, both of which are readily available to the general public.

Recognising withdrawal symptoms for what they are and developing coping strategies is important (Hajek 1994). It may be necessary to iniate a discussion to help group members develop their own strategy to prevent relapse in the future. The use of nicotine gum as an adjunct to patches may help during particularly stressful periods as a short term measure (Tonneson & Fagerstrom 1994). Stressing the positive aspects which have occurred since quitting and using the group to reinforce the individual's commitment to maintain abstinence should also help as well as emphasising that discomfort is transient and will pass.

In the early stages of quitting, smokers often report feeling hungrier than normal, as appetite is no longer suppressed by smoking. The therapist should approach this subject sensitively; putting on a few pounds in weight may be acceptable to some while others may use weight gain as a reason for returning to smoking. Advice to reduce fat and sugar intake while increasing fibre and vegetable content may help to satiate the initial pangs of hunger. Attempting to diet while quitting smoking is not to be recommended. Increasing exercise a little while still taking small treats may give a more positive response by helping to diminish the feelings of deprivation often experienced by smokers.

One to one intervention

Key points

The assessment of nicotine dependence and motivation to quit is based on the Fagerstrom test for nicotine dependence (Heatherton *et al.* 1991). The taking of a smoking history incorporates the following questions:

❑ Number of years as a smoker?
❑ How soon after waking is the first cigarette?

❑ Does the patient crave a cigarette when in a no smoking area or situation?

Then the procedure is:

❑ Examine any previous attempts to quit.
❑ Assess suitability for NRT, i.e. no contraindications (in certain cases written permission from the patient's GP may need to be obtained).
❑ Ensure the patient has realistic expectations of the efficacy of the treatment.
❑ Discuss concerns, e.g. withdrawal discomfort.
❑ Send a letter to the GP to inform them of the patient's quit programme.
❑ Measure expired carbon monoxide levels (ECO).

During the interview ground rules are discussed with the patient and a setting 'quit date' is agreed. It is beneficial during this session to allow the patient to express any anxieties regarding the quit attempt, to discuss previous failed attempts and to declare a serious commitment to quit. The type of NRT should be decided (patches or gum) and its use and limitations explained to the patient. NRT helps to relieve nicotine craving but withdrawal symptoms can still be quite strong for some people (Foulds & Ghodse 1995).

Carbon monoxide levels are an indicator of the amount of tobacco smoke inhaled by an individual smoker and it is important that the ECO level is assessed (Foulds 1996). ECO measurement is a quick, simple, non invasive test which can be used as a basis for interventions. The levels can be affected by the time elapsed since the last cigarette, for example, an afternoon readings will give a more accurate indication than a morning reading. It is important to point this out to the patient that ECO levels can also be affected by recent exercise and the way in which a cigarette is smoked, e.g. depth and frequency of inhalation. Carbon monoxide is excreted by the body quite rapidly and will reduce considerably within hours of giving up smoking. Use of an ECO monitor where patients can see and gain feedback on the positive effects of not smoking can also act as a major incentive towards quitting.

A second appointment should be made for the quit date and the individual is encouraged to make immediate preparations to quit, such as disposing of smoking equipment, and to prepare for difficult situations – for example, socialising with friends who are smokers or stress at work. In the early stages of quitting, smokers may be taken off guard and reach for a cigarette as a reflex action. It is during the assessment interview that the patient may decide not to join the next group or choose one to one counselling. Subsequent appointments, usually on a weekly basis for about 4 weeks, last on average 15 minutes. When planning follow up sessions it may be practical to book patients at 10–15 minute intervals, as approximately one third will fail to attend, almost all of whom will have returned to smoking and given up their quit attempt.

Generally, patients are encouraged to discuss how they have coped during the week since the last appointment and what has been difficult for them. For example, some describe the first week as 'not too bad', appearing to be almost euphoric and confident, while others describe cravings and physical discomforts such as sleeplessness, anxiety and difficulty concentrating (Foulds 1993). It is important to caution the overconfident that the euphoria may lessen somewhat, while pointing out the positive results of quitting to those who are perhaps viewing the prospect of being a non smoker as less attractive due to present discomfort. Where patients are unable to attend the clinic in person on a regular basis due to work commitments, etc., telephone contact may be a suitable alternative with the patient visiting clinic occasionally to have ECO measurements recorded.

Case vignette 1 One to one counselling

David is 56 years old and has smoked 25–30 cigarettes a day for 36 years. He has made numerous attempts to quit over the past 5 years using NRT patches and gum. The longest period of abstinence was 15 days while in hospital. He suffered a myocardial infarction 4 years ago and has had severe cardiovascular problems and asthma. David was referred to clinic by his GP who approved the use of NRT. David is retired due to ill health and also had a history of alcohol dependence from which he has been in remission for the last 5 years.

At the assessment interview, David's ECO level was measured as 34 parts per million (ppm) and he had smoked 15 cigarettes so far that day. David recognised that he was addicted to nicotine. His first cigarette was taken within 5 minutes of waking in the morning and he continued to smoke at regular intervals during the day, except when he took his dog for a walk. He particularly enjoyed a cigarette after meals and felt that he had to have them with him at all times. David said that he was desperate to quit for many reasons: health, financial and to break free from dependency. His wife did not smoke and objected to his smoking, which made him feel guilty. His main reason for wanting to quit smoking was the continuing deterioration of his health.

The determination he had shown in overcoming alcohol dependency illustrated his tenacity. However, he felt it was more difficult for him to quit smoking. During the interview he appeared a little nervous and apprehensive about quitting and explained that this was due to his previous failed attempts. To try to dispel these feelings the rationale behind weekly appointments and the efficacy of using NRT were explained. It was also pointed out that while NRT may help to overcome some of the discomfort of withdrawal symptoms, there may still be a craving to smoke. Unless this is made clear the smoker may believe the NRT is not working when such cravings occur. David preferred not to join a group as he felt nervous in such situations.

A quit day for David was decided for the following week and an appointment arranged for the same day. He had several days to prepare to quit and decided to use the first patch (15 mg) on the morning of his quit day after smoking up to going to bed the previous night. He decided to remove his ashtrays and dispose of all his cigarettes, thus ensuring that none remained in the house. He also paid to have his car valeted to remove the smell of stale tobacco. He intended to take the dog out for more walks as the exercise should help his overall level of fitness and help to take his mind off smoking. David had recently taken up water colour painting which he believed would help to take his mind off any craving for a cigarette. He decided to use 16 hour transdermal nicotine replacement, 15 mg (full strength), and was given detailed instruction on the use before leaving the clinic.

Appointment 2 Quit date

David had not smoked from 12 noon the previous day. He was very enthusiastic about his quit attempt and as his ECO was 12 this was a considerable boost for him. We discussed any possible difficulties which may occur over the next week. He intended to maintain a healthy diet, take a little more exercise and not socialise with friends who were smokers during the early part of the quit process. Before he left, David made a further commitment to remain a non smoker over the following week.

Appointment 3 One week follow up

David had not smoked the previous week and his measured ECO was 4. There had been several occasions during the week when the urge to smoke had been very strong. The craving had only lasted for a short period and he found that by distracting himself it made things easier. David continued to attend the clinic over the next few weeks and remained abstinent throughout. Six months after the quit date he remained abstinent, confirmed by an ECO of below 6 at all his follow up visits. He does not envisage a return to smoking.

Group interventions

Attendance at group sessions is often dependent upon patient choice: for example, it may be difficult to attend a daytime session due to work or family commitments. During the assessment interview the effectiveness of attending group sessions and using NRT can be discussed. An explanation of how the group sessions will proceed can dispel anxiety or nervousness. Because all those participating will be quitting on the same day, i.e. at the first group meeting, bonding between the group can be an effective adjunct to the quit process. Group sizes vary but are generally between 15 and 25. A practical reason for trying to start with at least 15 members is the expectation that by the last group session possibly half the members will have relapsed and may have stopped attending. A large starting group is more cost effective and avoids the risk of an extremely small number of successes.

Key points

- ❑ Assess nicotine dependence and motivation to quit.
- ❑ Assess patient's suitability for group therapy.
- ❑ Arrange venue and time and question whether the patient is able to attend all sessions.
- ❑ Send postal reminders to those accepted for group treatment including a map and directions to the venue. Reiterate the quit date and the importance of commitment.
- ❑ Two group therapists are necessary – one to lead the sessions, the other to provide emergency cover for sickness and to assist, particularly at the start of each session, when ECO levels are measured.

General points

- ❑ The group therapist should outline briefly how the course will proceed and provide positive but realistic expectations regarding quitting, e.g. that 50% of those attending the group will be successful in quitting (Foulds & Ghodse 1995).
- ❑ Reinforce their commitment to quit at the first group meeting.
- ❑ Instruct on the use of NRT.
- ❑ Emphasise that all smoking materials should be discarded prior to quitting.
- ❑ Some members may not be used to group situations and may be shy during the first session, needing encouragement.

Once the ground rules are described the group therapist should not take a major role in leading the group. Other group members should be encouraged to use their own expertise in supporting each other. In this way the group maintains both support and pressure for each other to maintain abstinence, helping to pull along those members who may be weakening in their resolve to quit (Hajek 1994). By allowing the group to form its own alliances this should ensure that the 'classroom' situation does not prevail. The role of the therapist should be to encourage goal focused discussion among members of the group while maintaining a 'low profile', and to facilitate group discussion rather than provide answers at every opportunity (Hajek 1994).

There may be a time lapse of up to one month from the time of the assessment interview to commencement of the next group. This can be beneficial as smokers are able to plan for their quit date and they are notified that this will coincide with the first group session. Quitting at the first session ensures that maximum support is available when withdrawal symptoms are at their peak in the early stages of the quitting process. Patients should be available to attend all five one-hour sessions of the group therapy. Patients should inform their GPs of their quit decision, particularly if they intend to use NRT. If an underlying medical condition exists, an explanatory letter is forwarded to the GP outlining the group's aims and NRT within this context. Before the session starts, ECO levels are measured and the previous week's smoking history recorded.

Format of session

In session one each member identifies themselves and gives a brief outline of their smoking history. In subsequent sessions, they report whether they have been abstinent and outline how the week has progressed with regard to withdrawal discomfort, craving to smoke and stressful situations which they have overcome. Longer discussion then follows where group interaction reinforces their commitment, particularly amongst those who may be finding it difficult to stay abstinent.

Case vignette 2 Group counselling

Susan is 50 years old with two children and has smoked for 30 years. Her total cigarette consumption is about 25–30 per day. Susan remarried 2 years ago and her partner is a non smoker. She now actively dislikes smoking and feels addicted and guilty. Her 19 year old son who also smokes will be returning to university during her initial quit period and she feels that this will help. Her particular concerns are that she is often alone during the day and has a coffee and a cigarette to relieve the boredom and relax. She and her partner entertain a lot and she does not wish to impose a smoking ban on her guests.

During the assessment interview Susan opted for group counselling. She felt that being required to face the group each week would deter her from smoking and reinforce her commitment to quit. Her ECO measured 31 which shocked her and this added a positive challenge to quit. She had tried several times over a 5 year period to quit and her longest tobacco free period lasted for 6 days. Susan's preference with NRT was to use patches. She decided to keep a diary of her smoking habit until the quit day. In preparation she intended to remove all smoking materials the night before the quit day, clean the car and begin to launder all her clothes. She determined that she would continue to smoke until the group met on the afternoon of the quit day.

Week one

Susan had her ECO level of 35 and her previous week's cigarette consumption of 300 recorded. She described to the group that she felt powerless to quit smoking and this in turn lowered her self-esteem so she smoked more and consequently was trapped in a cycle which she found impossible to break. During the session NRT was introduced and its use described and Susan, together with the rest of the group, applied a patch. During general discussion she said how she intended to cope with the 'difficult' periods during the day when alone. She was advised by some group members to give up coffee which she associated with 'time out' for a cigarette. However, giving up coffee would be difficult and she felt that too much deprivation would be the excuse to smoke. It was also suggested that Susan use an aromatherapy oil burner with a relaxing fragrance and that she listen to her favourite music during these periods.

Towards the end of the session the group was urged to discard any cigarettes, tobacco, lighters, etc. into a bin as a gesture of their intention to quit and for each person to make a commitment to the group that they would not smoke over the following week.

Week two

Susan had not smoked any cigarettes during the previous week; she had an ECO of 5 and was using 15 mg NRT patches. She was delighted with her ECO level and felt that this was a most encouraging result. However, her main craving to smoke came at the end of meals. She also found it very hard not to overeat. She had used the aromatherapy oil and had taken several relaxing baths to take her mind off smoking. A group member suggested that she got into the routine of eating a favourite fruit at the end of each meal to replace the cigarette. Susan said that she had gained 2 lb since quitting. She intended to swim three times per week and eat sensibly to counter this increase. The rest of the group provided positive feedback to Susan on her efforts and she made a further commitment not to smoke for the next week.

Week three

Susan had not smoked during the previous week and her ECO was 4; she was continuing with nicotine patches. She described feeling a little depressed during the week. Several members of the group expressed similar experiences and also irritability, anxiety, poor concentration and craving. Susan attended all five sessions and maintained her abstinence. She continued using NRT patches and also used 2 mg of nicotine gum during difficult periods.

Final session

During session five, group members who have remained abstinent from week one or at least during the past week (as confirmed by their ECO reading) receive a certificate which states the date when they stopped smoking. Although this is generally accepted as a 'fun ceremony', the certificates are particularly prized by some members as a reflection of the effort expended, and many say they will have it framed and displayed prominently as a reminder of this. Instruction and advice on the continuation of NRT is offered and members are encouraged to contact the smokers' clinic for help or advice in the future. The session ends with members making a commitment to remain non smokers.

Smokers' clinics

A well-publicised service which includes a mailshot to GPs and also accepts self-referrals will soon find it has more than enough patients. For example, in its first 6 months, St George's Smokers Clinic received 494 enquiries, of which 207 were assessed and commenced treatment. Most were heavy smokers averaging 24 cigarettes per day. A clinic run along the lines described should begin to achieve abstinence rates above 50% and longer term abstinence of 20–25%. The Lung Health Study (Anthonisen *et al.* 1994) recorded abstinence rates at 1 year of 35% in the intervention group compared with 9% in the no intervention control group; 22% of the intervention group sustained abstinence for 5 years compared with 5% of the control group, clearly indicating the impact of intensive treatment provided by a smokers clinic. The Smokers Clinic at St George's achieved a total abstinence rate of 26% at 3 months. Patients who were lost to the follow up were assumed to be smoking. The high drop out rate from the group means that recruiting large groups is vital. A larger group will have a higher number who remain abstinent initially and this may have the effect of carrying along those who are floundering somewhat. It adds to the positive 'feel' of the group generally and even adds a slightly competitive atmosphere which may help prevent relapse.

At follow up patients are asked to comment on what helped most in their quit programme and many say that using the ECO monitor is a boost as they see the initial dramatic reduction in levels and continue to maintain this by not smoking. However, the machines are expensive, costing approximately £400 each, so are not readily available to many health professionals working with smokers. Most health promotion units do have at least one machine and it may be possible to arrange to borrow this for the duration of the group sessions.

Conclusions

In maintaining a cost effective smokers cessation service, the resource could be developed to include a training programme for other health professionals. The training programme for professionals would include

- ❏ the nature of nicotine addiction
- ❏ motivation to quit
- ❏ assessment of potential quitters' motivation
- ❏ what questions to ask when planning group or one to one therapies
- ❏ the use of case studies to demonstrate the process of smoking cessation

It would be a relatively simple task to transfer the programme to health visitors, practice nurses, GPs, pharmacists and general hospital staff, initially targeting a particular speciality, e.g. the cardiothoracic unit. Key members could then 'cascade' the stop smoking information among staff. This could be particularly useful in helping prevent relapse as patients tend to have regular appointments at out-patients clinics after a serious medical episode such as a myocardial infarction, and would receive continuing support during the stopping process. The smoking clinic should act as resource centre, supporting those GP practices already offering help to potential quitters, whilst maintaining a pro-active role in training those health professionals endeavouring to initiate stop smoking programmes.

Acknowledgement

The author gratefully acknowledges the invaluable help and support of Dr Jonathan Foulds, lecturer in tobacco addiction, Centre for Addictive Studies, Department of Addictive Behaviour, St George's Hospital Medical School, London.

References

Anthonisen, N.R., Connet, J.E, Kiley J.P. *et al.* (1994) For the lung study research group. Effects of smoking intervention and the use of inhaled anticholinergic bronchodilator on the rate of decline of FEVI: the Lung Health Study. *JAMA*, **272**, 1497–1505.

Callum, C., Johnson, K. & Killoran, A. (1992) *The Smoking Epidemic: A Manifesto for Action in England*. Health Education Authority, London.

Foulds, J. (1993) Does nicotine replacement therapy work? *Addiction*, **88**, 1473–8.

Foulds, J. (1996) Strategies for Smoking Cessation. *British Medical Bulletin*, **52**, 157–73.

Foulds, J. & Ghodse, A.H. (1995) Treating tobacco dependence. *Advances in Psychiatric Treatment*, **1**, 116–23.

Hajek, P. (1994) Helping smokers to overcome tobacco withdrawal: background and practice of withdrawal orientated therapy. In: *Interventions for Smokers: An International Perspective* (ed. R. Richmond), pp. 29–43. Williams & Wilkins, Baltimore.

Heatherton, T.F., Kozlowski, L.T., Frecker, R.C. & Fagerstrom, K.O. (1991) The Fagerstrom tolerance questionnaire. *British Journal of Addiction*, **86**, 1119–27.

Tonneson, P. & Fagerstrom, K. (1994) Nicotine replacement. In: *Interventions for Smokers: An International Perspective* (ed. R. Richmond), pp. 3–25. Williams & Wilkins, Baltimore.

West, R. (1997) *Getting Serious About Stopping Smoking. A Review of Products, Services & Techniques. A Report for No Smoking Day 1997.* Health Education Authority, London.

Chapter 22
Working with Diverse Special Populations

G. Hussein Rassool and Bridget Kilpatrick

Introduction

This chapter addresses the contemporary health care issues and problems affecting the special populations. The term special population refers to groups or categories of people whose life circumstances and/or personal characteristics can create particular vulnerabilities to health problems (Litz & Platt 1995). In the context of this chapter, special population refers to groups whose needs are underrepresented, such as as ethnic minorities, young people, the elderly and the homeless. It is beyond the scope of this chapter to cover those special populations such as gay men and lesbians, women, refugees and immigrants, etc. The following sections provide an overview of the nature and extent of substance misuse and the issues and problems related to those diverse special populations. Nursing and other health and social care responses are also addressed. The order of presentation in no way reflects the priorities that should be accorded to any individual group.

Ethnic minorities

Ethnic minorities are a heterogeneous population with a diverse cultural entity and wide variations in life-style, health behaviour, religion and language. Approximately 6% of the total population of England and Wales, around a total of 3 million people represent ethnic minorities (Office of Population Censuses and Surveys (OPCS) 1992). The largest ethno-cultural group is Indian, followed by Caribbean, Pakistani, African, Bangladeshi and Chinese. These communities are largely established in the capital and metropolitan areas of London, the West Midlands, West Yorkshire, and Greater Manchester (OPCS 1992; Karmi 1995). One of the oldest ethnic minority groups in the UK is the traveller gypsies, and only recently have these been recognised as a separate ethnic group. Ethnic monitoring was established as a mandatory requirement with in-patient admission in England in April 1995 (National Health Service Executive 1994).

Nature and extent

There is a dearth of literature and a paucity of reliable data on the extent of the use and misuse of alcohol, tobacco and prescribed and illicit drugs among ethno-cultural groups in the UK. The reasons for the use and misuse of psychoactive substances by ethnic minorities are not essentially different from those of the British majority. However, different ethnic groups have their own preferences for a certain class or classes of substance and mode of consumption, which are linked with their historical and cultural characteristics (Oyefeso & Ghodse 1993).

Studies have shown high levels of alcohol use among Asian and Caribbean populations (Cochrane & Bal 1989; Clarke *et al.* 1990). Specifically looking at Asian male groups, Cochrane & Bal (1990) found over 90% of Muslims were alcohol abstainers and less than 1% were classed as heavy drinkers. Sikhs had the largest proportion of males drinking over 40 units of alcohol, particularly spirits, a week, while 11% of Hindus were drinking over 21 units a week. Taylor *et al.* (1986) found that 6% of all Afro-Caribbean hospital admissions were alcohol related compared with 10% of admissions in the British population. However, Cochrane and Howell (1993), in a comparison of white and Afro-Caribbean men, showed Afro-Caribbeans to have far lower levels of alcohol related problems than white men. The findings also suggested that of all men, Indian born men had the highest rates of admission to psychiatric hospital for alcohol related problems.

Studies concerning the use of tobacco smoking in ethno-cultural groups show varying results. Some have shown a low prevalence in Asian and Caribbean men (Balarajan & Yuen 1986; Waterson & Murray-Lyon 1989), while others report higher use (McKeigue *et al.* 1988, 1991). Heavy smoking is common among Bangladeshi and Chinese men (Karmi 1996). Among the Somali male population, the use of khat, a mild stimulant, is very common and is chewed in social gatherings. Injecting drug use behaviour has been largely uncommon among Asian and black people, but a recent study in Bradford showed that among the Asian people using heroin, a high percentage of the users were injecting (Patel 1993).

Special problems and issues

Recognising and addressing substance misuse is a problem among the indigenous population. This is also true for ethnic minorities, where additional factors are often present. Low rates of early presentation of health problems to, and utilisation of, services by ethnic minorities may be due to a multitude of factors: reliance upon or greater use of traditional medicine, cultural dissonance, lower education and literacy, earlier experience of persecution, language and communication difficulties, lack of knowledge about services, religio-cultural prescriptions and discrimination (Oyefeso & Ghodse 1993; Rassool 1995). These compound the difficulties of later recognition and presentation.

Nursing response

Nurses and other health care professionals are likely to encounter patients from different ethnic minorities within the health care system. The United Kingdom Central Council for Nursing, Midwifery and Health Visiting (UKCC) *Code of Professional Conduct* (1992) points out that 'each registered nurse is accountable for his or her practice, and in the exercise of professional accountability, shall take account of the customs, values and spiritual beliefs of patients/clients'. Health care professionals need to have an awareness of the existence of and health care needs of ethnic minorities within the community they serve. Patients from different cultural and ethnic backgrounds may present a special challenge to nurses and other health care professionals. Language barriers, cultural differences in pain response, sick role behaviour, denial due to stigma attached to alcohol or drug misuse in some ethnic groups, cultural and religious diversity and attitudes of professionals towards members of ethnic minorities may all act as barriers to meeting the holistic needs of client groups. In order to be culturally sensitive to the health care needs of ethnic minority clients, some of the above issues need to be addressed at all levels of the professional disciplines.

In the context of the misuse of psychoactive substances, nursing interventions should focus upon screening and health education responses as part of the overall treatment. It is essential when taking a substance misuse history with some ethnic minorities, for example Asians, to enquire about the use of complementary medicines obtained from traditional healers. This information will help avert the consequences of drug interactions. The health education activities will include teaching about self-medication and the provision of health information in their own language. Health education should also focus on the risk factors associated with key areas of health targets for ethnic minorities, for example coronary heart disease, stroke and hypertension.

Conclusions

It is debatable whether the National Health Service is adequately addressing the health care needs of ethnic minority communities and providing equitable access to services (Stokes 1991; Mello 1992; Murphy & Macleod Clark 1993). One area of concern is how to bridge the information gap on the health status of all ethno-cultural groups in the UK (Rassool 1995; 1997). To work effectively with ethnic minorities does not require one to become an expert in all ethno-cultural groups but to have cultural flexibility, acceptance and understanding and to perceive the patient as an individual (Rassool 1995). What is essential is to develop an openness to differing cultural experiences of particular client groups and to respond in a culturally sensitive way (Rassool 1997). Education and training of health professionals in multi-cultural nursing is a priority. Nursing needs a rigorous programme of education and research which can form the basis of nursing interventions and health policy decisions.

The elderly

Elderly individuals are not immune to drug and alcohol misuse but their problems are often missed, unaddressed or go untreated in clinical settings. The growing population over the age of 65 is predicted to increase from 20.8% to 26.0% by the middle of the twenty-first century (OPCS 1987). The health care system can expect an increasing number of elderly substance misusers in their practice settings. Elderly individuals misuse alcohol, prescribed psychoactive drugs and over-the-counter medications, but rarely illicit drugs. It is estimated that between 5% and 12% of men and 1–2% of women in their 60s are problem drinkers (Atkinson 1984), and drug related problems amongst the elderly may account for between 30% and 50% of admissions to hospital and nursing homes (Cooper 1990).

McInnes & Powell (1994) found that 41% of hospital patients aged 65 and over were defined by researchers as having a problem with substance misuse; these substances included benzodiazepines, alcohol and cigarettes. However, only 25% of this sample were identified as having substance misuse problems by the medical staff. Psychotropic drugs such as anxiolytics, hypnosedatives, tranquillisers and antidepressants are frequently prescribed to the elderly (Jones & Sweetnam 1980). Over-the-counter medications which are misused include analgesic preparations, cough medicines, antacids and vitamins. Szwabo (1993) reviewed the literature and concluded that it is the older women who are at risk for self-medicating with prescribed drugs and alcohol and have a greater risk for drug–alcohol interactions.

Issues and problems

Physical, psychosocial and economic reasons exist to explain substance misuse in the elderly. These include disabilities, physical limitations, sleep disturbances, decline of health, loss of social supports, withdrawal from social routines, loss of spouse and friends, retirement, relocation, role changes and economic hardships. Increased stress, anxiety and depression can result, possibly leading to or exacerbating an existing problem of substance misuse. The elderly have a higher rate of psychotropic drug use than the younger population. The elderly may not follow health information as well, and may not use medications as directed. This can result in the elderly:

❑ Increasing the quantity and frequency of use of medications
❑ Taking prescribed medications simultaneously with over-the-counter drugs
❑ Taking medications with alcohol

There are many health problems associated with alcohol and drug misuse. While these can also be present with the younger population, the elderly are more likely to have a number of health related problems and the difficulties directly caused by substance misuse can reduce the individual's ability to care for themselves independently and safely. In addition to the problems caused by substance misuse, dementia, depression and suicide have been highlighted with substance misuse in the elderly (Saunders *et al.* 1991; Wittington 1983).

Nursing response

The failure to identify and respond effectively to elderly substance misusers may be due to a variety of factors. There is the difficulty of recognising substance misuse in the elderly because presenting symptoms are often commonly associated with ageing itself. Taking a drug and alcohol history and using simple screening questionnaires such as the MAST and CAGE (see Chapter 8 on assessment and screening) are rarely carried out with the elderly. Health workers may adopt the attitude that the elderly have only a limited time of life left and they do not wish to deprive them of their 'recreational medication'.

The signs, symptoms and behaviour of elderly individuals with alcohol and drug problems can be different from those in younger age groups. There are warning signs that should alert nurses to the likelihood of substance misuse, for example patients who present with poor co-ordination, forgetfulness, gastro-intestinal disorders, incontinence, depression, self-neglect, falls, cognitive and affective impairment and social withdrawal. Nurses have an important role in the prevention, early recognition, detection and treatment of substance misuse in the elderly. Due to the complexities of medical and psychosocial problems associated with the elderly, an interdisciplinary collaboration and the involvement of key individuals in the social network is of prime importance in their management (Lindblom *et al.* 1992). An assessment including a detailed history of substance misuse needs to be taken routinely on admission. The health education of the elderly includes teaching about self-medication, explaining the effects of over-the-counter medicines, the provision of health information about prescribed drugs and advice on alcohol and other psychoactive drug use as part of the overall treament regime.

Conclusions

The promotion of non pharmacological remedies and a rational use of psychoactive substances in the elderly need to be implemented. Exercise, leisure pursuits and counselling are some of the activities that should be encouraged as alternatives to overuse of medication. The issue of appropriate service provision for elderly individuals with substance misuse problems has been neglected in the literature and in practice settings. A drug and alcohol liaison service linking with generic health care services would improve the service provision and elderly substance misusers may be referred to, or visited by, this service for specialist intervention. McInnes and Powell (1994) indicated that hospitals with drug and alcohol counselling services have become more effective in diagnosing substance misuse among elderly patients.

Young people

Substance misuse in young people encompasses legal and illicit drugs, ranging from tobacco, alcohol and volatile substances to stimulant, depressant and hallucinogenic drugs, such as cannabis, amphetamines, Ecstasy, cocaine, crack, heroin and LSD. Although the use of illicit drugs gives rise to greater concern, there is little doubt that excessive and prolonged cigarette smoking and alcohol consumption can have a far more deleterious effect on the health of young people. Cannabis, Ecstasy and amphetamines are popular among young people who go to clubs and 'raves', where the use of these drugs is seen as integral to the attainment of sustained energy, conviviality and emotional warmth of the setting.

Nature and extent

The use of alcohol and tobacco has often been regarded as a 'gateway' to the misuse of other substances. This link was confirmed in a 20 year follow up study of adolescents which suggested that alcohol and tobacco are important stepping stones to other drug use (Kandel *et al.* 1992). In this respect, tobacco seems to play a more important role for girls and alcohol for boys. A review of substance misuse by young people suggested that 3–5% of young people between the ages of 11 and 16 had used cannabis, rising to 17% for older adolescents (Health Education Authority 1992; Gilvarry *et al.* 1995). In one study (Miller & Plant 1996) of 7722 pupils aged 15 and 16, it was found that more than 40% of the sample had tried cannabis.

Since the 1970s, solvent or volatile substance abuse has emerged as a considerable problem; such substances include various types of adhesives, thinning fluids, petrol and aerosol gases. However, over the last 10 years there have been significant falls in the numbers of deaths associated with aerosols and glues, but not in those associated with gas fuels. Deaths associated with gas fuels and aerosols increased from 58 in 1994 to 68 in 1995 (Taylor *et al.* 1997). There is a preponderance of boys abusing solvents, with a peak age of abuse at between 13 and 15 years, and a tendency for this form of substance abuse to occur more frequently among children from lower socio-economic groups and disrupted or unstable families. Furthermore, the highest death rates continue to be in the northern areas of the British Isles (Taylor *et al.* 1997).

Issues and problems

Many factors contribute to the initiation and continuation of adolescent substance use and misuse: an early introduction to substances (i.e. early teens), peer influence, opportunities for use, alcohol or other drug problems in parents, family dynamics, school difficulties, social isolation, low self-esteem and unemployment. Adolescence is a time of experimentation, adventure risk taking, challenge to authority, formation of self-identity and development of independence. Establishment of a peer group membership and its approval is important, while at the same time there is a move away from family and parental dependence. Peer influence may exert greater influence in situations where a young person lacks familial support and understanding. This can lead to increased vulnerability and to the likelihood of substance abuse as a means of dealing with their feelings of sadness, distress and emotional confusion. Adolescence is the period for significant choices and decisions: development of sexuality, forming emotional and sexual relationships and the transition from school to further education, work or unemployment. The majority of people manage the transition from adolescence to adulthood satisfactorily. However, the majority of illicit drug users and problem drinkers begin their substance misuse in teenage years, suggesting that some are not able to make successful decisions at this crucial time. It is worth pointing out that adolescents perceive the use of drugs and alcohol as a recreational activity.

There is growing evidence that strong links exist between substance misuse and other antisocial and psychological problems (Swadi 1993). Whether behavioural or delinquency problems are the cause or the effect of substance misuse problems can be unclear but there is little doubt that substance misuse significantly exacerbates any underlying or existing difficulties. Misuse of solvents and volatile substances has physical and psychological risks. Euphoria, confusion, perceptual distortions such as hallucinations and delusions can occur, but subside as the effects wear off. Sudden death can occur due to associated trauma, anoxia and cardiac or respiratory failure. Effects of these drugs, including alcohol, vary depending on the degree of use, route of administration and the current mood or situation of the user. Regular, heavy or binge use can bring about a low mood or depressed episode when use of the substance ceases. Nurses should be alert to the possibility of substance misuse in an adolescent who is uncharacteristically depressed or low in mood. Reports such as that from Hawton *et al.* (1993) empasise the link between substance use and attempted and completed suicide in young age groups. While the use of stimulant 'designer' drugs and their associated risks including fatalities have been prominently reported, the problems linked with more commonly used alcohol should not be underestimated. It is widely used, seen as socially acceptable and can occasionally lead to disastrous and tragic outcomes, for example acute alcoholic poisoning, intoxication leading to inhalation of vomit and increased risk of accidents, fights and injuries.

Nursing response

There is a trend towards the use of combinations of substances, rather than the sole use of a single substance, and this is often referred to as 'polydrug' use. This may make the task of identification and accurate diagnosis even more difficult and means that assessment needs to be carried out very carefully. There are many reasons why young people may be reluctant to discuss their use of psychoactive drugs with others. Several explanations (Association of Nurses in Substance Abuse (ANSA) 1997) have been given:

❑ they do not believe that a problem exists
❑ they are worried about the consequences of disclosure
❑ they do not share the same jargon or vocabulary with the other person (nurse, teacher, counsellor, parent, etc.)
❑ they are rebellious and reluctant to speak to authority
❑ they have poor previous experience, and do not consider, for example, the school nurse to have the legitimate authority in addressing issues related to substance misuse

Zeitlin and Swadi (1991) argued that adolescent substance experimenters and users should be considered vulnerable and a potential source of future social difficulties with major implications for health service planning. Thus, general and primary health care services, accident and emergency units and school health care professionals should be prepared to identify and respond to substance misuse problems in young people, as well as being involved with health education and preventative initiatives.

Conclusions

There is a strong argument for a more active part to be played by teachers, school nurses, probation officers and all those involved with young people, especially as it appears that only about 20% of young people with emotional problems are in contact with health services (Fergusson *et al.* 1993). Credible preventative and educational programmes are of the utmost importance, as well as the adoption of identification and assessment skills, the use of brief intervention techniques, family work and social skills training. These serve to help young people to make informed choices and to be assertive when confronted with offers of drugs or peer pressure.

The homeless

Homelessness is an increasing problem in the UK and it is a collective term that encompasses a variety of different settlements, including rooflessness, temporary accommodation, hostel accommodation and sleeping in friends' or relatives' homes (ANSA 1997). Several factors, either by themselves or existing concurrently, may contribute to people becoming and remaining homeless. These factors include:

❑ unemployment
❑ financial problems
❑ mental illness
❑ alcohol or drug dependency
❑ physical disability
❑ social disruption as a result of substance misuse

The term 'skid row' has been associated with the homeless and usually refers to a place where homeless individuals, primarily men, congregate after dropping out from normal societal functions (Segal 1991).

Nature and extent

There is ample evidence to suggest that a significant and increasing minority of homeless individuals do have substance misuse problems. Fischer (1989) estimated that alcohol misuse is about nine times more prevalent among homeless individuals than it is amongst the home-based population. Other studies (Shanks *et al.* 1994; Newton & Geddes 1994) have found a high prevalence of substance misuse among homeless people, with rates between 25% and 75%. It is estimated that alcohol misuse is six to seven times higher among homeless men and 15 to 30 times higher in homeless women than in the general population (Fischer & Breakey 1992). The co-existence of mental health problems and substance misuse has been found in 20% of homeless people (Ridgely & Dixon 1993). This figure may be an underestimate of the range of mental health problems such as affective disorders and schizophrenia that may be associated with homeless individuals. An increasing trend is the number of young homeless people who are misusing both alcohol and illicit psychoactive drugs (Ritson 1990).

Issues and problems

In addition to their social, economic and psychological problems, homeless substance misusers suffer from a high incidence of physical problems and have a mortality rate that is three times higher than homeless people who are not substance misusers (Gafoor 1997). Physical problems include such conditions such as bronchitis, tuberculosis, peripheral vascular disease, peptic ulcers and accidental injuries. Other complications as a result of substance misuse may include overdose, withdrawal, delirium tremens, abscesses, septicaemia, etc. It has been suggested that homeless drug users are more likely to be involved in HIV risk taking behaviour through increased sharing of injecting equipment and casual, unprotected sex (Klee & Morris 1995).

Unless individuals have secure accommodation, it may not be possible to gain access to specialist treatment facilities. In some instances, the homeless individual may be refused admission to night shelters or hostels and may end up in the local accident and emergency department for a non emergency situation. Many homeless individuals are not registered with their GP and, while it is possible that many GPs are reluctant to take on this unpopular group of clients, an alternative explanation might be that the homeless do not perceive health care as a priority over more pressing needs such as food, clothing and shelter (Gafoor 1997). Many of the homeless with substance misuse problems find it difficult to keep hospital appointments or fail to comply with institutional rules, and as a result they are less likely to be referred to specialist services (Finn 1985).

Nursing response

Primary health care team and outreach workers are those who may have direct access to the homeless substance misusers, in responding to their diverse needs and problems. Because of the reluctance of the homeless to engage in traditional treatment programmes, it would be helpful to forge links with homeless agencies and help staff both to recognise and manage individuals with drug and alcohol problems, so ensuring that care is provided in a setting most suited to their needs (Gafoor 1997). In some inner city areas, specialist outreach teams, which are nurse led, have been established in an attempt to access this special population. Some individulals may require hospital emergency care and treatment or detoxification, and this can be facilitated by liaison with the appropriate generic or substance misuse services. General nursing interventions, beside physical care, should include health information, health education and harm minimisation. In addition, health care professionals need to liaise with other agencies *a propos* other needs of the homeless substance misuser, including housing, welfare benefits and employment.

Conclusions

Homeless people represent one of the most marginalised groups in our society. With the new National Health Service reforms, it has been suggested that homeless individuals have been excluded from the health care system as many health authorities responsible for comissioning health care services for the resident population have 'disowned' the homeless as residents (Black & Scheuer 1991). Gafoor (1997) suggested that policy planners and health care workers need to be more imaginative and innovative in order to access this group by setting up satellite health clinics and the use of community health workers. The implementation of a shared care approach among mental health, substance misuse and primary care services agencies is the way forward in meeting the diverse and complex needs of the homeless substance misusers. As Gafoor (1997) rightly pointed out 'homeless people are a microcosm of our society: being homeless should not equate with being healthless'.

References

Association of Nurses in Substance Abuse (1997) *Substance Use: Guidance on Good Clinical Practice for Nurses, Midwives and Health Visitors. Working with Alcohol and Drug Users.* ANSA, London.

Association of Nurses in Substance Abuse (1997) *Substance Use: Guidance on Good Clinical Practice for Nurses, Midwives and Health Visitors. Working with Children and Young People.* ANSA, London.

Atkinson, R.M. (1984) Substance use and abuse in late life. In: *Alcohol and Drug Abuse in Old Age* (ed. R.M. Atkinson), pp. 1–21. American Psychiatric Press, Washington DC.

Balarajan, R. & Yuen, P. (1986) British smoking and drinking habits: variations by country of birth. *Community Medicine*, **8**, 237–9.

Black, M.E. & Scheuer, M.A. (1991) Utilisation by homeless people of acute hospital services in London. *British Medical Journal*, **303**, 958–61.

Clarke, M., Ahmed, N., Romaniuk, H., *et al.* (1990) Ethnic differences in the consequences of alcohol misuse. *Alcohol and Alcoholism*, **25**, 9–11.

Cochrane, R. & Bal, S.S. (1989) Mental hospital admission rates of immigrants to England: a comparison of 1971 and 1981. *Social Psychiatry and Psychiatric Epidemiology*, **24**, 2–11.

Cochrane, R. & Bal, S.S. (1990) The drinking patterns of Sikh, Hindu and Muslim and White men in the West Midlands: a community survey. *British Journal of Addiction*, **85**, 759–69.

Cochrane, R. & Howell, M. (1993) *A Survey of Drinking Patterns among Afro-Caribbean Men.* University of Birmingham, Birmingham.

Cooper, J.W. (1990) Drug-related problems in the elderly at all levels of care. *Journal of Geriatric Drug Therapy*, **4**, 79–83.

Fergusson, D.M., Horwood, L.J. & Lynskey, M.T. (1993) Prevalence and comorbidity of DSM-III-R diagnoses in a birth cohort of 15 year olds. *Journal of the American Academy of Child and Adolescent Psychiatry*, **32**, 1127–34.

Finn, P. (1985) Decriminalization of public drunkenness: response of the health care system. *Journal of Studies on Alcohol*, **46**, 7–23.

Fischer, P. (1989) Estimating the prevalence of alcohol, drug and mental health problems in the contemporary homeless population. *Contemporary Drug Problems*, **16**, 333–89.

Fischer, P.J. & Breakey, W.R. (1992) The epidemiology of alcohol, drug and mental disorder among homeless persons. *American Psychologist*, **46**, 1115–28.

Gafoor, M. (1997) Homelessness and addictions. In: *Addiction Nursing: Perspectives on Professional and Clinical Practice* (eds G.H. Rassool & M. Gafoor), pp. 139–42. Stanley Thornes, Cheltenham.

Gilvarry, E., McCarthy, S. & McArdle, P. (1995) Substance use among school children in the North of England. *Drug and Alcohol Dependence*, **37**, 255–9.

Gomberg, E.S.L. (1990) Drugs, alcohol and aging. In: *Research Advances in Alcohol and Drug Problems* (eds L.T. Kozlowski, H.M. Annis, H.D. Cappell, *et al.*), Vol. 10, pp. 171–213. Plenum, New York.

Hawton, K., Fagg, J., Platt, S. & Hawkins, M. (1993) Factors associated with suicide after parasuicide in young people. *British Medical Journal*, **306**, 1641–4.

Health Education Authority (1992) *Tomorrow's young adults 9–15 year olds look at alcohol, drugs, exercise and smoking.* MORI, London.

Jones, D. & Sweetnam, P.M. (1980) Drug prescribing by general practitioners in England and Wales. *Journal of Epidemiology and Community Health*, **34**, 119–23.

Kandel, D. Yamaguchi, K. & Chen, K. (1992) Stages of progression in drug involvement from adolescence to adulthood: further evidence for gateway theory. *Journal of Studies on Alcohol*, **53**, 447–57.

Karmi, G. (1996) *The Ethnic Health Handbook. A Factfile for Health Care Professionals.* Blackwell Science, Oxford.

Klee, K. & Morris, J. (1995) Factors that characterize street injectors. *Addiction*, **90**, 837–41.

Lindblom, L., Kostyk, D., Tabisz, E., *et al.* (1992) Chemical abuse: an intervention program for the elderly. *Journal of Gerontological Nursing*, **18**, 6–14.

Litz, V. & Platt, J.J. (1995) Substance misuse in special populations. *Current Science*, **8**, 189–94.

McInnes, E. & Powell, J. (1994) Drug and alcohol referrals: are elderly substance abuse diagnoses and referrals being missed? *British Medical Journal*, **308**, 444–6.

McKeigue, P.M., Marmot, M.G., Syndercombe Court, Y.D., *et al.* (1988) Diabetes, hyperinsulinaemia, and coronary risk factors in Bangladeshis in East London. *British Heart Journal*, **60**, 390–96.

McKeigue, P.M., Shah, B. & Marmot, M.G. (1991) Relation of central obesity and insulin resistance with high diabetes prevalence and cardiovascular risk in South Asians. *Lancet*, **337**, 382–6.

Mello, M. (1992) Plugging the gap ... diabetes ... UK's ethnic minorities ... provision for them is limited and reflects wider racial issues. *Nursing Times*, **88**, 34–6.

Miller, P. & Plant, M. (1996) Drinking, smoking and illicit drug use among 15–16 year olds in the United Kingdom. *British Medical Journal*, **313**, 394–7.

Murphy, K. & Macleod Clark, J. (1993) Nurses' experiences of caring for ethnic-minority clients. *Journal of Advanced Nursing*, **18**, 442–50.

National Health Service Executive (1994) *Collecting Ethnic Group Data for Admitted Patient Care.* Department of Health, London.

Newton, J.R. & Geddes, J.R. (1994) Mental health problems of the Edinburgh 'roofless'. *British Journal of Psychiatry*, **165**, 537–40.

Office of Population Censuses and Surveys (OPCS) (1987) *Population Projections, 1985–2041*. HMSO, London.

Office of Population Censuses and Surveys (OPCS) (1992) *1991 Census: Outline Statistics for England and Wales. National Monitor CEN 91 CM 58*. HMSO, London.

Oyefeso, A. & Ghodse, A.H. (1998) Addictive behaviour. In: *Assessing the Health Needs of People from Minority Ethnic Groups* (eds S. Rawaf & V. Bahl), pp. 137–51. Royal College of Physicians, London.

Patel, J. (1993) Ethnic minority access to services. In: *Race, Culture and Substance Problems* (ed. L. Harrison). Department of Social Policy and Professional Studies, University of Hull.

Rassool, G.H. (1995) The health status and health care of ethno-cultural minorities in the United Kingdom: an agenda for action. Editorial. *Journal of Advanced Nursing*, **21**, 199–201.

Rassool, G.H. (1997) Ethnic minorities and substance misuse. In: *Addiction Nursing: Perspectives in Professional and Clinical Practice* (eds G.H. Rassool & M. Gafoor), pp. 99–107. Stanley Thornes, Cheltenham.

Ridgely, M.S. & Dixon, L.B. (1993) *Integrating Mental Health and Substance Misuse Services for Homeless People with Co-curring Mental and Substance Use Disorders*. Federal Center for Mental Health Services, Washington DC.

Ritson, B. (1990) *Mental health and homelessness: report of the Royal College of Psychiatrists*. Occasional Paper OP9. RCP, London.

Saunders, P., Copeland, J., Dewey, M.E., *et al*. (1991) Heavy drinking as a risk factor for depression and dementia in elderly men. *British Journal of Psychiatry*, **159**, 213–16.

Segal, B. (1991) *Homelessness and Drinking: A Study of a Street Population*. The Haworth Press, New York.

Shanks, N.J., George, S.L., Westlake, L. & Al-Kalai, D. (1994) Who are the homeless? *Public Health*, **108**, 11–19.

Stokes, G. (1991) A transcultural nurse is about. *Senior Nurse*, **11**, 40–42.

Swadi, H. (1993) Adolescent substance misuse. *Current Opinion in Psychiatry*, **6**, 511–15.

Szwabo, P.A. (1993) Substance abuse in older women. *Clinics of Geriatric Medicine*, **9**, 197–208.

Taylor, C.L., Kilbane, P., Passmore, N. & Davies, R. (1986) Prospective study of alcohol-related admissions in an inner-city related hospital. *Lancet*, **2**, 265–8.

Taylor, J.C., Norman, C.L., Bland, J.M., *et al*. (1997) *Trends in Deaths associated with Abuse of Volatile Substances 1971–1995*. Department of Public Health Sciences and the Toxicology Unit Department of Cardiological Sciences, St George's Hospital Medical School, London.

Thibault, J.M. & Maly, R.C. (1993) Recognition and treatment of substance abuse in the elderly. *Primary Care, Clinics in Office Practice*, **20**, 155–65.

United Kingdom Central Council for Nursing, Midwifery and Health Visiting (1992) *Code of Professional Conduct*, 3rd edn. UKCC, London.

Waterson, E.J. & Murray-Lyon, I.M. (1989) Alcohol, smoking and pregnancy: some observations on ethnic minorities in the United Kingdom. *British Journal of Addiction*, **84**, 323–5.

Wittington, F.J. (1983) Consequences of drug use, misuse and abuse. In: *Drugs and the Elderly* (eds M.D. Glantz, D.M. Peterson & F.J. Wittington). Research Monograph 32. NIDA, Rockville, MD.

Zeitlin, H. & Swadi, H. (1991) Adolescence: the genesis of addiction. In: *The International Handbook of Addiction Behaviour* (ed. I.B. Glass), pp. 163–7. Tavistock/Routledge, London.

Chapter 23
Working with Dual Diagnosis Clients

Mike Gafoor and G. Hussein Rassool

Introduction

In the UK the increase in the number of mentally ill patients who misuse psychoactive substances is currently receiving growing attention by mental health professionals including addiction nurses. The term dual diagnosis has been coined to describe this group of patients whose mental health problems co-exist with substance misuse. In the UK, the recent closures of long stay psychiatric institutions and increasing emphasis on care and treatment in the community have meant that mentally ill patients are perhaps becoming more exposed to a wider range of illicit drugs than previously (Gafoor & Rassool 1998). Furthermore, those individuals in the community with mental health problems may be drawn into a substance using culture that appears more attractive and less stigmatised for social interactions.

Several theories have been put forward to explain why some mentally ill patients misuse drugs and alcohol. It has been suggested that some patients may self-medicate in an effort to treat their psychiatric symptoms, and stimulant type drugs such as amphetamines and cocaine have been used by some patients to counteract distressing extrapyramidal side effects (Schneider & Siris 1987; Dixon *et al.* 1990). Compared to other psychiatric patients, dual diagnosis patients are regarded as more problematic during treatment because of poor compliance with treatment regimes and higher levels of violence, suicide and homelessness (Ridgely *et al.* 1990). In addition, their risky life-styles and behaviour make them more susceptible to HIV infection and overall make greater demands on services.

The aims of this chapter are to examine briefly the concept of dual diagnosis and address the nature and extent of problems relating to dual diagnosis. It also outlines the main nursing interventions and treatment strategies that may be used for this cohort of patients.

What is dual diagnosis?

Health care professionals have used the term dual diagnosis to refer to individuals who were mentally retarded or had a learning disability and who also had co-existing psychiatric disorder (Evans & Sullivan 1990). Dual diagnosis can be defined as the concurrent existence of both substance abuse or dependency and one or more psychiatric disorders (NIDA 1991). More recently, clinicians in the UK have begun to use the term to refer to the 'co-existing diagnoses of mental illness and substance use' (Institute for the Study of Drug Dependence 1996). The dual diagnosis patient meets the DSM-IV (Diagnostic Statistical Manual) criteria for both substance abuse or dependency and a co-existing psychiatric disorder. The concept of dual diagnosis can be seen as an umbrella term that incorporates a wide range of co-existing problems, including addictive behaviours such as drug, alcohol, gambling and eating disorders with concurrent mental health problems. Individuals may develop a wide range of psychiatric disorders depending on the drug of choice being used. For example, a cocaine user may experience depressive symptoms and paranoid delusions. It is stated that with dual diagnosis patients, the psychiatric disorders and the substance misuse are separate, chronic disorders, each with an independent course, yet each able to influence the properties of each other (Carey 1989).

Nature and extent

The problems associated with dual diagnosis have attracted little interest in the UK by both researchers and clinicians alike. It has been noted that 'to date there has been no published research in the UK on dual diagnosis' (Smith & Hucker 1994). In a recent study by Menzes *et al.* (1996) prevalence rates of approximately 32% for alcohol misuse and 16% for drug misuse were found among individuals with severe mental illness in south London. However, this figure may not be truly representative of the prevalence rates of co-morbidity in the UK population as a whole. By contrast, in the USA, where the co-morbidity of substance misuse and psychiatric disorders has received greater interest during the past decade, research data indicate that approximately 50% of severely mentally ill patients misuse drugs or alcohol at some point in their lives. It is argued that as the term dual diagnosis refers to an extremely heterogeneous population, any research findings need to be considered with caution because of a lack of consensus regarding methodology and biased samples (Alber 1997). However, a study by Reiger *et al.* (1990), with samples from both community and residential settings, found the highest co-morbidity rate for those with drug dependence.

Individuals with psychiatric disorders have an increased risk of developing an alcohol or drug related problem or dependence. For example, people with schizophrenia have a three-fold risk of developing alcohol dependence compared with individuals without a mental illness (Crawford 1996). The most common psychiatric disorder among injecting drug users is antisocial personality disorder (ASPD). Drake & Noordsy (1994) found a prevalence rate of approximately 61% lifetime personality disorder among Australian opiate addicts. It is worth pointing out that even though an epidemiological association exists between personality disorder and drug misuse, no deductions can be made about cause (Ghodse 1995). Dual diagnosis patients, like most substance misusers, are a heterogeneous group and any defining features or diagnostic profiles evident may change over time. However, they are more likely to come from one of the following categories whereby the patient has:

- ❑ A primary psychiatric disorder with a secondary substance misuse disorder;
- ❑ A primary substance misuse disorder with psychiatric complications;
- ❑ A concurrent substance misuse and psychiatric disorder; for example, alcohol dependency and depression;
- ❑ An underlying traumatic experience, for example post traumatic stress disorder (PTSD), resulting in both substance misuse and mood disorders.

Problems and issues for mental health nurses

Patients with a co-existing psychiatric disorder and substance misuse problem present many challenges for nurses and other health care professionals. As a group, dual diagnosis patients are more difficult to treat and manage in view of higher levels of physical, social and psychological impairment. Schizophrenic patients who misuse alcohol or other psychoactive substances, for example, have more delusions, hallucinations, suicidal behaviour, hostility, aggression and homelessness (Wilen *et al.* 1993). Furthermore, co-morbidity of alcohol dependence and schizophrenia have been shown to be associated with poor self-care, worsening of symptoms and disruptive behaviour and higher recidivism (Miller 1994). Compliance with taking prescribed medication is also a problem for dual diagnosis patients (Pristach & Smith 1990), and this can lead to a worsening of mental health symptoms and an unnecessarily prolonged stay in hospital. This is an obvious problem for service providers given the current shortage of acute psychiatric beds within the National Health Service.

There is a reluctance by substance misusers to admit to being physically or psychologically dependent on drugs and alcohol and many go to great lengths to conceal their substance misuse from mental health staff and also other health care professionals. Some nurses may lack the confidence to ask patients about their substance misuse or may have pessimistic views regarding treatment. Failure to recognise and treat substance misuse at an early stage will not only lead to ineffective management and treatment outcomes, but may also result in a deterioration of the patient's symptomatology. The mental state of the patient may act as a barrier to recognition as some patients may not be able to understand the nature of the symptoms they experience or adequately describe them in a way that enables clinical staff to make an accurate assessment. This task of diagnosis is further compounded if the patient is a polydrug user and is taking a combination of psychoactive substances at the same time.

Even when substance misuse is identified it is often difficult to distinguish between symptoms that are related to substance misuse and a psychiatric disorder. A typical example is that of an alcohol dependent patient who manifests depressive features. There may be several possible explanations for the patient's condition. First, dependency on alcohol may have developed against a background of an underlying depression which predated his/her misuse of alcohol. Second, the patient's depression may be related to the negative physical, social and psychological sequelae associated with alcohol misuse. Finally, a psychiatric disorder and substance use disorder may occur independently of each other.

In summary, the major problems associated with dual diagnosis patients are:

- ❑ Violence, homelessness, suicide, poor compliance with treatment
- ❑ Higher rates of recidivism
- ❑ Problems of diagnosis
- ❑ Denial of substance misuse by patients
- ❑ Negative attitudes of health care professionals

Working with dual diagnosis patients

Substance misuse among mentally ill patients is more likely to be the norm than the exception and it is necessary for mental health nurses to play a more active role in meeting the health needs of this group of patients. Hitherto, many nurses have tended to assume that dealing with substance misuse is a specialist's job, and have seen their role mainly as referring patients to specialist services (Rassool 1993) . Research has shown that dual diagnosis patients are best treated by the general psychiatric services (Minkoff 1989). Such patients may find specialist drug and alcohol services too confrontational and stress provoking, and in treatment groups may be pressurised by other patients to abstain from any prescribed medication (Gafoor & Rassool 1998). This could result in a relapse of their mental illness.

Concurrent treatment under the two systems may also be problematic due to different treatment philosophies and often results in fragmented and contradictory care (Ridgely *et al.* 1990). Patients often appear to lack motivation and are difficult to engage in out-patient treatment or rehabilitation programmes. Motivation is not a fixed attribute and can be influenced by various psychological and behavioural strategies. Developing a trusting and non judgmental relationship with the patient will help to increase his/her motivation for change. The use of motivational interviewing techniques (Miller 1985) has been shown to increase patients' insight into the nature and severity of their substance misuse and to facilitate positive behavioural changes.

Assessment and screening

Mental health nurses should ensure that a full assessment of drug and alcohol history is undertaken on psychiatric patients presenting for treatment, especially those with a history of violence, homelessness, poor compliance and repeated admissions. The assessment should aim to acquire information on the following areas:

- ❑ Drugs: types, dose (amounts, cost), frequency, duration and mode of use, effects, complications (physical, social and psychological) and presence of any withdrawal symptoms.
- ❑ Alcohol: number of units, frequency and duration of use, withdrawal symptoms and complications.
- ❑ Psychiatric history: nature of illness and details of any previous treatment, and whether illness was related to drug and alcohol.
- ❑ Mental state: appearance/behaviour (withdrawal or intoxication), speech (slurred or rapid), mood and thought disorder, suicidal thoughts/intent, sleep, appetite, perceptual disturbances, insight of problem.

Assessment is an ongoing process aimed at identifying substance misuse so that the patient may receive the most appropriate treatment and intervention. It should not be used as a method of identifying the substance misuser for punitive reasons such as discharge from hospital or refusal of psychiatric care. Where substance misuse is identified, the nurse should explore with the patient the circumstances behind the use of substances and educate him/her on the psychological, social and physical consequences that may occur. Some patients may be too psychiatrically ill to undertake an assessment interview and may require a period of stabilisation of their mental state before addressing issues relating to substance misuse.

Physical examination for injecting 'track' marks may be carried out to confirm the mode of use among drug users or to detect signs of a swollen liver among an alcohol misuser. In addition, urine screening and collateral information from family members and other professionals should be carried out. The use of screening instruments, for example CAGE (Mayfield *et al.* 1974), Short Michigan Alcoholism Screening Test (SMAST) (Selzer *et al.* 1975), Substance Abuse Assessment Questionnaire (SAAQ) (Ghodse 1995), can be used to identify the nature and severity of drug and alcohol use. A summary of the assessment and nursing interventions for dual diagnosis patients includes the following:

- ❑ Physical examination for signs of injecting marks, enlarged liver;
- ❑ Observation for mental health symptoms relating to intoxication and

withdrawal of drugs and alcohol, e.g. tremors, slurred speech, irritability, paranoid ideas;
- ❑ Urine screen; use of screening questionnaires and collateral information from friends and relatives;
- ❑ Establishing trust and a non judgmental approach, which will increase motivation for change;
- ❑ Development of a shared care approach with the specialist substance misuse service.

Shared care

In some cases it may be necessary to link up with the local substance misuse service and to develop a shared care approach, with the substance misuse nurse acting as a specialist resource to ensure that a good assessment and care plan are achieved. Mental health nurses do possess the core therapeutic skills required to work with substance misusers, such as assessment and counselling skills as well as the skills of stress management and relapse prevention. However, they may be reluctant to intervene due to a lack of confidence in their ability to effect any change or they may hold negative views towards the outcome of any interventions on their part (Gafoor & Rassool 1998). As patients begin to experience improvement in their symptoms and their trust in the psychiatric staff increases, they are more likely to demonstrate positive changes in attitudes and behaviour regarding their use of drugs and alcohol.

The government has issued recommendations for service planners to implement shared care arrangements and for the primary health care workers to develop their role in the management of drug users (Department of Health 1995). On discharge from hospital, the involvement of a community psychiatric nurse can also help to increase patients' compliance with taking prescribed medication. The following case history describes the assessment and management of a dual diagnosis patient.

Case vignette

Peter is a 22 year old unemployed man who was arrested by the police for shouting at passers by. He was admitted to the local psychiatric unit under section 136 of the Mental Health Act 1984. He had a previous psychotic episode 2 years ago which was thought to be drug induced. On admission, Peter was restless and agitated. He was expressing paranoid ideas and believed that his thoughts were being broadcast on the Internet. He was reassured by the staff and nurses in a quiet part of the ward. He reported heavy amphetamines and cannabis use over the past 5 years and had recently ended a 3 year relationship with his partner. Peter's drug use dates back to his late teens and is confined mainly to weekend use of cannabis,

Ecstasy and LSD. His use of these drugs became more regular when he dropped out of university 2 years ago.

According to information later provided by his mother, Peter had always been a rather sensitive person who found it difficult to interact socially. As a child, he tended to isolate himself from the rest of the family, choosing instead to spend long periods on his computer and build model aeroplanes. Peter's mother herself was treated for a post-natal depression, shortly after he was born. During his stay in hospital, Peter responded well to general nursing care and to the antipsychotic medication. His symptoms subsided over the following 6 weeks. He attended a series of drug education groups held on the ward by the addiction specialist nurse and also completed a social skills programme. Peter left hospital and was followed up by the community psychiatric nurse who monitored his antipsychotic medications and helped him to develop skills in relapse prevention.

Case discussion

Peter's symptoms such as paranoid ideas and thought broadcasting are common in both schizophrenia and drug induced psychotic states. It is extremely diffult to distinguish the two conditions. However, there is some evidence to suggest that Peter is suffering from a schizophrenic illness which is exacerbated by the use of drugs such as cannabis, amphetamines and Ecstasy. His tendency to be socially withdrawn as an adolescent and the family history of mental ilness are both factors associated with schizophrenia. Additionally, his mental health problems and symptoms persisted longer than would have been the case in a drug induced psychosis, where the symptoms usually disappear when the drug is cleared from the system. Peter's mental state improved after he commenced an antipsychotic medication and is likely to deteriorate if this is stopped regardless of whether he returns to illicit drug use. It is also possible that Peter self-medicates with stimulant drugs such as amphetamines and Ecstasy to overcome his lack of social skills. This would suggest a dual diagnosis of substance misuse and mental illness which, although linked, may occur independently of each other.

Implications for nursing

Because of their close involvement with patients in both residential and community settings, mental health nurses are in a unique position to develop effective interventions and management strategies for dual diagnosis patients. The magnitude of substance misuse and psychiatric disorders in the community and increased hospital admissions highlight the pressing need for mental health nurses to intervene effectively. However, it is not feasible for this cohort of patients to be dealt with exclusively by staff from specialist drug and alcohol agencies. Moreover, only a minority of dual diagnosis patients are likely to come into contact with such specialist addiction services.

A recent survey showed that awareness of the problems of dual diagnosis among mental health nurses was low (McKeown & Liebling 1995). Nurses may be reluctant to intervene with substance misuse problems, due either to lack of knowledge and expertise regarding substance misuse or because they have negative attitudes towards the substance misuser (Rassool 1993). Overtly self-abusive behaviour, particularly when it involves illicit drugs, is dealt with in a suppressive and moralistic way by many health care workers, not least of all nurses, probably out of a sense of frustration or inadequacy about their ability to effect any change (Gafoor 1985). It would be fruitful to raise the awareness of nurses and others and to provide adequate training in areas of substance misuse and mental health problems. However, it is argued that, at present, much professional education and training of health care professionals reinforces the view that dealing with substance misuse is a specialist's job (Rassool & Oyefeso 1993).

The argument for raising the profile of both substance misuse and mental health problems is challenging for both addiction nurses and mental health workers with the prospect of meeting the health targets as identified in *The Health of the Nation* documents (Department of Health 1992, 1993). Since substance misuse is more likely to be the norm than the exception among mentally ill patients, there is a pressing need for mental health nurses and other health care professionals to develop their knowledge and clinical expertise in substance misuse in order to respond effectively to the needs of this group of patients (Gafoor & Rassool 1998). It has been suggested that education and training on substance misuse and addictive behaviour can enhance positive attitudes and increase confidence and skills in identifying and working with substance misusers (Cartwright 1980; Kennedy & Faugier 1989; Rassool 1993; Rassool *et al.* 1994).

The need for education and training of mental health nurses in order to provide therapeutic responses to those with dual diagnosis is beyond dispute. The curriculum content at both pre-registration and in continuing professional education programmes needs to be modified to incorporate aspects of substance misuse and mental health problems. Rassool and Oyefeso (1993) have suggested the use of a vertical-integration approach for integrating substance use and misuse within existing nursing and health sciences curricula. Guidelines for good practice in education and training of nurses, midwives and health visitors on substance use and misuse are outlined elsewhere (English National Board for Nursing, Midwifery and Health Visiting 1996). These guidelines are for use by programme planners and are useful indications for the content of both pre-registration and continuing professional education programmes.

Conclusions

There are complex links between substance misuse and psychiatric disorders. Intoxication and withdrawal from drugs and alcohol can produce psychiatric symptoms, while on the other hand some patients with psychiatric disorders such as antisocial personality disorders and schizophrenia are more susceptible to substance misuse (Gafoor & Rassool 1998). Dual diagnosis patients tend to be more problematic to treat and manage as the result of higher rates of non compliance, violence, homelessness and suicide. The therapeutic skills of mental health workers can be harnessed to respond effectively to the needs of the dual diagnosis patient with clinical support and consultancy from specialist substance misuse services and addiction nurses.

The changing patterns and prevalence of substance misuse in the UK necessitate new and innovative responses from health care workers. Mental health nurses should forge closer links with addiction nurses and, whenever possible, develop joint working relationships in caring for patients with dual diagnosis. Additionally they should aim to identify the extent of the problem locally and bring this to the attention of service planners and health care purchasers. Purchasers and providers should ensure that health care professionals working in specialist substance misuse and mental health agencies are aware of the need to identify and respond to the problems of combined substance misuse and psychiatric disorders (Department of Health 1996).

References

Alber, C. (1997) Dual diagnosis. *Drug News. Maudsley/Regional Drug Training Unit*, Summer, 12–18

Carey, K.B. (1989) Emerging treatment guidelines for mentally ill chemical abusers. *Hospital and Community Psychiatry*, **40**, 341–2, 349.

Cartwright, A. (1980) The attitude of helping agents towards the alcoholic client: the influence of experience, support, training and self-esteem. *British Journal of Addiction*, **75**, 413–31.

Crawford, V. (1996) Comorbidity of substance misuse and psychiatric disorders. *Current Opinion in Psychiatry*, **9**, 231–4.

Dixon, L., Haas, J., Weiden, P., *et al.* (1990) Acute effects of drug abuse in schizophrenic patients: clinical observation and patients' self reports. *Schizophrenia Bulletin*, **16**, 69–79.

Department of Health (1992) *The Health of the Nation. A Strategy for Health in England.* HMSO, London.

Department of Health (1993) *The Health of the Nation: Key Area Handbook – Mental Illness.* HMSO, London.

Department of Health (1995) Reviewing shared care arrangements for drug users. *Circular No EL (95) 114.* NHS Executive.

Department of Health (1996) *The Task Force to Review Services for Drug Misusers.*

Report of an Independent Survey of Drug Treatment Services in England. HMSO, London.

Drake, R. & Noordsy, D. (1994) Case management for people with co-existing severe mental disorder and substance abuse disorder. *Psychiatric Annals*, **24**, 427–31.

Drake, R.E., Haas, J., Teague, G.B., *et al.* (1993) Treatment of substance abuse in severely mentally ill patients. *Journal of Nervous and Mental Disease*, **181**, 69–79.

English National Board for Nursing, Midwifery and Health Visiting (1996) *Substance Use and Misuse: Guidelines for Good Practice in Education and Training of Nurses, Midwives and Health Visitors*. ENB, London.

Evans, K. & Sullivan, J.M. (1990) *Dual Diagnosis: Counselling the Mentally Ill Substance Abuser*. The Guilford Press, New York.

Gafoor, M. (1985) Nurses' attitudes to the drug abuser. Letter to *Nursing Times*, 30 October.

Gafoor, M. & Rassool G.H. (1998) The co-existence of psychiatric disorders and substance misuse: working with dual diagnosis patients. *Journal of Advanced Nursing*, **27**, 497–502.

Ghodse, A.H. (1995) *Drugs and Addictive Behaviour: A Guide To Treatment*, 2nd edn. Blackwell Science, Oxford.

Institute for the Study of Drug Dependence (1996) Dual diagnosis factsheet 17. *Druglink*, **112**, 2.

Kennedy, J. & Faugier, J. (1989) *Drug and Alcohol Dependency Nursing*. Heinemann Nursing, London.

Mayfield, D., Mcleod, G. & Hall, P. (1974) The Cage questionnaire: validation of a new alcoholism screening instrument. *American Journal of Psychiatry*, **13**, 1121–3.

McKeown, M. & Liebling, H. (1995) Staff perceptions of illicit drug use within a special hospital. *Journal of Psychiatric and Mental Health Nursing*, **2**, 343–50.

Menzes, P.R., Johnson, S., Thornicroft, G., *et al.* (1996) Drug and alcohol problems among individuals with severe mental illnesses in South London. *British Journal of Psychiatry*, **168**, 612–19.

Miller, W.R. (1985) Motivation for treatment: a review with special emphasis on alcoholism. *Psychological Bulletin*, **98**, 84–107.

Miller, N.S. (1994) Prevalence and treatment models for addiction in psychiatric populations. *Psychiatry Annals*, **24**, 399–406.

Minkoff, K. (1989) Integrated treatment models of dual diagnosis of psychosis and addiction. *Hospital Community Psychiatry*, **40**, 1031–6.

NIDA (National Institute on Drug Abuse) (1991) *Third biennial report to Congress: drug abuse and drug abuse research*. DHSS Publication No. ADM 91-1704. Government printing Office, Washington DC.

Pristach, C.A. & Smith, C.M. (1990) Medication compliance and substance abuse among schizophrenic patients. *Hospital Community Psychiatry*, **41**, 1345–8.

Rassool, G.H. (1993) Nursing and substance misuse: responding to the challenge. *Journal of Advanced Nursing*, **18**, 1401–7.

Rassool, G.H. & Oyefeso, N. (1993) Substance misuse in health studies curriculum: a case for nursing education. *Nurse Education Today*, **13**, 107–10.

Rassool, G.H., Oyefeso, A. & Ghodse, A.H. (1994) Linking theory to practice: the impact of a course on the competence of nurse practitioners. Paper presented at the *First International Nursing Conference*, Negara, Brunei Darussalam, 6–9 November.

Ridgely, M.S., Goldman, H.H. & Willenbring, M. (1990) Barriers to the care of persons with dual diagnosis: organisational and financial issues. *Schizophrenia Bulletin*, **16**, 123–32.

Rieger, D.A., Boyd, J.H. & Burke, J.D. (1988) One-month prevalence of mental disorders in the United States. *Archives of General Psychiatry*, **45**, 977–86.

Schneider, F.R. & Siris, S.D. (1987) A review of psychoactive substance use and abuse in schizophrenia: patterns of drug choice. *Journal of Psychiatry*, **165**, 13–21.

Selzer, M.S., Vinoku, A. & Rooijien, E.V. (1975) A self-administered Short Michigan Alcoholism Screening Test (SMAST). *Journal of Studies on Alcohol*, **36**, 117–26.

Smith, J. & Hucker, S. (1994) Schizophrenia and substance abuse. *British Journal of Psychiatry*, **165**, 13–21.

Wilen, T.E., O'Keefe, J & O'Connell, J.J. (1993) A public dual diagnosis detoxification unit, part one: organisation and structure. *American Journal of Addictions*, **2**, 91–8.

Chapter 24

Contemporary Issues in Addiction Nursing

G. Hussein Rassool

Introduction

In the UK, there has been an expansive governmental, societal and professional interest in the prevention, treatment and rehabilitation of substance misusers. The health and social care policies (Department of Health 1992, 1993a, 1994; Tackling Drugs Together 1995; Advisory Council on the Misuse of Drugs 1988, 1989) instigated by the government, coupled with the changing health care needs of the population and educational initiatives (English National Board for Nursing, Midwifery and Health Visiting 1996) have provided added impetus in the care and management of a significant proportion of the population with substance misuse problems. Although psychoactive drug misuse is given relatively little prominence in *The Health of the Nation* (Department of Health 1992) document, except in relation to lifestyle and HIV\AIDS (Ghodse 1993), it does, however, signal a shift in emphasis towards accessible treatment, prevention and health education.

Thus, the growing demand for increased access to health care provision for substance misusers has resulted in some innovations in service provision such as the development of community drug teams, alcohol liaison teams, day care programmes, street agencies, outreach work, needle exchange schemes and residential rehabilitation. Most of these innovations in service development have been nurse led (Rassool & Gafoor 1997) and have heralded the development of addiction nursing. The rationale for the development of addiction nursing as an academic and clinical speciality can be attributed to four major factors (Rassool 1997a):

(1) Harm and costs of substance misuse
(2) Policy development
(3) Professional initiatives
(4) Societal attitudes

There are also political and socio-economic variables that have shaped both service provision and clinical development.

This chapter aims to provide an overview of contemporary issues in addiction nursing. The concept of addiction nursing and aspects of addiction nursing such as nursing roles, nursing diagnosis, nursing models, clinical supervision, research in addiction nursing and professional and educational development will be briefly examined.

Concept of addiction nursing

In the UK, although nurses have been the major component of the work force, working as specialists in both alcohol and drug fields for the past two decades (Kennedy & Faugier 1989, Advisory Council on the Misuse of Drugs 1990; Rassool 1996; Rassool & Gafoor 1997), addiction nursing is a recent clinical speciality within the branch of mental health nursing. Historically, occupational labels such as alcohol nurse, drug dependency nurse, chemical substance nurse, specialist nurse in addiction and community psychiatric nurse have been ascribed to those working with substance misusers (Rassool 1997a).

Addiction nursing may be defined as

'a clinical speciality concerned with the care and treatment interventions aimed at those individuals whose health problems are directly related to the use and misuse of psychoactive substances and to other addictive behaviours such as eating disorders and gambling.'

(Rassool 1997a)

Furthermore, according to Rassool (1997a), the components of addiction nursing incorporate the activities of policy development, clinical practice, education and research through which the addiction nurses contribute to the care of the patients.

In the context of the USA, addiction nursing has been defined as

'an area of speciality practice concerned with care related to dysfunctional patterns of human response that have one or more of these characteristics: loss of self-control capability, episodic or continuous maladaptive behaviour or abuse of some substance, and development of dependence patterns of a physical and/or psychological nature.'

(American Nurses' Association *et al.* 1987)

The concept of addiction nursing has been adopted by professional organisations and statutory bodies with the production of two major documents on addiction nursing addressing the rationale, scope, functions, roles and preparation for practice (American Nurses' Association *et al.* 1987; American Nurses' Association and National Nurses' Society on Addictions 1988). Rassool (1997a) has argued that although the concept of addiction nursing may be criticised on the grounds that it is too medically orientated and substance focused, other labels ascribed to the work practices of nurses working within this speciality are too generic and lack the distinctive professional representation of what addiction nurses do.

The conceptual framework of addiction nursing is inherently a multi-disciplinary business with a multi-disciplinary perspective of assessment and intervention strategies. However, the scope of professional practice is based upon

❑ Understanding the nature and extent of substance misuse and addictive behaviour (alcohol, drugs, eating disorders, gambling and excessive sexual appetites);
❑ Understanding the different health, social, psychological, economic and legal problems associated with substance misuse;
❑ Possessing nursing skills and a range of specialist skills and competencies.

Nursing roles

The changing health needs of the population and natural history of substance use and misuse make new demands on existing services and delivery of care. The roles of nurses, midwives and health visitors, in relation to substance misuse, within the health care system are changing to meet the changing health needs of the population (Rassool 1996). Working as an autonomous practitioner, the addiction nurse has been able to respond to the changing health care needs by exploring new alternatives and adapting to changes in treatment approaches. The new approach for addiction nurses' work is aimed at the health promotion of communities via public health initiatives as well as direct care of communities, families or significant others and individuals (Coyne & Clancy 1996).

The roles of addiction nurses include provider of care, educator/resource, counsellor/therapist, advocate, promoter of health, researcher, supervisor/leader and consultant (World Health Organization/International Council of Nurses (WHO/ICN) 1991). The roles go far beyond those suggested here, as there is a role differentiation between registered nurse practitioner and clinical nurse specialist working within a residential or community based setting (Rassool 1997a). Due to the multi-disciplinary nature of the work and the composition of many community substance misuse teams, the blurring of roles among the disciplines is highly apparent (Rassool 1997a; Gafoor 1997). The nursing and psychosocial intervention skills utilised by addiction nurses include assessment, dealing with physical aspects of care, counselling and motivational interviewing, harm minimisation, relapse prevention, teaching and coaching skills. More research is needed to validate the role of the addiction nurse in both residential and community settings.

Nursing diagnosis

Nursing diagnosis originated in North America in the 1970s in an effort to provide nursing theory and practice a framework which is distinctive from other professional disciplines. The nursing professions and professional organisations in many American and European countries adopted the nursing diagnosis framework as part of a key component of the nursing process. In the UK, the concept of nursing diagnosis is not included as part of the component of the nursing process but it is slowly emerging in the nursing literature, especially in addiction nursing (Rassool 1997c). The main difference between nursing diagnosis and medical diagnosis is that the former describes the patient's current health problems and identification of health needs and the latter focuses on the patient's disease.

The North American Nursing Diagnosis Association (NANDA 1990) defines nursing diagnosis as

'a clinical judgement about the individual, family or community responses to actual and potential health problems/life processes. Nursing diagnoses provide the basis for the selection of nursing interventions to achieve outcomes for which the nurse is accountable.'

The International Council of Nurses, for the purposes of the International Classification for Nursing Practice (ICNP), defines nursing diagnosis as 'terms for nursing factors, recorded as diagnoses or problems, indicating a reason for nursing care' (*International Nursing Review* 1994). The above definitions and explanation of the concept seem to be congruent for the substitution of patient's needs or problems identified with 'nursing diagnosis'. It is apparent that the identification of needs or problems as part of the nursing care plan is expedient upon making clinical judgement. Roper *et al.* (1986) have pointed out that making a clear statement of the patient's problems as confirmed from the nursing assessment is increasingly being referred to as nursing diagnosis.

The rationale for the incorporation and implementation of nursing diagnosis has been related to the following factors: the paradigm shift from a medically dominated model of care to a care plan which has a nursing focus; organising and planning of nursing care and the provision of a common language (taxonomy) in nursing for communication and evaluation of quality of care, and for sharing clinical innovations and research. Nursing diagnosis is based on the four categories:

- ❑ Biological or physical responses
- ❑ Cognitive responses
- ❑ Psychosocial responses (psychological-emotional, social)
- ❑ Spiritual belief responses

In addiction nursing, 26 nursing diagnoses that are common to addiction nursing have been identified and described with their defining characteristics (American Nurses' Association and National Nurses' Society on Addictions 1988).

Nursing models

Following from the use of nursing diagnosis in addiction nursing, the application of nursing models to clinical practice has been slow in implementation in this clinical speciality. Hence, in addiction nursing, a limited number of models have been used in the nursing care of addicted clients in both in-patient and community settings (Rassool 1993). These models include Roy's (1980) adaptation model, Orem's (1985) self-care model, Roper and colleagues' (1983) activities of daily living model, Andersen and Smereck's (1989) personalized nursing light model and Peplau's (1988) interpersonal relationship model. The focus of the use of a nursing model is the provision of a flexible framework upon which to base the assessment, planning, implementation and evaluation, thus underpinning the clinical practice of addiction nursing. However, Rassool (1996, 1997a) argues that no single nursing model, currently in use, is applicable to meet the diverse health needs of substance misusers and the focus for clinicians and academics should be directed towards the adaptation and refinement of existing nursing models or the development of an integrated model of care applicable to the complexities and nature of substance misuse and addictive behaviour.

Education and training

The professional development of addiction nurses has been hampered by the lack of adequate preparation of nurses in drug and alcohol misuse at both pre-registration and post-registration level (Advisory Council for the Misuse of Drugs 1982, 1984, 1988, 1989, 1990; Alcohol Concern 1994; Rassool & Oyefeso 1993; WHO/ICN 1991; English National Board for Nursing, Midwifery and Health Visiting (ENB) 1996). Addiction nurses should have specialist professional education programmes to meet the changing nature in the use and misuse of psychoactive substances. The English National Board for Nursing, Midwifery and Health visiting (1996) called for an increase in the education and training of specialist nurses in the addiction field. Due to the changes in continuing professional development (United Kingdom Central Council for Nursing, Midwifery and Health Visiting (UKCC) 1994) coupled with current policy (Department of Health 1992; Tackling Drugs Together 1995) and educational initiatives (ENB 1996), addiction nurses must engage in continuing education and professional development as a statutory requirement to maintain their professional competence.

In its recommendations for nurses in relation to substance abuse, the WHO/ICN (1991) document states that nurses should be educated about substance misuse, starting at the basic training levels, and that continuing education and training should be provided for those working in this field. The Advisory Council on the Misuse of Drugs report (1990) recommended that specialist training should equip those who are directly involved in the management of drug related problems to embrace a whole range of knowledge and skills, including interventions, counselling, knowledge of drink/drugs interaction, research and evaluation. The practitioners should also have a solid theoretical background on the theories of substance misuse and addictive behaviour. In response to the changes in health and social policy over recent years, there has been an emergence of a few academic courses, professional journals and networking groups which aim to educate, guide and support health and social care staff in adjusting to their changing roles.

At the post-registration level, the development of education and training of clinical nurse specialists in substance misuse and addictive behaviour has been restricted to a few centres. Courses at undergraduate level include Drug and Alcohol Dependency Nursing (course 612), Alcohol Dependency Nursing (course 620), Recognition and Management of Substance Abuse (course 962) and the Short Course on the Recognition of and Nursing Responses to the Problem Drinker.

Clinical supervision

The nature of the clinical practice and the multiple roles that addiction nurses perform in statutory and non statutory organisations give rise to the need for clinical supervision. Faugier (1994) argues that, despite increasing recognition of the importance of clinical supervision, few mental health nurses have access to skilled, sensitive and formal supervision. Staff (1997) states that

> 'the opportunity for independent autonomous working practices in a specialism where the patient is frequently operating in an illegal under-world or sub-culture is a danger ... and becoming over involved, overstresses or stretching the boundaries of professional conduct.'

The need for clinical supervision for addiction nurses can no longer be ignored. Nurses, midwives and health visitors should embrace the concept of clinical supervision and incorporate it as an integral part of their practice (Department of Health 1993a, 1994; UKCC 1995; ENB, 1995).

The definitions of supervision are often conflicting and contradictory and this is augmented by the negative connotations attached to the concept. In its simplest form clinical supervision refers to a process of practising, experiencing and reflecting upon clinical practice. The reality of clinical supervision is that it is seldom clear-cut in the context of addiction nursing and substance misuse. Clinical supervision can be seen as a formal process whereby a worker and an experienced practitioner meet to examine and reflect on the management of clients and the refinement of therapeutic skills (Rassool 1997b). For a comprehensive account of clinical supervision, the reader is referred to Butterworth & Faugier (1992), Loganbill *et al.* (1982) and Hawkins and Shohet (1993).

Nurse practitioners, with the help of clinical supervision, would be able to develop professional competence in their specific areas of work and, with adequate supervision and support, stress and burnout would be reduced. It is argued that practitioners who are well supported, up to date and professionally aware as a result of having access to effective clinical supervision will benefit the organisation (UKCC 1995). In summary, the purpose of clinical supervision includes the maintenance of clinical standards, development of professional competence, reduction of stress and burnout, provision of support and consequent job satisfaction. Although some form of supervision is grounded in mental health nursing, it remains underdeveloped in the addiction field. Existing models of clinical supervision, either integrated or developmental, could be adapted to fulfil the gap.

Nursing research

There is a dearth of nursing research in addiction nursing in the UK, thus there is a window of opportunity and potential for clinicians, practitioners and academics to initiate and undertake research programmes. Although there is a variety of research in substance misuse by nurses, mainly from North America, the studies have mainly focused on prevalence, clinical specialities and education (Sullivan & Handley 1992). However, areas of research in addiction nursing interventions and conceptual development are relatively barren. The need for evidenced based practices is becoming more necessary with the introduction of the National Health Service reforms relating to professional competence, effective delivery and standards of care, clinical audit and health outcomes.

The focus of nursing research, according to the *Report of the Task Force on the Strategy for Research in Nursing, Midwifery and Health Visiting* (Department of Health 1993b) is related to

'nursing practices; nursing services and service delivery; the nursing professions and issues concerned with the workforce; health promotion; complex health care procedures or patterns of intervention; and service systems within which nursing plays but a part along with other health care professions.'

Nursing research should be at the forefront of this drive, both in broadening the research base of nursing care and in furthering the development of nursing science (Byrne & Kilpatrick 1997)

Nurses working in custodial settings, non statutory services, rehabilitation and detoxification units, within community or in-patient settings, can all contribute to the general body of knowledge by researching and reporting on their own particular aspect (Byrne & Kilpatrick 1997). For example, some of the areas that addiction nurses may research include:

- Evaluation of health education programmes in smoking cessation;
- Development and empirical testing of nursing models appropriate to addiction nursing;
- Critical examination of the role of the addiction nurse in residential and community settings;
- Process, outcomes and impact of educational programmes in the preparation of addiction nurses;
- Developing and testing nursing diagnosis appropriate to addiction nursing in the UK context;
- Relationship of clinical supervision and patient outcomes;
- Reviewing the effectiveness of detoxification in residential and community settings;
- Effectiveness of harm minimisation programmes for patients with HIV and substance misuse, etc.

Knowledge of nursing research and research methodologies are increasingly becoming an integral part of postgraduate educational programmes in addiction nursing and addictive behaviour (diploma and MSc courses) and this state of affairs should be welcomed as both an essential part of personal development and as a potential means to enhance the professional status of addiction nursing as a clinical speciality.

Conclusions

While this chapter has introduced some aspects of the contemporary issues pertaining to addiction nursing, it is beyond its scope to examine all relevant clinical and professional perspectives of addiction nurses. What is at stake is the dual development and integration of the subject of substance misuse at both pre- and post-registration levels in the nursing curriculum (Rassool 1996; 1997d). Currently, substance misuse is back on the political and professional agenda and the opportunity remains for educationalists, practitioners and researchers to 'grasp the nettle' and strive to develop a theoretical framework and research based practice in addiction nursing (Rassool 1996). The shared vision and practice of addiction nursing should be part and parcel of the parallel process of change.

References

Advisory Committee on Alcoholism (1978) *The Pattern and Range of Services for Problem Drinkers*. HMSO, London.

Advisory Council for the Misuse of Drugs (1982) *Treatment and Rehabilitation*. HMSO, London.

Advisory Council on the Misuse of Drugs (1984) *Prevention*. HMSO, London.

Advisory Council on the Misuse of Drugs (1988) *Aids and Drug Misuse*. Part 1. HMSO, London.

Advisory Council on the Misuse of Drugs (1989) *Aids and Drug Misuse*. Part 2. HMSO, London.

Advisory Council on the Misuse of Drugs (1990) *Problem Drug Use: A Review of Training*. HMSO, London.

Alcohol Concern (1994) *A National Alcohol Training Strategy*. Alcohol Concern, London.

American Nurses' Association, Drug and Alcohol Nursing Association, and National Nurses' Society on Addictions (1987) *The Care of Clients with Addictions: Dimension of Nursing Practice*. American Nurses Association, Kansas City.

American Nurses' Association and National Nurses' Society on Addictions (1988) *Standards of Addictions Nursing Practice with Selected Diagnoses and Criteria*. American Nurses' Association, Kansas City.

Andersen, M.D. & Smereck, G.A.D. (1989) Personalized nursing light model. *Nursing Science Quarterly*, **2**, 120–30.

Butterworth, T. & Faugier, J. (eds) (1992) *Clinical Supervision and Mentorship in Nursing*. Chapman & Hall, London.

Byrne, S. & Kilpatrick, B. (1997) Projects and research: an agenda for action. In: *Addiction Nursing: Perspectives on Professional and clinical practice* (eds G.H. Rassool & M. Gafoor). Stanley Thornes, Cheltenham.

Coyne, P. & Clancy, C. (1996) Out of sight, out of mind. In: *Aids: The Nursing Response* (eds J. Faugier & I. Hicken). Stanley Thornes, Cheltenham.

Department of Health (1992) *The Health of the Nation: A Strategy for Health in England*. HMSO, London.

Department of Health (1993a) *A Vision for the Future. The Nursing, Midwifery and Health Visiting Contribution to Health and Healthcare*. HMSO, London.

Department of Health (1993b) *Report of the Task Force on the Strategy for Research in Nursing, Midwifery and Health Visiting*. HMSO, London.

Department of Health (1994) *Working in Partnership: A Collaborative Approach to Care: A Report of the Mental Health Review Team*. HMSO, London.

English National Board for Nursing, Midwifery and Health Visiting (1996) *Substance Use and Misuse: Guidelines for Good Practice in Education and Training of Nurses, Midwives and Health Visitors*. ENB, London.

Faugier, J. (1994) Thin on the ground ... clinical supervision in mental health nursing. *Nursing Times*, **90**, 64–5.

Gafoor, M. (1997) Development of the role of the specialist nurse in substance misuse. *Psychiatric Care*, **4**, 132–4.

Ghodse, A.H. (1993) Substance misuse, health objectives and gains. Editorial. *Substance Misuse Bulletin*, **4**, 1–2.

Hawkins, P. & Shohet, R. (1993) *Supervising in the Helping Professions*. Open University Press, Milton Keynes.

International Nursing Review (1994) News: nursing classification moves into new phase. *International Nursing Review*, **41**, 164–5.

Kennedy, J. & Faugier, J. (1989) *Drug and Alcohol Dependency Nursing*. Heinemann Nursing, Oxford.

Loganbill, C., Hardy, H. & Delworth, U. (1982) Supervision: a conceptual model. *Counselling Psychologist*, **10**, 3–42.

NANDA (1990) NANDA definition. *Nursing Diagnosis*, **1**, 50.

Orem, D. (1985) *Nursing: Concepts of Practice*. McGraw-Hill, New York.

Peplau, H.E. (1988) *Interpersonal Relations in Nursing: A Conceptual Frame of Reference for Psychodynamic Nursing*. Macmillan, London.

Rassool, G.Hussein. (1993a) Substance misuse: responding to the challenge. *Journal of Advanced Nursing*, **18**, 1401–7.

Rassool, G.H. & Oyefeso, A. (1993b) The need for substance misuse education in health studies curriculum: a case for nursing education. *Nurse Education Today*, **13**, 107–10.

Rassool, G.H. (1996) Editorial. Addiction nursing and substance misuse: a slow response to partial accommodation. *Journal of Advanced Nursing*, **24**, 3.

Rassool, G.H. (1997a) Addiction nursing – towards a new paradigm: The United Kingdom experience. In: *Addiction Nursing: Perspectives on Professional and Clinical Practice* (eds G.H. Rassool & M. Gafoor). Stanley Thornes, Cheltenham.

Rassool, G.H. (1997b) Clinical supervision. In: *Addiction Nursing: Perspectives on Professional and Clinical Practice* (eds G.H. Rassool & M. Gafoor). Stanley Thornes, Cheltenham.

Rassool, G.H. (1997c) Addiction nursing: the relevance and appropriateness of nursing diagnosis in the United Kingdom context. *Journal of the Association of Nurses in Substance Abuse*. Summer, 34–8.

Rassool, G.H. (1997d) Professional education and training. In: *Addiction Nursing: Perspectives on Professional and Clinical Practice* (eds G.H. Rassool & M. Gafoor). Stanley Thornes, Cheltenham.

Rassool, G.H. & Gafoor, M. (1997) Themes in addiction nursing. In: *Addiction Nursing: Perspectives on Professional and Clinical Practice* (eds G.H. Rassool & M. Gafoor). Stanley Thornes, Cheltenham.

Roper, N., Logan, M, & Tierney, A. (1986) *The Elements of Nursing*, 2nd edn. Churchill Livingstone, Edinburgh.

Roy, C. (1980) The Roy adaptation model. In: *Conceptual Models for Nursing Practice*, 2nd edn (eds J.P. Riehl & C. Roy), pp. 179–88. Appleton-Century-Crofts, New York.

Staff, A. (1997) Community substance misuse team: management and practice. In: *Addiction Nursing: Perspectives on Professional and Clinical Practice* (eds G.H. Rassool & M. Gafoor). Stanley Thornes, Cheltenham.

Sullivan, E.J. & Handley, S.M. (1992) Alcohol and drug abuse. In: *Annual Review of Nursing Research* (eds J.J. Fitzpatrick, R.L. Taunton & J.Q. Benoliel), Vol. 11. Springer, New York.

Tackling Drugs Together (1995) *A Strategy for England 1995-1998*, HMSO, London.

United Kingdom Central Council for Nursing, Midwifery and Health Visiting (1994) *The Future of Professional Practice: The Council's Standards for Education and Practice Following Registration*. UKCC, London.

United Kingdom Central Council for Nursing, Midwifery and Health Visiting (1995) *Clinical Supervision for Nursing and Health Visiting*. Registrar's letter, 4/95. 24 January. UKCC, London.

World Health Organization/International Council of Nurses (1991) *Nurses Responding to Substance Abuse*. WHO/ICN, Geneva.

Appendix 1
UK Self-Help Groups and Helplines

Organisation	Address	Tel/Fax/Internet sites
Action on Smoking and Health (ASH)	Devon House, 12–15 Dartmouth Street, London SW1H 9BL	Tel: 0171 314 1360 Fax: 0171 222 4343
Adfam National	5th Floor, Epworth House, 25 City Road, London EC1Y 1AA	Tel: 0171 638 3700 Fax: 0171 256 6320
Al-Anon (24-hour helpline)	c/o Al-Anon Family Groups, 61 Great Dover Street, London SE1 4YF	Tel: 0171 403 0888
Alcoholics Anonymous (AA)	England & Wales General Service Office of AA, PO Box 1, Stonebow House, York YO1 2NJ	Tel: 01904 644026 Fax: 0190 462 9091
Al-Teen (24 hour helpline)	c/o Al-Anon Family Groups, 61 Great Dover Street, London SE1 4YF	Tel: 0171 403 0888
Drink-Line National Alcohol Helpline	Weddel House, 7th Floor, 13–14 West Smithfield, London EC1A 9DL	Tel: 0171 332 0202 0345 32 1202 (11am–11pm) Freephone: 0500 801 802 (24 hour)
Drug-Line	Maudsley Regional Drug Training Unit	Tel: 0800 776600
Drug and Alcohol Women's Network (DAWN)	c/o Greater London Association of Alcohol Services (GLASS), 30–31 Great Sutton Street, London EC1V 0DX	Tel: 0171 253 6211 Fax: 0171 250 1627
Drugs in Schools Helpline	388 Old Street, London EC1V 9LT	Tel: 0345 36 6666 Fax: 0171 729 2599

Organisation	Address	Tel/Fax/Internet sites
Families Anonymous (FA)	The Doddington and Rollo Community Association, Charlotte Despard Avenue, Battersea, London SW11 5JE	Tel: 0171 498 4680
Narcotics Anonymous (NA)	UK Service Office, PO Box 1980, London N19 3LS	Tel: 0171 730 0009 (helpline) 0171 272 9040 (publications)
Quit Helpline (Smokers)	170 Tottenham Court Road, London W1P 0HA	Tel: 0171 487 3000
Release (24 hour helpline)	388 Old Street, London EC1V 9LT	Tel: 0171 729 9904 0171 603 8654 (24 hour emergency helpline)
The Terence Higgins Trust (HIV/AIDS)	52–54 Gray's Inn Road, London WC1X 8JU	Tel: 0171 831 0330 Fax: 0171 242 0121

Appendix 2

International Organisations:
Professional Information and Resources

Organisations	Address	Tel/Fax/Internet sites
Alcohol Concern	Waterbridge House, 32–36 Loman Street, London SE1 0EE, UK	Tel: 0171 928 7377 Fax: 0171 928 4644 http://www.alcoholconcern.org.uk
Alcohol Action Wales/ Gweithredu Alcohol Cymru	4 Dock Chamberrs, Bute Street, Cardiff CF1 6AG, UK	Tel/Ffon: 01222 4888000 Fax/Ffacs: 01222 488000
Alcohol Education and Research Council	Room 143, Horseferry House, Dean Ryle Street, London SW1P 2AH, UK	Tel: 0171 217 8393
Association of Nurses in Substance Abuse (ANSA)	120 Wilton Road, London SW1V 1JZ, UK	Tel: 0171 233 8322 Fax: 0171 233 7779
English National Board For Nursing Midwifery and Health Visiting	Victory House, 170 Tottenham Court Road, London, W1P 0HA, UK	Tel: 0171 388 3131 Fax: 0171 383 4031 http://www.enb.org.uk
European Association for the Treatment of Addiction (EATA)	6th Floor, 25–27 Oxford Street, London W1R 1RF, UK	Tel: 0171 439 3229 Fax: 0171 494 1764
Health Education Authority	Hamilton House, Mabledon Place, London, WC1H 9TX, UK	Tel: 0171 383 3833 Fax: 0171 387 0550 Library: 0171 387 0550
Health Education Board for Scotland	Wooburn House, Canaan Lane, Edinburgh, UK	Tel: 0131 447 6180 Fax: 0131 452 8140
Health Promotion Agency for Northern Ireland	18 Ormeau Avenue, Belfast BT2 8HS, Northern Ireland	Tel: 01232 311611 Fax: 01232 311711
Health Promotion Wales/ Hybu Iechyd Cymru	Ffynnon-las, Ty Glas Avenue, Llanishen, Cardiff, UK	Tel/Ffon: 01222 752222 Fax/Ffacs: 01222 756000
Institute for the Study of Drug Dependence	Waterbridge House, 32–36 Loman Street, London SE1 0EE, UK	Tel: 0171 928 1211 Library: 0171 803 4720

Organisations	Address	Tel/Fax/Internet sites
International Council on Alcohol and Addictions (ICCA)	Case Postale 189, 1001 Lausanne, Switzerland	Tel: 021 320 98 65
RCN Substance Misuse Forum, Royal College of Nursing	20 Cavendish Square, London, W1M 0AB, UK	Tel: 0171 409 3333 Fax: 0171 409 1379 http://www.the biz.co.uk/rcn.htm
Scottish Council on Alcohol (SCA)	2nd Floor, 166 Buchanan Street, Glasgow G1 2NH, UK	Tel: 0141 333 9677 Fax: 0141 333 1606
Scottish Drug Forum	5 Oswald Street, Glasgow G1 4QR, UK	Tel: 0141 221 1175 Fax: 0141 248 6414
Society for the Study of Addiction to Alcohol and Other Drugs	Department of Forensic Psychiatry, Institute of Psychiatry, De Crespigny Park, London SE5 8AF, UK	
Standing Conference on Drug Abuse (SCODA)	Waterbridge House, 32–36 Loman Street, London SE1 0EE, UK	Tel: 0171 928 9500 Fax: 0171 928 3343
The Advisory Council on Alcohol and Drug Education (TACADE)	1 Hulme Place, The Crescent, Salford, Manchester M5 4QA, UK	Tel: 0161 745 8925 Fax: 0161 745 8923
World Health Organisation (WHO)	CH-1211, Geneva 27, Switzerland	Tel: 22 791 2111 Fax: 22 791 0746 http://www.who.ch/

Appendix 3

UK Education and Training Resources (Addiction Studies)

Institutions	Address	Tel/Fax/Internet sites
Anglia Polytechnic University	Faculty of Health and Social Work, Broomfield Hospital, Chelmsford, Essex GM1 5 LG, UK	Tel: 01245 440334 Fax: 01245 443034
Aquarius Education and Training	6th Floor, The White House, 111 New Street, Birmingham B2 4EU, UK	Tel: 0121 632 4727 Fax: 0121 633 0539
HIT (former Mersey Drug Training and Information Centre)	Cavern Walks, 8 Mathew Street, Liverpool L2 6RE, UK	Tel: 0151 227 4012 Fax: 0151 227 4023
Leeds Addiction Unit	19 Springfield Mount, Leeds LS2 9NG, UK	Tel: 0113 2926930 Fax: 0113 2926950
Liverpool John Moores University	Social and Human Sciences Department, Trueman Building, 15–21 Webster Street, Liverpool L3 2ET, UK	Tel: 0151 231 4029 Fax: 0151 258 1224
North West Region Drug Misuse Training Programme	University College Chester, Cheyney Road, Chester, Cheshire CH1 4BJ, UK	Tel: 01244 375 444
Maudsley/Regional Drug Training Unit	National Addiction Centre, 4 Windsor Walk, Camberwell, London SE5 8AF, UK	Tel: 0171 703 0269 Fax: 0171 703 0269
Redwood College of Health Studies/South Bank University	Education Centre, Harold Wood Hospital, Gubbins Lane, Harold Wood, Romford RM3 0BE, UK	Tel: 0171 815 5959
Ruskin College	Dunstan Hall, Old Headington, Oxford O73 9BZ, UK	Tel: 01865 63437 Fax: 01793 825583

Institutions	Address	Tel/Fax/Internet sites
St George's Hospital Medical School Centre for Addiction Studies	Department of Addictive Behaviour (University of London), Hunter Wing, Cranmer Terrace, Tooting, London SW16 0RE, UK	Tel: 0181 725 2637 Fax: 0181 725 2914 http://www.sghms.ac.uk/ depts/psychaddbe.htm
South West Drugs Training Service (NACRO)	29A Southgate, Bath BA1 1TP, UK	Tel: 01225 336766 Fax: 01225 466495
The Centre for Research and Health	200 Seagrave Road, London SW6 1RQ, UK	Tel: 0181 846 6565 Fax: 0181 846 6555
University of Huddersfield	The Willows, Queensgate, Halifax HX3 0DH, UK	Tel: 0442 357222, ext 2393/2240
University of Kent	School of Continuing Education, Keynes College, Canterbury, Kent CT2 7NP, UK	Tel: 01227 764000 Fax: 01227 458745
University of Nottingham	B Floor, Queen's Medical Centre, Nottingham NG7 2UH, UK	Tel: 0115 924 9924 Fax: 0115 942 3876
University of Paisley	Centre for Alcohol and Drug Studies, Westerfield House, 25 High Calside, Paisley PA2 6BY, UK	Tel: 0141 848 3141 Fax: 0141 848 3000
University of Stirling	Drugs Training Project, Department of Sociology, Stirling FK9 4LE, UK	Tel: 0176 467732 Fax: 01786 467979
West Midlands Regional Drugs Training Unit	6 Unity Place, Albert Street, Oldbury, West Midlands B69 4DB, UK	Tel: 0121 544 3939 Fax: 0121 544 2094

Index

abuse
  child, 132–3
  misuse distinction, 14
Accident and Emergency (A&E)
    departments, 73–4, 117, 168–75
acid, *see* LSD
acupuncture, 113, 212
addiction
  addictive behaviour, 15
  group therapy, 110
  medical/disease model, 21
  nicotine, 29, 225–35
  personality approaches, 22
  prevention services, 119
  screening, 99
addiction nursing, 189–269
  alcohol, 191–9
  benzodiazepines, 200–7
  complementary therapies, 113
  contemporary issues, 260–9
  definition, 261
  dual diagnosis patients, 249–59
  nicotine addiction, 225–35
  opiates and polydrug use, 217–24
  special populations, 236–48
  stimulants, 208–16
adolescence, 160, 241–2
agencies, 120, 140–1
AIDS (acquired immunodeficiency
    syndrome), 176–7
alcohol, 54–67
  A&E departments, 170, 173–4
  alcoholism, 5, 21–2, 55, 70
  brief interventions, 108–9
  CATS, 116, 119
  dependence, 55–6, 61–2
  detoxification, 171, 191–9, 222
  ethnic minorities, 237
  'gateway' effect, 160, 241
  GP attendance, 145
  head injuries, 171–2
  health care professionals' use of, 92
  historical overview, 5–6
  homelessness, 244
  mental health realationship, 251–2

  pregnancy, 60, 137
  screening, 98–9, 100–101, 103
  withdrawal, 16, 61–2, 112, 171, 173–4,
    193
  young people, 10, 243
alcopops, 10, 191
amphetamine, 8–9, 41–3, 208–10, 214–15,
    see also methamphetamine
amyl nitrate, 48–9
anabolic steroids, 47–8
antenatal care, 127–30
antidepressants, 213–14
assessment, 96–105, *see also* nursing
    diagnosis; screening
  A&E departments, 172–3
  community detoxification, 193–4, 197
  dual diagnosis patients, 251–4
  health visitors, 138–9
  nicotine dependence, 226–7
  polydrug users, 220–1, 223
  practice nurses, 148–50, 154–5

barbiturates, 43–4
benzedrine, 209
benzodiazepines, 43–4, 200–7, 218, 222–3,
    see also diazepam; temazepam
brief interventions, 108–9, 211
butyl nitrate, 48–9

caffeine, 9
cancer, 29, 31
cannabis, 6–7, 18, 40–1
carbon monoxide, 30, 227–9, 231–3
cardiovascular disease, 30
case studies
  A&E departments, 173–4
  alcohol detoxification, 196–7
  benzodiazepines, 205–6
  dual diagnosis patients, 254–5
  health visitors, 141–2
  HIV, 185–6
  polydrug users, 223
  practice nurses, 154–6
  pregnancy, 133
  school nurses, 165–6

smoking cessation, 228–9, 231–2
stimulants, 214–15
CATs, *see* Community Alcohol Teams
CDTs, *see* Community Drug Teams
children, 76, 90–1, 118, 136–42, 159–67, *see also* young people
    parental smoking, 32–3
    protection of, 132–3
    solvent abuse, 49–50, 165, 241–2
cigarettes, *see* tobacco
clinical supervision, 265–6
coca, 7
cocaine, 7, 41–3, 208–13
coffee, 9, 18
Community Alcohol Teams (CATs), 116, 119
community approach, 88
community detoxification, 191–9
Community Drug Teams (CDTs), 116, 118–19
community mental health nurses, 75–6, 92, 173, 254–5
complementary therapies, 112–13, 206
confidentiality, 129, 131, 133, 140, 163, 180
contraception, 126, 132
counselling, 109–11, 120, 222, 228–33
couples therapy, 110
crack, 41–3, 209
craving, 17, 210, 212, 228–9
crime, 219–20
crisis intervention, 119
cross tolerance, 16
cultural factors, 22–3, *see also* ethnic minorities

DALTs, *see* drug and alcohol liason teams
dance culture, *see* rave/dance culture
DDUs, *see* drug dependence units
dependence, 15–17, 20, 29, 55–6, 61–2, 220
depressants, *see* barbiturates; benzodiazepines
designer drugs, 10
detoxification, 112–13, 119, 140–1, 156
    alcohol, 171, 191–9, 222
    stimulants, 211–12
diagnosis, nursing, 262–4
diazepam, 112, 171, 195, 204–5
disease model, 21, 24
district nurses, 77
drinking, *see* alcohol
drug and alcohol liason teams (DALTs), 119–20
drug dependence units (DDUs), 116, 118
dual diagnosis patients, 249–59

ECO levels, 227–9, 231–3

Ecstasy, 4, 8, 10, 45–7, 208–9
education, *see* health education
elderly, the, 168–9, 202, 239–41
ethnic minorities, 22–3, 57, 236–9
experimental users, 19

family interaction model, 22
family planning, 77
FRAMES, 108
freebasing, 41

gas inhalation, *see* solvents
'gateway effect', 160, 241
GBH, 51
general nurses, 73
general practitioners (GPs), 28, 117, 145–6, 153, 194
generic interventions, 72–7, 107, 117–18, 122–88
    A&E departments, 168–75
    health visitors, 136–44
    HIV and hepatitis, 176–88
    practice nurses, 145–58
    pregnancy, 125–35
    school nursing, 159–67
genito urinary nurses, 74
GHB, 51
group therapy, 110, 229–33

hallucinogens, 8, 44–5, *see also* LSD; mushrooms
harm minimisation, 86–7, 139–40
hashish, *see* cannabis
head injuries, 171–2
health care professionals, 5, 11, 68–79, 106, *see also* general practitioners; health visitors; nurses; primary care workers
    attitudes towards misusers, 69–70, 168–9, 174–5
    ethnic minorities, 238
    homelessness, 245
    prevention, 83, 87–9, 92–3
    screening, 96–104
    smoking, 35
    substance misuse by, 92
    the elderly, 240
    training programmes, 142, 234, 256, 264–5, 267
health education, 69, 83–95, 139–40, 151–2
    ethnic minorities, 238
    HIV/hepatitis sufferers, 184–5
    schools, 160–1, 163–4
    smoking, 28, 35
    the elderly, 240
health promotion, 69, 83–4, 89–92, 162
health visitors, 76, 136–44

heart disease, 30
hemp, *see* cannabis
hepatitis, 176, 182–6
heroin, 16, 38–40, 128–9, 169, 218–20, 223
high risk behaviour, 97–8
history-taking, 96–8, 100–3, 253
HIV (human immunodeficiency virus), 74, 87, 176–81, 184–8, 218, 245
homelessness, 57, 244–6
hospitals, 73, 89–90, 117, 168–75
hypnosedatives, 43–4, *see also* barbiturates; benzodiazepines

in-depth assessments, 149
Indian hemp, *see* cannabis
individual counselling, 109–10
infection control, 181, 184
inhalation, 18
injection, 17–18, 20, 39, 140, 181, 237
    HIV risk, 176, 179, 202, 218, 245
intervention strategies, 106–15, *see also* generic interventions; specialist interventions
intrapartum care, 130–1
intravenous use, *see* injection

ketamine, 10, 52
khat, 10, 52, 208–9, 237

laudanum, 6
LSD (lysergic acid diethylamide), 8, 10, 44–5

'magic mushrooms', *see* mushrooms
marijuana, *see* cannabis
maternity, *see* pregnancy
MDMA, *see* Ecstasy
medical/disease model, 21, 24
mental health, 72, 75–6, 173, 219, 244, 249–59
mescaline, 44
metabolic tolerance, 16
methadone, 39, 112, 128–30, 132, 169, 221–2
methamphetamine, 8, 209
midwives, 74
models, 20–26, 264
moral model, 21, 24
morphine, 38–9
motivational interviewing, 111, 212, 215, 221, 252–3
multiple drug taking, *see* polydrug use
mushrooms, hallucinogenic, 8, 44–5

National Curriculum, 159–61
national organisations, 121

nicotine, 16, 29–30, 225–35
nicotine replacement therapy (NRT), 225, 227–8, 231–2
nurses, 68–79, *see also* addiction nursing; community mental health nurses; health visitors; practice nurses; psychiatric nurses; school nurses
    alcohol misuse, 65
    attitudes towards misusers, 70, 168–9, 174–5
    health education, 83–4, 88, 91–2
    roles, 71–2, 147, 156, 262
    training, 256, 264–5, 267
nursing assessment, 100
nursing diagnosis, 262–4

obstetric nurses, 74
occupational health departments, 77, 118
opiates, 38–40, 112, 128–31, 137, 217–24, *see also* heroin; morphine; opium
opium, 6, 9, 38
oral administration, 17
over-the-counter drugs, 50–1, 239–40
overdoses, 44, 168–70, 172–4, 219

paranoia, 42, 210
parents, 21–2, 32–3, 136–42
passive smoking, 27–8, 32–3
patient-centred interventions, 151, 184
personality, 18, 22, 250–1
peyote, 8, 40
pharmacodynamic tolerance, 16
pharmacological therapy, 112
physical dependence, 16
policy, 23, 85, 260, 264–5
    alcohol, 63
    health promotion, 68–9
    homelessness, 246
    schools, 164
    tobacco, 27–8
polydrug use, 217–24, 243
'poppers', 48–9
postpartum care, 131
practice nurses, 76, 145–58
pregnancy, 125–35
    alcohol effect on, 60, 137
    benzodiazepines, 129
    detoxification, 140–1
    health visitors, 138
    HIV risk, 180
    opiate use, 128–31, 137, 219
    tobacco effect on, 31–2, 136–7
    withdrawal, 127–9, 130–1, 137–9
prescribed medication, 88–9, 102, 164, 200–1, 239–40
prevention, 83–95, 151

primary health care workers, 5, 65, 69, 75–7, 103–4, *see also* health visitors; nurses
primary prevention, 86, 90
prison nurses, 70, 74–5
private sector services, 120–1
problem drinkers, 56–7, 61–2, 98–9, 145, 191–8
problem drug user definition, 14–15, 20
psychedelics, *see* hallucinogens
psychiatric disorders, *see* mental health
psychiatric nurses, 72, 92, 251–7, *see also* community mental health nurses
psycho-social support, 140, 222–3
psychological dependence, 16
psychological model, 21–2, 24
psychosis, 210
psychosomatic reactions, 16

questionnaires, 98–9, 148

rave/dance culture, 4, 8, 23, 45–6, 208–9, 241
recreational user definition, 19–20
rehabilitation, 87, 120–1
relapse prevention, 111, 196, 213–15
research, 266–7
residential rehabilitation services, 120
respiratory diseases, 30–1

schizophrenia, 250–51, 255
school nurses, 76, 91, 159–67
schools, 90–1
screening, 96–105, 148–9, 194, 253–4
secondary prevention, 86–7
self-help groups, 21, 120, 204
service provision, 116–22, 260
sexual health, 31, 132, 219
shared care, 146, 153, 246, 254
smoking, *see* inhalation; nicotine; tobacco
social learning theory, 21–2, 24, 111, 192, 196
social services, 132–3
sociocultural model, 22–4
solvents, 49–50, 165, 241–2
specialist interventions, 97, 106–8, 118–21, 146, 153, 189–269
  alcohol, 191–9
  benzodiazepines, 200–7
  contemporary issues, 260–9
  dual diagnosis patients, 249–59
  nicotine addiction, 225–35
  opiates and polydrug use, 217–24
  special populations, 236–48
  stimulants, 208–16

special populations, 236–48
speed, *see* amphetamine
steroids, 47–8
stimulants, 41–3, 128, 208–16, *see also* amphetamine; cocaine
street agencies, 120
stress, 92
suicide, 168–70, 173, 212
supervision, 265–6
support, 140, 152, 194, 222–3

tar, 29
temazepam, 43, 202, 223
tertiary prevention, 87
therapy, *see* intervention strategies
tobacco, 27–37, 225–35, *see also* nicotine
  dependence, 29
  effect on children, 32–3, 137
  ethnic minorities, 237
  'gateway' effect, 160, 241
  health care professionals' use of, 92
  historical overview, 9
  pregnancy, 31–2, 136–7
  schools, 164–5
  withdrawal, 34, 226
tolerance, 15–16, 220
training, professional, 142, 234, 256, 264–5, 267
tranquilisers, *see* barbiturates; benzodiazepines
triage, 96, 150, 172
tuberculosis (TB), 181–2

valium, *see* diazepam
volatile substances, 49–50, 241–2

withdrawal
  alcohol, 16, 61–2, 112, 171, 173–4, 193
  barbiturates, 44
  benzodiazepines, 44, 112, 201–6
  dependence, 16–17
  heroin, 16, 39–40
  opiates, 112, 220–2
  pharmacological therapy, 112
  pregnancy, 127–9, 130–1, 137–9
  stimulants, 210–14
  tobacco, 34, 226
women, *see also* pregnancy
  alcohol consumption, 57–60
  benzodiazepines, 202
  psycho-social support, 140
work places, 77, 91, 118

young people, 10, 90–1, 118, 159–67, 191, 241–4, *see also* children